AF874260

SYMPOSIUM
ON
CLINICAL PHARMACOLOGY

SYMPOSIUM

ON

CLINICAL PHARMACOLOGY

Sponsored by the National Cancer Institute

CANCER CLINICAL INVESTIGATION REVIEW COMMITTEE

Clinical Investigation Branch

Held at the
Hotel Robert Mayer
Jacksonville, Florida
March 12 – 13, 1973

Symposium Committee:

WILLIAM A. CREASEY
MONTAGUE LANE
ALAN C. SARTORELLI, CHAIRMAN

PERGAMON PRESS

PERGAMON PRESS INC.
Maxwell House, Fairview Park, Elmsford, N.Y. 10523

PERGAMON OF CANADA LTD.
207 Queen's Quay West, Toronto 117, Ontario

PERGAMON PRESS LTD.
Headington Hill Hall, Oxford

PERGAMON PRESS (AUST.) PTY. LTD.
Rushcutters Bay, Sydney, N.S.W.

PERGAMON GmbH
Burgplatz 1, Braunschweig

Copyright © 1975, Pergamon Press Inc.

Library of Congress Cataloging in Publication Data

Symposium on Clinical Pharmacology, Jacksonville, Fla., 1973.
Symposium on Clinical Pharmacology.

(Biochemical pharmacology : Supplement ; v. 23, 1974, no. 2)

1. Cancer--Chemotherapy--Congresses. I. Creasey, William A., ed. II. Lane, Montague, ed. III. Sartorelli, Alan Clayton, 1931- ed. IV. United States. National Cancer Institute. Cancer Clinical Investigation Review Committee. V. Series: Biochemical pharmacology : Supplement ; 1974, no. 2.

RC271.C5S93 1973 616.9'94'061 74-31005
ISBN 0-08-018949-0 (paper)
ISBN 0-08-018950-4 (case)

All Rights Reserved. No part of this publication may be reproduced, stored in a retrieval system or transmitted in any form, or by any means, electronic, mechanical, photocopying, recording or otherwise, without prior permission of Pergamon Press Inc.

Printed in the United States of America

SYMPOSIUM ON CLINICAL PHARMACOLOGY

Sponsored by the National Cancer Institute

CANCER CLINICAL INVESTIGATION REVIEW COMMITTEE

Clinical Investigation Branch

Held at the
Hotel Robert Meyer
Jacksonville, Florida
March 12–13, 1973

Symposium Committee: WILLIAM A. CREASEY
MONTAGUE LANE
ALAN C. SARTORELLI, CHAIRMAN

PROGRAM

FACTORS INFLUENCING DRUG SELECTIVITY
THOMAS C. HALL, CHAIRMAN

MECHANISMS OF CLINICAL DRUG RESISTANCE
MONTAGUE LANE, CHAIRMAN

COMBINATION CHEMOTHERAPY
F. STANLEY PORTER, JR., CHAIRMAN

NEW INFORMATION ON MECHANISMS OF DRUG ACTION
WILLIAM A. CREASEY, CHAIRMAN

INTRODUCTORY REMARKS
WILLIAM A. CREASEY

I WOULD like to express our appreciation to Doctors Alan C. Sartorelli and William G. Hammond for organizing this Symposium. We are all aware that arranging this type of meeting requires considerable effort in terms of making contact with prospective speakers and urging them to agree to cover specified areas.

Those of us who work in the broad area of cancer chemotherapy are only too painfully aware of the shortcomings of drug therapy that is currently available. There is a wide gap between the promise held out by experimental systems and the actual achievement seen in the clinic. We can, of course, speculate as to the reasons for this discrepancy. Three factors come to mind.

First, the screening systems used to identify active agents are in themselves highly selective. It is no accident that the human cancers most responsive to current therapy are those that are similar to the rapidly growing, soft-tissue mouse tumors used as primary screens. It is with choriocarcinoma, the lymphomas, Wilm's tumor and the acute leukemias of childhood that the greatest successes of chemotherapy have been achieved. These cancers are in many ways analogous to transplanted murine tumors. Awareness of this factor is now fairly general, and steps are being taken to broaden the screening systems.

Second, most chemotherapeutic approaches have neglected or ignored the host immunologic system. Successful therapy frequently may depend upon delivery of damage to tumor cells, followed by destruction of those cells by immune processes. Drugs that suppress this second step actually may be defeating their own purpose. A large fraction of the cancer chemotherapeutic armamentarium consists of immunosuppressive drugs.

Third, there is the pharmacologic factor. Much pharmacologic knowledge about currently used agents has been accumulated. However, on the one hand, this knowledge often does not extend to the human system, while on the other hand, all too little attention is paid to utilizing this information in developing drug schedules. It is possible that if our knowledge of clinical pharmacology and biochemistry were greater, and the determination to make use of it were more prevalent, cancer chemotherapy might achieve a new impetus. In holding this Symposium, it is our hope that by collating the available knowledge and pointing out the deficiencies, we can aid in materially improving the efficacy of cancer chemotherapy.

Pp. 1—8, Supplement Number 2, 1974.
Biochemical Pharmacology. Printed in the U.S.A.

PHARMACOKINETICS AND DRUG EFFECT

DANIEL S. ZAHARKO

Laboratory of Chemical Pharmacology, NCI, Bethesda, Md. 20014, U.S.A.

ALTHOUGH I have been asked to talk about pharmacokinetic models, I have taken the liberty to diverge somewhat from the formal presentation of equations and data fitting of curves usually conjured by such a topic. Instead, after a very brief summary of the different kinds of pharmacokinetic models currently used, I hope to show by specific examples how detailed kinetic investigations of a drug in animals may provide further insight into modes of its clinical use.

Classical pharmacokinetic models

Those of you who have ever measured timed plasma concentrations of any substance have used a pharmacokinetic model, for when one reports a plasma half-life, he commits himself to a model as illustrated in Fig. 1. A single half-life after a single intravenous injection means the body is behaving as if it were a single well mixed

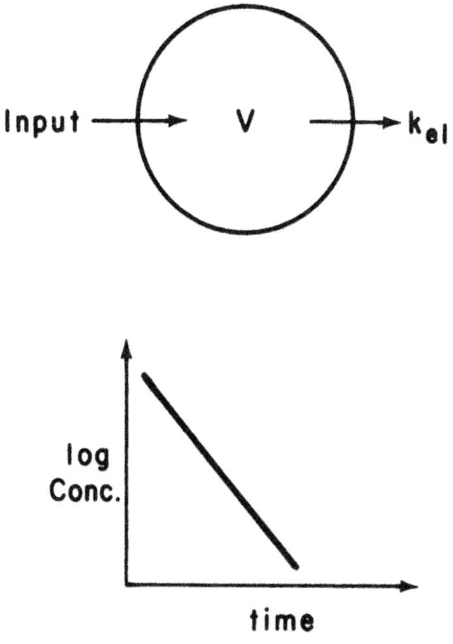

FIG. 1. One-compartment model with first-order removal rate that will fit plasma drug kinetics with a single half-life.

compartment, with rate of removal being a constant fraction of the concentration present at any time. Sometimes plasma drug kinetics suggest two half-lives and, therefore, two compartments can be used to explain mathematically the plasma and urinary data, as illustrated in Fig. 2. As the number of apparent plasma half-lives increases, so does the number of compartments that are used to aid mathematically in designing equations of best fit. These types of compartmental models are statistical fits of data. They have been used most often to predict plasma drug concentrations after multiple dosing and constant infusions. Plasma and urine data after a single dose first must be collected in the same species in order to use such a model.[1,2] It is important to realize in the above models that the compartments are mathematical tools and should not be equated with anatomical compartments, even though the often-called "central compartment" is fitted with plasma concentration data.

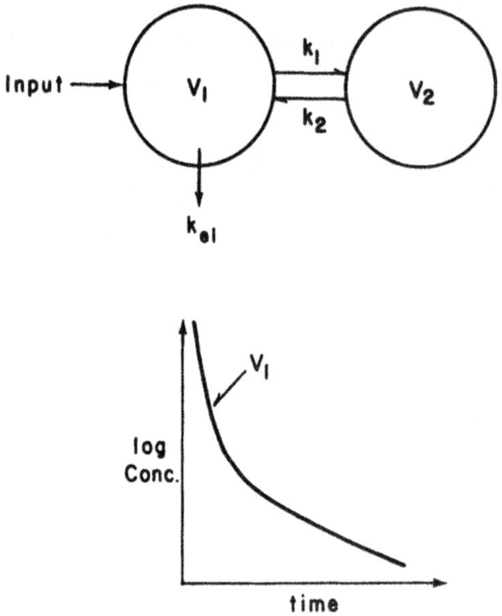

FIG. 2. Two-compartment model with first-order rate constants that will fit plasma drug kinetics with two phases of decline.

Physiological pharmacokinetic model

A pharmacokinetic model that is based on anatomical compartments is illustrated in Fig. 3. It uses anatomically discrete compartments that can be adjusted from species to species according to differences among species in organ size, blood flow, protein binding, membrane permeability and enzyme kinetics.[3,4] The inclusion or exclusion of a compartment (organ) in this model is determined by the importance of the organ in influencing the kinetics of drug behavior, or in being influenced by the drug, so that a knowledge of the drug kinetics in that tissue is desired by the modeler. This kind of model requires extensive kinetic distribution studies in one species. Then with appropriate adjustments for physiological differences and drug-metabolizing enzyme kinetics

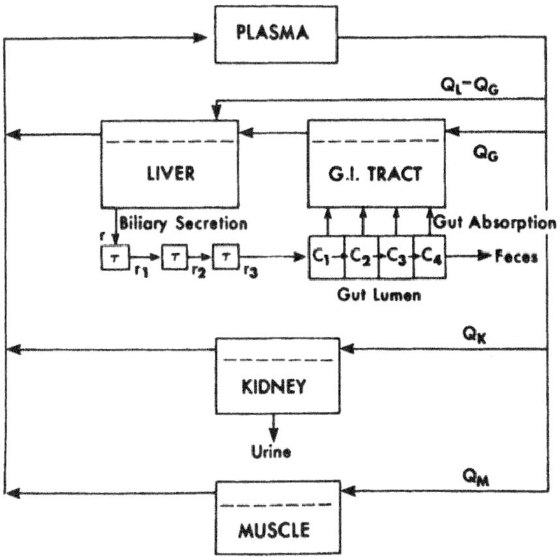

FIG. 3. Body compartments important in methotrexate distribution. Q = flow rate. Subscripts: G = gut; L = liver; K = kidney; M = muscle.

in each organ, it can be used to extrapolate to other species.[3,5] The limitation of such a pharmacokinetic approach is the extensive drug kinetic data – which Dr. Oliverio will review in the following paper – that must be collected before a realistic model can be constructed. These data are often limited by the availability and sensitivity of analytical methods and by the complexity of metabolic processes of certain drugs. For such a model, it is essential to know the K_m and V_{max} for each important drug metabolite in each organ.[4]

Methotrexate kinetics and effect

So much for a review of pharmacokinetic models. Now I would like to give an example to illustrate why the use of such models can be helpful to cancer chemotherapists. A survey of the cancer chemotherapy literature both in animals and man with respect to toxicity and tumor therapy gives the impression that a lot of emphasis is placed on the dose of the drug administered, with some little attention placed on schedule of administration, and with very little attention placed on the time course of drug action. We have recently attempted to concentrate on this latter somewhat neglected area.

Dose effect. Table 1 shows that dose alone, at least with a cell cycle specific drug, is really quite meaningless. Knowing that we had available a pharmacokinetic model that used all the available data on the kinetic behavior of methotrexate (MTX), we sought to explain single-dose toxicity and multiple-dose toxicity in mice on the basis of model-predicted plasma concentrations, proposed mechanism of drug action and intestinal cell kinetics.[6] We were able to do so only after postulating additional factors not included in the pharmacokinetic model.

TABLE 1. RELATIONSHIP OF TOTAL CUMULATIVE DOSE OF METHOTREXATE TO TOXICITY IN MICE*

Individual dose (mg/kg)	Total dose (mg/kg)	Schedule	Effect
350	350	*q*.(1X)	LD_{50}
25	50	*q.d.*(2X)	LD_{50}
3	24	*q*.3 hr (5X) rest 8 hr (3X)	$>LD_{50}$
0.5	10	*q*.3 hr (20X)	$>LD_{50}$
0.6 μg/hr	2.4	infusion 96 hr	$>LD_{50}$

*Injections were made intraperitoneally. Infusion was by a micro-infusion cell placed subcutaneously.

Plasma kinetics and effect. Using a sensitive enzyme assay to measure inhibition of dihydrofolate reductase in terms of MTX equivalents *in vitro*, we discovered a low persistent plasma level of MTX after a very high single dose that was inexplicable by all the factors included in the model. (Fig. 4).[7] These findings, coupled with recent literature reports, indicated that recovery of mouse small intestine from DNA inhibition occurs at very low MTX plasma concentrations.[8] Studies by Chabner and Young[9] at NCI laboratories confirmed this to be so, and showed that marrow recovery of DNA synthesis after a variety of doses occurred at different times but at the same plasma MTX concentration (Fig. 5). The plasma concentration of 2×10^{-8} M MTX for

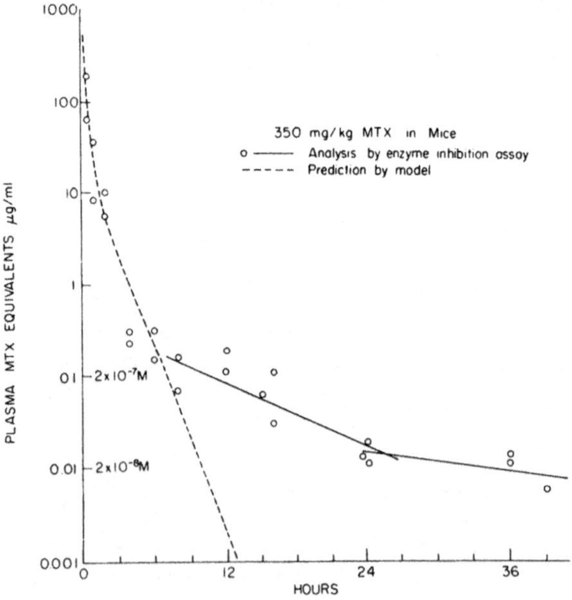

FIG. 4. Comparisons of enzyme assay of MTX equivalents in mouse plasma to model predictions.

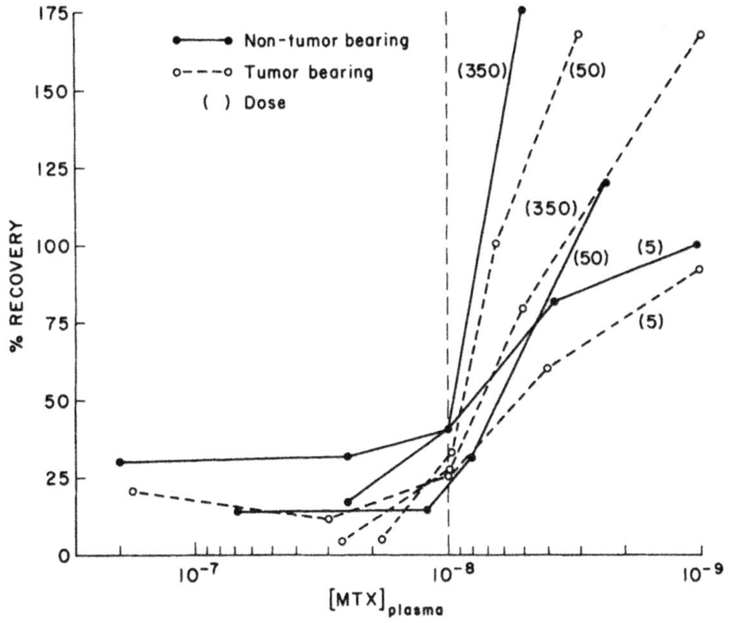

FIG. 5. Recovery of DNA synthesis in mouse bone marrow as a function of plasma MTX concentration after several doses (mg/kg) of MTX in mice.[9]

marrow cells *in vivo* is lower than those concentrations usually reported for studies on cell kill *in vitro*, where the usual figures are 1×10^{-7} M or higher.[10,11] Chabner also has shown that human marrow begins to recover from DNA inhibition at a plasma concentration of 2×10^{-8} M MTX, the same concentration at which mouse marrow recovers, but at a different time. The question can be raised whether the recovery occurred because of plasma dropping below a critical concentration of 2×10^{-8} M or because of delayed recovery due to earlier exposure at very much higher concentrations after single parenteral injections.

Micro-infusion cells and effect. With the aid of some recently designed micro-infusion cells, which are transplanted into mice and which give plasma MTX kinetics similar to those achieved by a constant intravenous infusion, we have conducted some preliminary studies. These studies (Fig. 6) show that lethality in mice can be achieved by coming up to a plasma plateau concentration of approximately 2×10^{-8} M MTX. The time of exposure at this concentration is a critical factor in determining the drug's lethal effect. Exposure times of 48 hr or less manifest little toxicity, whereas exposures above approximately 96 hr are lethal to all mice. Constant infusions, which resulted in plasma plateau concentrations of less than 1×10^{-8} M MTX, did not cause lethal effects when maintained for periods up to 3 weeks in mice. Preliminary calculations based on model predictions of the rate of entry of MTX into small intestine cells [12] and the rate of synthesis of enzyme dihydrofolate reductase in these cells,[8] suggest that at plasma plateau concentrations of less than 1×10^{-8} M MTX the rate of enzyme synthesis exceeds the rate of drug entry into the small intestine tissue of the

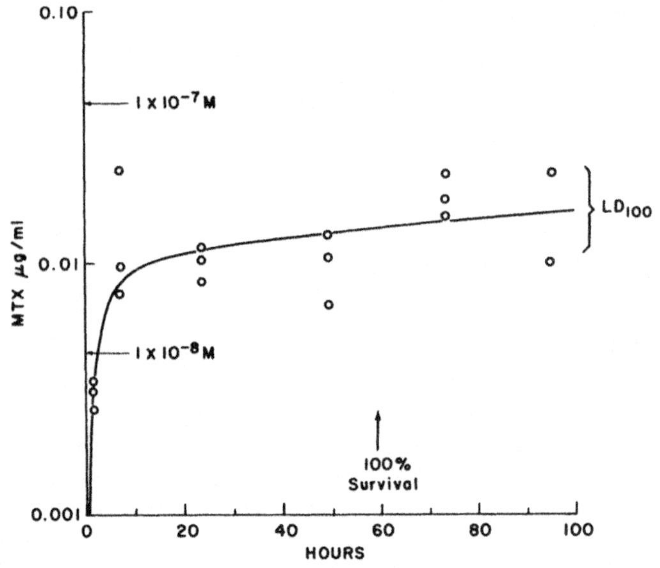

FIG. 6. Plasma concentration of MTX by enzyme assay after subcutaneous implant of a microdiffusion cell.

mouse (Table 2). It is likely that each tissue (either normal or neoplastic) has characteristic drug permeability rates and enzyme synthesis rates that in part determine its sensitivity to constantly held plasma MTX levels.

Additional studies in mice show that, at high doses, compartments in certain organs may act as storage depots for MTX and then release the drug at a very slow rate. This causes the persistence of MTX in plasma not predicted by the model (Fig. 4). The importance of such low persistent plasma concentrations in causing toxicity in mice has been demonstrated. From the DNA inhibition studies in man, it is evident that these low MTX concentrations may be a significant factor in marrow toxicity in

TABLE 2. CALCULATION OF STEADY STATE PLASMA MTX NEEDED IN ORDER TO BIND ALL THE NEW ENZYME SYNTHESIS TAKING PLACE IN MOUSE SMALL INTESTINE

Rate constant for small intestine permeability in linear phase = $0.03\ \text{min}^{-1}$

Initial synthesis rate of dihydrofolate reductase after 0.5 mg/kg of MTX = 0.007 µg/g/hr in MTX equivalent

Therefore, for the rate of drug entry to be equal to the rate of enzyme synthesis:

$$(0.03\ \text{min}^{-1})\ (60\ \text{min/hr})\ \begin{pmatrix}\text{steady state plasma}\\ \text{MTX concentration}\\ (\mu\text{g/ml})\end{pmatrix} = 0.007\ \mu\text{g/g/hr}$$

and therefore

Plasma steady state MTX = 0.004 µg/ml ($\sim 1 \times 10^{-8}$ M) clinical situations. These findings confirm the importance of using citrovorum factor after high doses of MTX and suggest a reason for its effectiveness – that is, counteracting low persistent plasma MTX.[13,14] Alternate methods to lower plasma MTX concentration rapidly after a critical time of exposure are available. The use of an enzyme, carboxypeptidase G, has recently been introduced to lower rapidly the extracellular MTX concentrations *in vivo*.[15] The use of long-term constant infusions at critical effective concentrations for discrete critical time periods could also be employed, as illustrated in Fig. 7. On stopping the infusion, plasma concentration falls rapidly (within 6 hr) to nontoxic levels (below 1×10^{-8} M) in mice. This kind of controlled time exposure at critical concentrations may enable a greater exploitation of the differences in cell cycle times and drug permeabilities among tumors and normal tissues.

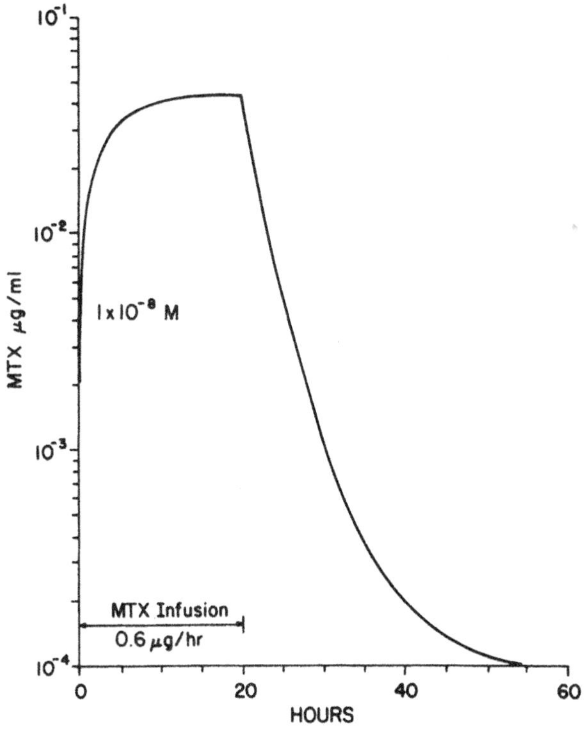

FIG. 7. Prediction of mouse plasma kinetics during and after stopping a slow infusion of MTX.

Acknowledgement – I thank Dr. R. L. Dedrick for supplying the micro-infusion cells and for his cooperation in some of these studies, Dr. R. Lutz for computer simulations, Miss Ann Peale and Mr. James Drake for technical assistance, and Dr. Bruce Chabner for the use of some of his data.

REFERENCES

1. E. KRUGER-THIEMER and P. BUNGER, *Chemotherapia* **10**, 61 (1966).
2. J. G. WAGNER, *Biopharmaceutics and Relevant Pharmacokinetics*, pp.237–246. Drug Intelligence Publications, Hamilton, Illinois (1971).
3. K. B. BISCHOFF, R. L. DEDRICK, D. S. ZAHARKO and J. A. LONGSTRETH, *J. pharm. Sci.* **60**, 1128 (1971).

4. R. L. DEDRICK, D. D. FORRESTER and D. H. W. HO, *Biochem. Pharmac.* **21**, 1 (1972).
5. D. S. ZAHARKO, R. L. DEDRICK and V. T. OLIVERIO, *Comp. Biochem. Physiol.* **42A**, 183 (1972).
6. D. S. ZAHARKO and R. L. DEDRICK, in *Pharmacology and the Future in Man* (Ed. G. H. ACHESON), Vol. 3, p. 316. S. Karger, Basel (1973).
7. D. S. ZAHARKO and D. G. JOHNS, *Pharmacologist* **13**, 260 (1971).
8. S. MARGOLIS, F. S. PHILIPS and S. S. STERNBERG, *Cancer Res.* **31**, 2037 (1971).
9. B. A. CHABNER and R. C. YOUNG, *J. clin. Invest.* **52**, 1804 (1973).
10. J. BORSA and G. F. WHITMORE, *Molec. Pharmac.* **5**, 303 (1969).
11. N. M. BRASLOW and R. L. BOWMAN, *Science, N.Y.* **175**, 1436 (1972).
12. R. L. DEDRICK, D. S. ZAHARKO and R. J. LUTZ, *J. pharm. Sci.* **62**, 882 (1973).
13. J. R. BERTINO and D. G. JOHNS, in *The Twenty-second Hahnemann Symposium: Cancer Chemotherapy II*, p. 9. Grune & Stratton, New York (1972).
14. A. GOLDIN, J. M. VENDITTI, I. KLINE and N. MANTEL, *Nature, Lond.* **212**, 1548 (1966).
15. B. A. CHABNER, D. G. JOHNS and J. R. BERTINO, *Nature, Lond.* **239**, 395 (1972).

Pp. 9—20, Supplement Number 2, 1974.
Biochemical Pharmacology. Printed in the U.S.A.

ABSORPTION, PROTEIN BINDING, DISTRIBUTION AND EXCRETION OF ANTINEOPLASTIC DRUGS

VINCENT T. OLIVERIO and ANTHONY M. GUARINO

Experimental Therapeutics, Division of Cancer Treatment, National Cancer Insititute, NIH, Bethesda, Md. 20014, U.S.A.

ZAHARKO[1] has dealt primarily with the quantitative aspects of drug disposition, the study of drug kinetics and the development of mathematical pharmacokinetic models. When this is combined with actual measurement of the absorption, distribution, metabolism and excretion of foreign compounds, the preliminary assessment of the likely physiological performance and disposition of a compound in the body is more easily made. In discussing the chief factors in determining the effective concentration of a drug at a receptor site, the duration and intensity of drug effect, we will use antineoplastic agents as examples.

However, before considering these factors which govern a drug's sojourn and action within the body, it should be pointed out that clinicians employing cancer chemotherapeutic agents are faced with a special problem not commonly met with ordinary drugs employed for therapy of other diseases, i.e. they are faced with the problem that antitumor agents as a rule, rather than the exception, have a narrow therapeutic index, thus requiring extra skill and knowledge on the part of the therapist to employ these agents effectively. This places the added burden upon the clinician of not only being thoroughly informed concerning the biologic effects of these drugs, particularly with respect to the host, but also of having a more than usual understanding of the qualitative and quantitative aspects of the pharmacologic disposition of these agents.

Figure 1 depicts the various body compartments and major physiological barriers which cancer chemotherapeutic agents, as well as most other xenobiotics, must negotiate from the time of administration until reaching the target, in this case, the tumor.

In order for a drug to act, it must first enter the blood or plasma pool to be distributed throughout the body and thus reach the appropriate target site. This is usually accomplished either by absorption across the cell membrane barriers along the GI tract, after oral administration, or by direct injection into blood vessels. The body compartments shown in Fig. 1 represent potential sites of action for a drug, but in the case of an antitumor drug, it is hoped that the tumor compartment is selectively penetrated and acted upon without undue expense to the other body tissues. The rate at which a drug reaches the target site or other organs and tissues is determined primarily by blood flow. The effective concentration of the drug at the reactive site also is related to its concentration in the plasma and the duration of time that the effective level is maintained. This is commonly referred to as the $C \times T$.[2] It is one of the purposes of pharmacological studies to adivse the physician on how to maintain most effectively a $C \times T$ sufficient to bring about an optimal drug effect. In a

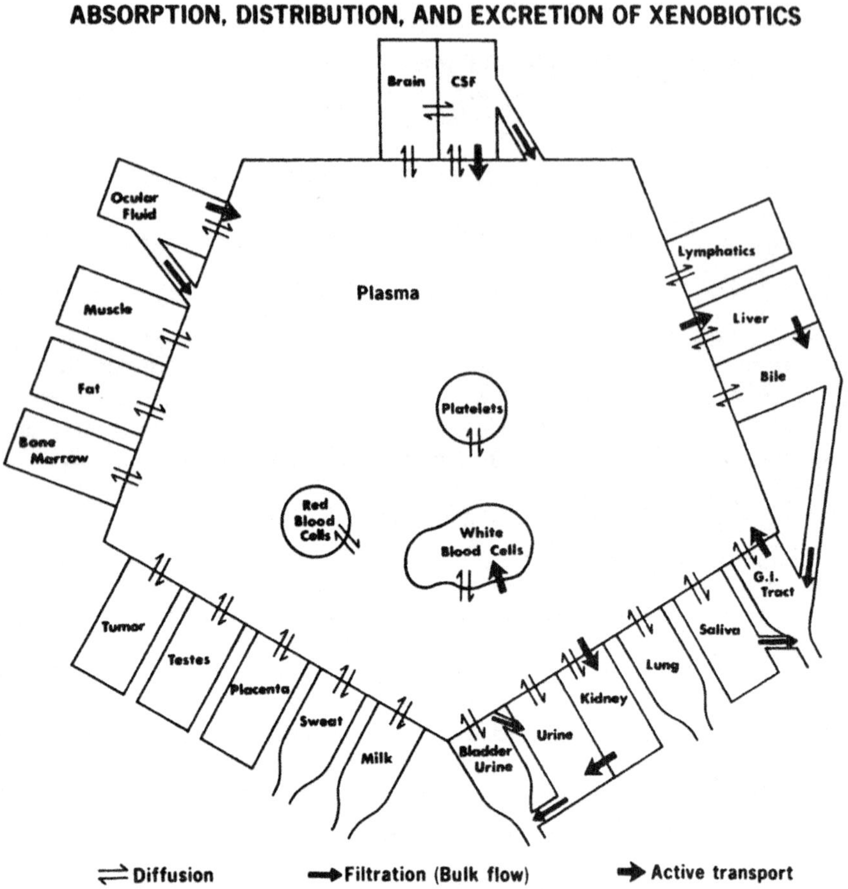

FIG. 1. Body compartments and physiological barriers involved in the disposition of cancer chemotherapeutic agents and other xenobiotics.

subsequent presentation, Mellett[3] will delve into the implications of the $C \times T$ concept in maintaining drug plasma levels for more effective chemotherapy.

As shown in Fig. 1, in addition to the target tumor tissue compartment, an antitumor drug may be simultaneously distributed to a number of other tissues or organs, bound or stored, metabolized to inactive or active products, or excreted. Tissue storage, binding, metabolism or excretion are called sites of loss because they usually decrease a drug's primary effect, whether it be therapeutic or toxic.

In this paper, we will focus on the particular body compartments shown in Fig. 1 which have been implicated in recent or current studies of investigators primarily in the Experimental Therapeutics Program of the Division of Cancer Treatment of the National Cancer Institute to illustrate generally the physiological processes of absorption, distribution, binding and excretion. It is felt that, because of our involvement and firsthand knowledge of these studies, this sort of approach would be better than a general review of the work of many others.

To exert its action in the body, a drug must cross one or more semipermeable cellular membranes in either entering the body, entering intracellular sites of action, or in being removed by excretion mechanisms. The cell membrane is best considered to be a bimolecular lipid layer sandwiched by two monomolecular protein layers. The membrane contains pores and is capable of accepting nonpolar (lipid-soluble) substances and excluding polar molecules. The transfer of drug molecules across the cell membrane can take place in four general ways: simple diffusion, filtration, active transport and pinocytosis.

Most drugs enter cells by simple diffusion through the lipoidal membrane under the influence of a concentration gradient to the aqueous phase. Hence, nonpolar drugs pass through the membranes more freely than polar compounds because the rate of passage through the membrane depends on the drug's partition coefficient. Thus, compounds with a high lipid-to-water partition coefficient and which are nonionized pass through the cell membrane fastest.

Absorption and the rate of diffusion of drugs across cell membranes are also markedly influenced by the degree of ionization. For highly ionized molecules, it may be necessary for transfer across membranes to occur by specialized transport processes, or if they are small enough, transfer might take place by filtration through membrane pores. In any event, many drugs are weak acids or weak bases which are often imcompletely ionized at physiological pH. The degree of ionization is related to this pH and to the p*K*a value, the fraction of the drug present in the ionized form. For certain organic acids and bases in the ionized form, absorption has been shown to be related to their p*K*a values (for further details see Ref. 4).

The penetration of cell membranes by filtration is limited to drug molecules whose equivalent pore radius is less than 4Å, although the glomeruli of kidneys and the blood capillaries have larger pores to permit the passage of higher molecular weight compounds. As Brodie[5] has stated, the latter membrane barriers act like four-lane highways to pass large molecules from the plasma to the extracellular fluid. For a number of drugs, simple filtration or diffusion does not account for their passage across membranes. Special transport mechanisms have been postulated for these compounds such as "carrier-mediated transport," in which the drug forms a complex with a carrier capable of crossing a membrane because of its lipid solubility. On the other side of the membrane, the complex breaks down and the transported drug is released. When the drug moves across the membrane against a concentration gradient, energy is required and the process is termed "active transport." These specialized transfer processes are largely involved with the transfer of sugars and amino acids and foreign molecules which are very similar in chemical structure to a natural substrate. For example, methotrexate (MTX) and 5-fluorouracil (5-FU), antimetabolites to naturally occurring folic acid and uracil, respectively, have both been shown to cross membrane barriers by active transport processes.

Finally, it should be mentioned that the process of pinocytosis, in which substances are engulfed by invaginations of the membrane, is a mechanism proposed to explain how certain proteins, macromolecules or macromolecular complexes cross a membrane.

The principles which have been outlined above govern the passage of drugs across various membrane barriers and are also operative in the absorption of drugs from the GI tract. This route is particularly used for drugs of low aqueous solubility, which are not irritating to the GI tract nor subject to hydrolysis or the destructive action of digestive enzymes. Drugs absorbed across the membranes of the GI tract are carried in the portal vein to the liver, where they may be exposed to the action of various enzymes in the liver, resulting in less potent or more active substances which are then secreted into the bile. A number of variables can regulate absorption after oral administration, such as dosage form, species differences in pH and size of GI tract, physico-chemical characteristics of the drug, and even the dose. This latter variable has been shown to influence the extent of absorption of MTX in man. This is illustrated in Fig. 2.

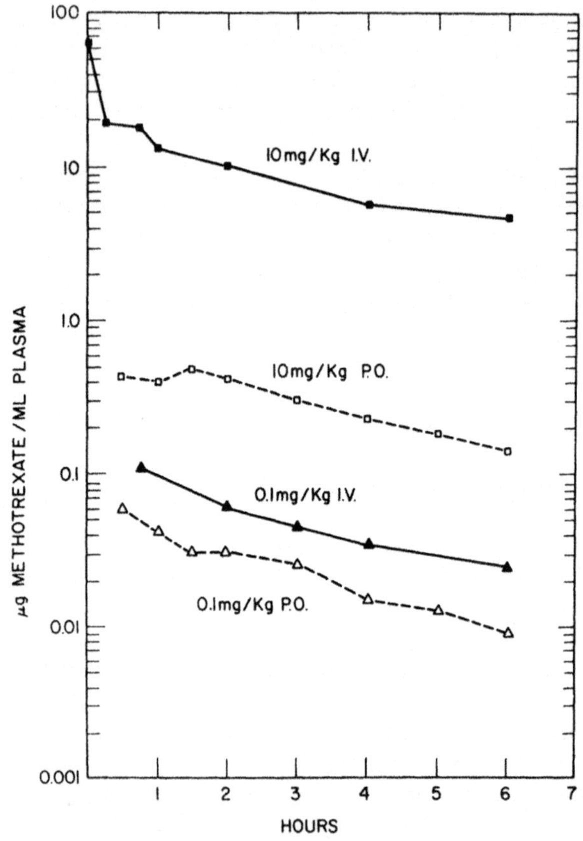

FIG. 2. Plasma disappearance of ^{3}H-methotrexate after oral and intravenous administration in patients.[6]

Henderson *et al.*[6] showed that 0.1 mg/kg of MTX resulted in plasma levels of the drug which were virtually indistinguishable whether the dose was given orally or parenterally. This is shown in the disappearance curve where the drug was given orally, compared with the curve where the same dose was given intravenously. Thus, for MTX, absorption from the GI tract of man appears to be a saturable process, and similar data exist in lower species of mammals.

An excellent example of increasing the lipid solubility of a drug to increase its rate of absorption comes from studies reported by Creasey *et al.*[7] of the pyrimidine analog 6-azauridine (AzUR). Figure 3 shows that while intravenous AzUR resulted in an initially higher blood level of AzUR and its metabolites, oral triacetyl-AzUR gave blood levels which were sustained for a longer period than either with intravenous or oral AzUR. The urinary excretion data also showed that intravenous AzUR and oral triacetyl-AzUR were similar in terms of rate of excretion and the total excreted.

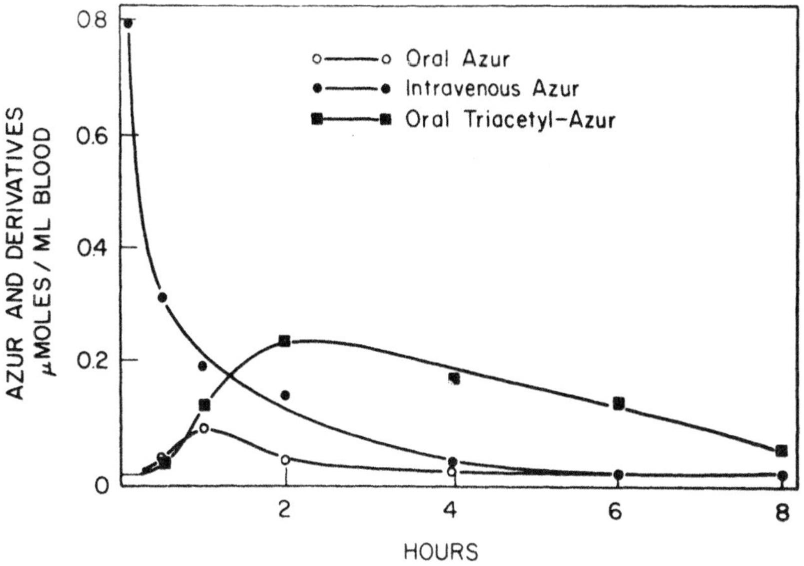

FIG. 3. Blood levels of 6-azauridine (AzUR) and metabolites after oral administration of triacetyl-6-azauridine or oral and intravenous administration of AzUR in patients.[7]

After a drug has been absorbed from the GI tract or injected intravascularly, it may remain in the plasma, usually bound to plasma proteins. Let us first consider the phenomenon of plasma protein binding in the distribution of drugs. Several kinds of plasma proteins will interact with drugs, but albumin appears to be the principal protein which accounts for most drug binding. This binding is usually reversible but in some cases may be used to advantage in prolonging low plasma levels of drug after a single dose. The presence of several drugs in the blood, especially molecules with similar structural characteristics, may have a profound effect on the distribution of each drug because of the competition for the same binding sites. The plasma protein binding of MTX has been extensively studied at the NCI[6] and elsewhere in man and laboratory animals (Table 1).

Binding primarily to the albumin fraction was approximately 50 per cent in human plasma and was comparable in the rodent and somewhat lower in dogs. In man, Liegler *et al.*[8] demonstrated that co-administration of the organic acids sodium salicylate or sulfisoxazole (Gantrisin), both of which are highly bound to plasma protein, reduced by 30 per cent the binding to protein of therapeutic plasma concentrations of MTX. The implication here is that either the purposeful or inadvertent co-administration of commonly employed drugs, in and of themselves relatively nontoxic, may cause significant alterations in the cytotoxicity of an antineoplastic agent such as MTX.

TABLE 1. PLASMA PROTEIN BINDING OF METHOTREXATE

	Per cent bound (0.1–1000 μg/ml)
Man	49
Dog	38
Rat	65
Mouse	52

Guarino *et al.*[9] have made some interesting observations of the plasma protein binding characterists of camptothecin, a plant alkaloid which recently underwent trials in clinical cancer. Plasma protein binding of sodium camptothecin (SC) was studied in 24 different species. In species with the greatest interest to experimental therapeutics – human, monkey, dog and mouse – the per cent binding was 98–74 per cent. Not only was the degree of binding high for many species, but by use of a newer technique, i.e. fluorescence polarization, we have determined that the association constant, K for SC is $7.9 \times 10^6 M^{-1}$ as calculated from the slope of the line in Fig. 4. This is the highest constant recorded for any drug and is approximately 8-fold higher than that of dicoumarol, previously reported to have the highest association constant.

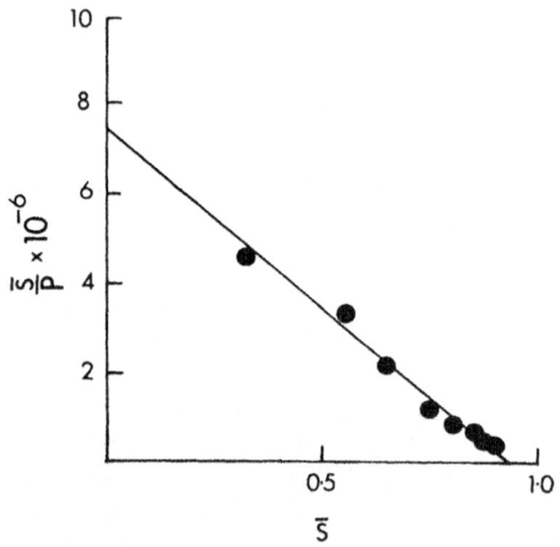

FIG. 4. Modified Scatchard plot of the binding of sodium camptothecin to human plasma albumin calculated from the polarization data in Fig. 2 of Ref. 9. $\bar{S}$ = saturation fraction of camptothecin; P = concentration (M) of free plasma albumin.

The passage of some drugs across the "blood–brain barrier" constitutes a special aspect of drug distribution but is of considerable importance in the clinical use of antineoplastic agents. Fenstermacher[10] discusses the pharmacologic and physiological aspects of this special barrier elsewhere.

In Fig. 5, two of the compartments indicated in Fig. 1, brain and tumor, are

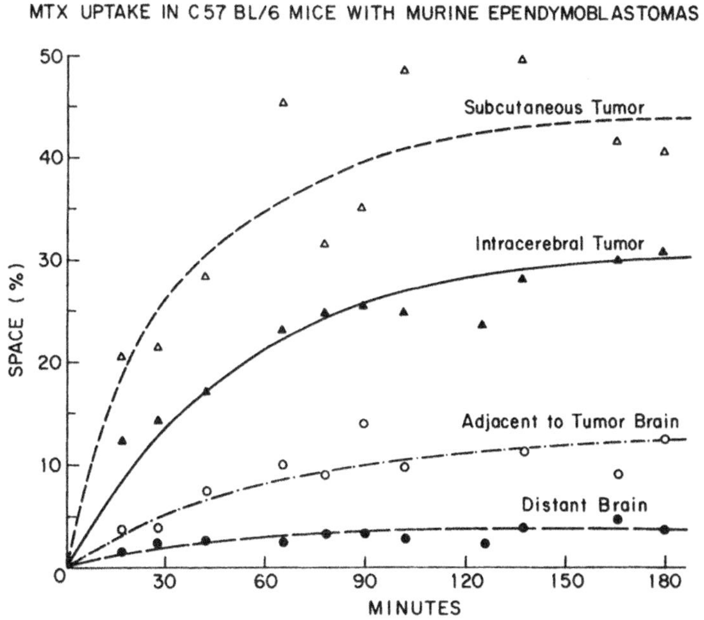

FIG. 5. Mean ^{3}H-methotrexate (MTX) spaces in C 57 BL/6 mice implanted with ependymoblastoma after intraperitoneal injection at three dose levels: 0.12, 1.4 and 42.8 m-moles/kg. Distribution space measurements for tumor and brain were calculated from radioactivity in tissue and plasma (plasma water for inulin).[11] Space (%) = (cpm/mg tissue) (cpm/mg plasma) × 100.

covered. Experimentally, Levin *et al.*[11] measured ^{3}H-MTX tissue levels in mice implanted with an intracerebral glioma. Here we will consider the results of their measurements of plasma, tumor and brain levels of MTX. In this figure, the term "space" is simply the (cpm/mg tissue)/(cpm/mg plasma) × 100 and, therefore, higher numbers represent elevated tissue/plasma ratios. It can be seen that when the tumor is carried subcutaneously, i.e. there is no blood–brain barrier, the upper curve shows the greatest penetrance of MTX. The distribution space for MTX is still large for intracerebral tumor, followed by brain adjacent to tumor (a mixture of normal brain plus approximately 20 per cent tumor) and lastly, the normal brain ("distant brain") in Fig. 5. At early times after administration, these space values are about equal to that of inulin (an indicator of the extracellular space), but at 24 hr, tumor/plasma ratios for MTX are 5-fold greater than those of inulin.

The placenta, testes and bone marrow also constitute special membrane barriers which a drug must negotiate in its entry and exit from various body compartments during its distribution. Thus, a blood–testes barrier has been proposed,[12,13] and since some anticancer agents have been reported to alter spermatogenesis, it is obvious that these agents are crossing this barrier. In Table 2 the tissue–plasma ratios for testes in the rabbit do not suggest anything more than simple diffusion with no evidence of selective bindings of the carcinostatic nitrosourea derivative, 1-(2-chloroethyl)-3-cyclohexyl-1-nitrosourea, CCNU.[14] One can compare the information for testes with

TABLE 2. TESTICULAR FAT AND PLASMA LEVELS OF CCNU IN THE RABBIT*

Time post i.v. injection (hr)	CCNU (μg equiv./g or ml)			Ratio	
	Testes	Fat	Plasma	Testes/plasma	Fat/plasma
1	0.47	0.85	0.47	1.00	1.80
4	0.29	0.37	0.38	0.76	0.97

*Mean value for N = 5. Animals were treated with 1 mg/ml of ^{14}C-ring-labeled CCNU in intralipid vehicle.

that obtained in fat[14] under the same conditions (Table 2). At 1 hr, the fat contained almost twice as much drug as the plasma contained. The clearance from this substernal fat depot was efficient, as indicated by the 4-hr values.

Drugs absorbed into the body or injected intravascularly are carried in the bloodstream to the liver, the principal organ where biotransformations may occur. The parent compound and metabolites produced in parenchymal cells can be eliminated via the hepatic vein to the kidney or via the bile duct to the intestine, the latter being most often the route for elimination of drug conjugates.

The most important route of excretion for drugs and their metabolites is the kidney. Renal excretion occurs by three different, but complementary mechanisms: glomerular filtration, tubular secretion of ionized substances, and tubular reabsorption of non-ionized substances.

Drugs that are bound to plasma proteins are not filtered by the glomeruli; thus, plasma protein binding retards the rate of filtration. Inulin and creatinine are classic examples of compounds that are excreted by pure glomerular filtration. Very few antineoplastic agents approach this ideal mechanism for renal clearance.

Classic examples of drugs which are excreted primarily by tubular secretion include the anions penicillin, probenecid, chlorothiazide and *p*-aminohippuric acid (PAH), and the cations hexamethonium and *N*-methylnicotinamide. PAH clearance rate from the kidney has been used as an estimate of renal flow or renal tubular secretion. It is also filtered by the glomeruli but is secreted more efficiently.

Once again we turn to MTX as an example of an antineoplastic agent primarily eliminated from the body by the kidney. MTX is a moderately weak dibasic organic acid (p*K*a 4.8 and 5.5), which in man was found by Liegler *et al.*[8] not only to be filtered by the kidney glomeruli but also, as might be suspected, to be actively secreted by the renal tubules. Table 3 shows that in 15 patients studied at the NCI, MTX exceeded the glomerular filtration (C_{MTX}/C_{Inulin}) rate by 26 per cent (average). The next line shows the influence of PAH loading on the glomerular filtrate of MTX (C_{MTX}/C_{Inulin}) in three patients. This was markedly curtailed by about 50 per cent. Sodium salicylate, in four patients, also reduced the glomerular filtration of MTX as well as its secretion by the tubules (C_{MTX}/C_{PAH}). Polar lipid-insoluble molecules, such as metabolites of many drugs, are more readily cleared through the kidneys, permitting more rapid elimination of drugs once they have been altered. For example, cyclophosphamide and procarbazine are extensively metabolized in the liver into more polar metabolites and excreted by the kidney. These are lipid-soluble drugs which

TABLE 3. RENAL CLEARANCE OF MTX IN MAN*

	Average†		Decrease (%)	No. of patients
	C_{MTX}/C_{Inulin}	(C_{MTX}/C_{PAH})		
Control	1.26	(0.26)		15
Control	1.35			
PAH	0.64		52	3
Control	1.32	(0.25)		
Sodium salicylate	0.86	(0.13)	35 (48)	4

*Data are from Liegler *et al.*[8]
†C = ml/min/1.73 m^2 body surface area.

could remain in the body for a long time if hepatic enzymes did not act upon them to produce more polar substances.

The bile represents another important pathway for the excretion of drugs and many antitumor agents. Both methotrexate and its halogenated derivative, dichloromethotrexate (DCM), are excreted into the bile and undergo enterohepatic circulation.[15] In the case of DCM, however, its metabolite, 7-OH-DCM, is not extensively reabsorbed in the gut after biliary excretion and appears in the stool. The extensive role of biliary excretion in the handling of DCM is shown in Fig 6 for a number of laboratory animals and man. DCM is not metabolized by the dog as it is by other mammals and man. Analogous data are not readily available for the biliary excretion of MTX in man, although if we are to accept the pharmacokinetic model developed for the mouse,[16] and which can predict for man, we would expect extensive biliary excretion of MTX in *Homo sapiens*.

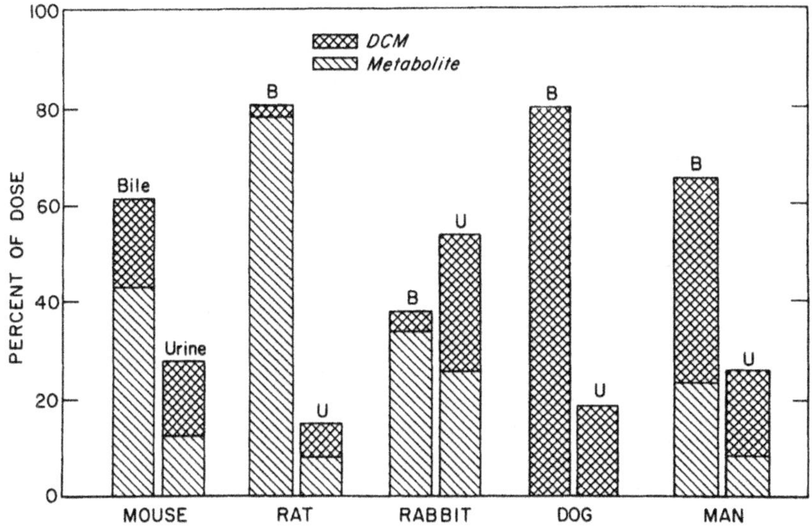

FIG. 6. Comparative distribution of dichloromethotrexate (DCM) and its metabolite (7-OH-DCM) in bile and urine of a variety of species.[15]

Because of reported preclinical and clinical toxic manifestations of SC in the gastrointestinal tract, we thought the possibility of biliary transport of this drug should be investigated (Fig. 7). Rats with ligated renal pedicles were treated with over a 1000-fold range of doses of SC. The double logarithmic plot in Fig. 7 shows the parallelism of the plasma and tissue curves and clearly demonstrates simple diffusion processes throughout this range of plasma levels. Bile concentrations exceed those of plasma by 1000-fold and, at the higher levels, demonstrate some evidence of saturation.

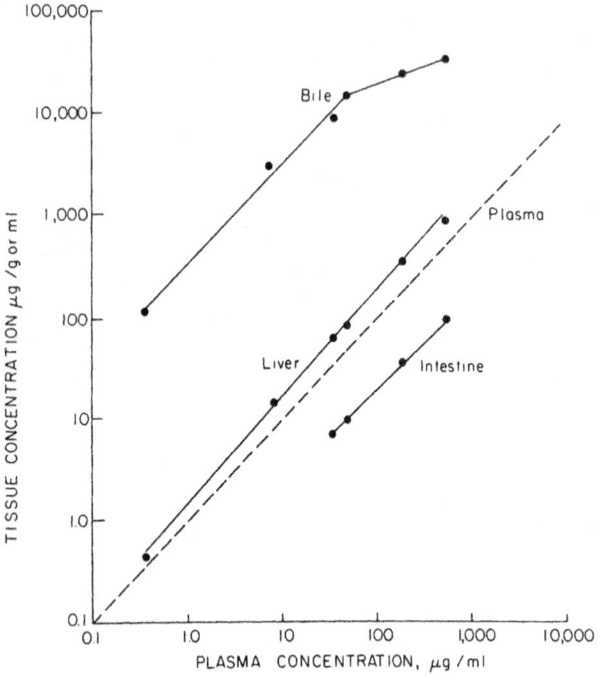

FIG. 7. Double logarithmic plot of tissue levels of sodium camptothecin vs. plasma levels. Rats were treated with intravenous doses from 0.4 to 400 mg/kg.

While urinary and biliary excretion mainly account for the elimination of drugs and their metabolites from the body, in some cases, other routes of elimination are important. For example, a significant proportion of the excretory products of nitrogen mustard and procarbazine appear in expired air. Some drugs are excreted in the gastrointestinal tract, saliva, sweat and milk.

Recently Johns *et al.*[17] measured the excretion of MTX in an African female. The top part of Fig. 8 compares the plasma level of MTX with the levels of MTX found in the milk over a 12-hr period after administration of an oral dose of 15 mg/m^2. Note that there is a 10-fold difference between the scale on the right representing milk-MTX and the scale on the left representing plasma-MTX. The bottom part of the figure shows a plot of the milk to plasma concentration ratio of MTX over this 12-hr period. Since MTX is ionized at body pH and is lipid insoluble, it is therefore excreted into the milk at a very low but detectable and non-harmful level. Excretion into the milk as

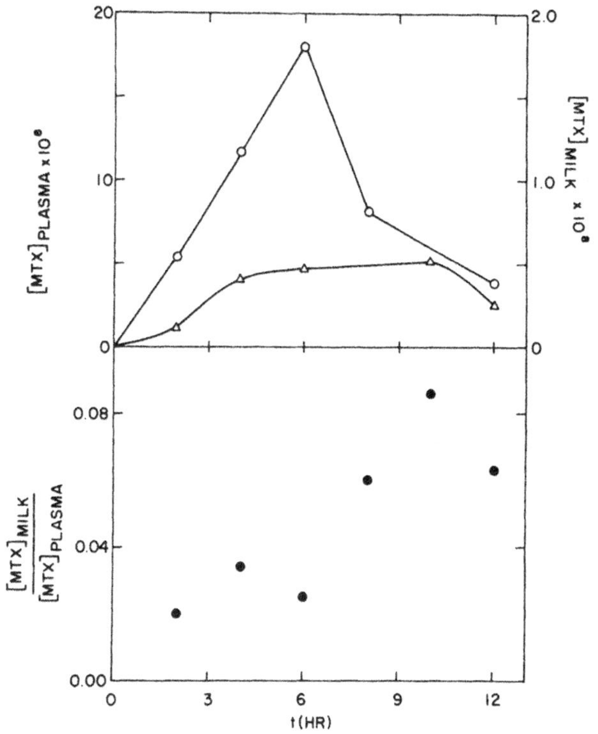

FIG. 8. Top, MTX (moles/litter) in plasma (○——○) and milk (△——△) after oral dose of 15 mg/m² in patient. Bottom, milk/plasma concentration ratio.[17]

well as expired air, sweat and saliva occurs mainly by simple diffusion of non-ionized molecules.

In summary, we have attempted to sketch a very simplistic picture of the general principles governing the absorption, protein binding, distribution and excretion of drugs within the various body compartments shown in Fig. 1. We have used the folate antagonist, methotrexate, primarily as the model drug to discuss these principles. The reason for this is clear. As a class of anti-tumor drugs, the folic acid antagonists, which includes MTX, have probably been the most extensively studied as pertains to pharmacological disposition. As acidic molecules, however, they do not represent the majority of antineoplastic agents, which are basic in character. Despite this difference, the principles which we have outlined apply equally well to both classes of drug.

REFERENCES

1. D. ZAHARKO, *Biochem. Pharmac.* Suppl. 2, 1–8 (1974).
2. A. J. CLARK, *General Pharmacology, Handbuch der Experimentellen Pharmakologie*, Vol. IV, pp. 123–142. Berlin (1973).
3. L. B. MELLETT, *Biochem. Pharmac.* Suppl. 2, 35–45 (1974).
4. L. S. SCHANKER, *Pharmac. Rev.* **14**, 501 (1962).
5. B. B. BRODIE, in *Absorption and Distribution of Drugs* (Ed. T. B. BINNS), p. 16. Williams & Wilkins, Baltimore (1964).

6. E. S. HENDERSON, R. H. ADAMSON and V. T. OLIVERIO, *Cancer Res.* **25**, 1018 (1965).
7. W. A. CREASEY, M. E. FINK, R. E. HANDSCHUMACHER and P. CALABRESI, *Cancer Res.* **23**, 444 (1963).
8. D. G. LIEGLER, E. S. HENDERSON, M. A. HAHN and V. T. OLIVERIO, *Clin. Pharmac. Ther.* **10**, 849 (1969).
9. A. M. GUARINO, J. B. ANDERSON, D. K. STARKWEATHER and C. F. CHIGNELL, *Cancer Chemother. Rep.* **57**, in press.
10. J. D. FENSTERMACHER and R. G. BLASBERG, *Biochem. Pharmac.* Suppl. 2, 51–56 (1974).
11. V. A. LEVIN, T. P. CLANCY, J. I. AUSMAN and D. P. RALL, *J. natn. Cancer Inst.* **48**, 875 (1972).
12. P. P. H. DEBRUYN, R. C. ROBERTSON and R. S. FARN, *Anat. Rec.* **108**, 27 (1960).
13. M. DYN and D. W. FAWCETT, *Biol. Reprod.* **3**, 308 (1970).
14. C. L. LITTERST, E. G. MIMNAUGH, S. EDELMAN and T. E. GRAM, *Pharmacologist* **15**, in press (1973).
15. V. T. OLIVERIO and D. S. ZAHARKO, *Ann. N.Y. Acad. Sci.* **186**, 387 (1971).
16. D. S. ZAHARKO, R. L. DEDRICK, K. B. BISCHOFF, J. A. LONGSTRETH and V. T. OLIVERIO, *J. natn. Cancer Inst.* **26**, 775 (1971).
17. D. G. JOHNS, L. D. RUTHERFORD, P. C. LEIGHTON and C. L. VOGEL, *Am. J. Obstet. Gynec.* **112**, 978 (1972).

Pp. 21—33, Supplement Number 2, 1974.
Biochemical Pharmacology. Printed in the U.S.A.

FACTORS AFFECTING BIOTRANSFORMATION AND ACTIVITY OF ANTITUMOR DRUGS

SILVIO GARATTINI, M. G. DONELLI and F. SPREAFICO

Instituto di Recerche Farmacologiche "Mario Negri", Via Eritrea 62, 20157 Milano, Italy

IN THE continuing effort to improve chemotherapy of human cancer, it is obviously necessary that we search for new effective agents as well as for new approaches to tumor treatment. However, while pursuing these objectives, we should not ignore the possibility that the already available antineoplastic compounds may be used more rationally, effectively and safely. Therefore, it is important to obtain more precise information on various aspects of these agents such as metabolism, absorption, tissue distribution and excretion, since, as is the case with most other drugs, these factors may decisively influence the clinical effectiveness of antitumoral compounds.

A very general scheme of the processes which control the availability of antineoplastic drugs to malignant tissue is presented in Fig. 1. Evidence from various sources has accumulated to indicate that, for a given drug, the relative importance of these processes may vary depending on a number of different factors, which range from the genetical constitution of the host to sex, age or nutritional status, from the presence of pathological conditions (e.g. liver damage caused by metastatic infiltration), to the concomitant or previous use of other drugs, etc. These variables, apart from the intrinsic sensitivity of the tumor to the drug, may all markedly influence the degree of antitumoral activity of the treatment employed. This presentation will deal with some experimental results chosen to illustrate the influence of some of the factors mentioned above.

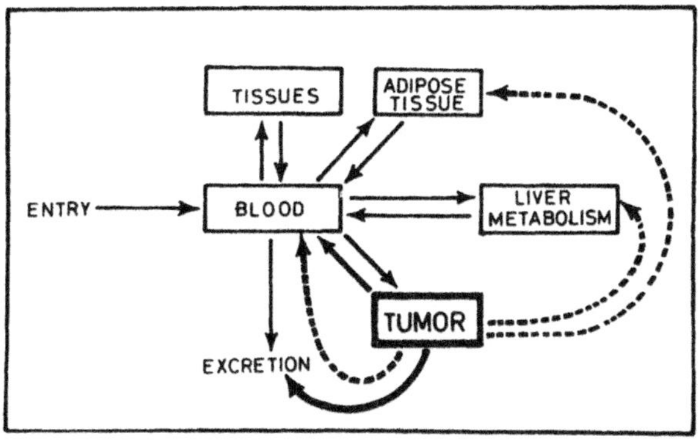

FIG. 1. Schematic outline of the processes governing availability of antineoplastic drugs to neoplastic tissues.

Table 1 shows the levels of alkylating activity, as measurable with the *p*-nitrobenzylpyridine test,[1] detectable in the serum after i.v. injection of 50 mg/kg of cyclophosphamide (cyclo-P) in CD_1 and (Balb/c x DBA/2)F_1 hybrid mice. It is evident that the peak level as well as the half-life of alkylating activity is significantly higher in the CDF_1 mice than in CD_1 animals. In the same table, the differential leukopenic activity of cyclo-P in the two strains is also presented, showing the correlation between the pharmacokinetic parameters and the activity *in vivo* present in this case. This type of finding also suggests that, in comparing the effectiveness of a given drug on tumors growing in different animal strains, consideration should also be given to the possibility that the drug may be distributed and/or metabolized in variable manners in the different hosts.

TABLE 1. PHARMACOKINETIC PARAMETERS AND LEUKOPENIC ACTIVITY OF CYCLOPHOSPHAMIDE (cyclo-P) IN CD_1 AND (Balb/c X DBA/2)F_1 MICE

Cyclo-P (50 mg/kg, i.v.)	CD_1	CDF_1
T_{10} plasma level (nmoles HN_2-equiv./ml ± S. E.)	118 ± 7	153 ± 10*
$T_{1/2}$ plasma alkylating activity (min ± 95% CL†)	18(16–20)	50(43–60)*
Vd (l/kg ± 95% CL†)	0.22(0.19–0.29)	0.30(0.26–0.34)
Leukopenic activity (% of controls)	73 ± 2	43 ± 7*

*$P<0.05$.
†CL = confidence limits.

Circadian rhythmicity may also play a role in modifying metabolism of drugs. As shown in Table 2, significantly lower peak serum levels of 6-mercaptopurine (6-MP) were found in rats when this agent was injected i.v. in the morning rather than in the afternoon. Table 2 also shows one effect of the sex of the host, since this difference in drug levels is observable only in female and not in male rats. Another example of this rhythmicity is illustrated in Table 3, where the plasma half-lives of hydrocortisone in humans injected with the drug at different times of the day are presented.[2]

It is expected that different types of tumors may have a varying capacity to take up anticancer drugs, but even for the same tumor a given drug may accumulate in different degrees, depending on many variables such as size, extent of necrosis and vascularization, and also on the site of the tumor growth. The possible importance of the latter factor is indicated in Table 4, which shows the peak levels and $T_{1/2}$ of alkylating activity in the tumor after administration of cyclo-P to mice bearing Ehrlich carcinoma growing subcutaneously, intraperitoneally or intracerebrally. In these conditions, the lowest levels of alkylating metabolites are found when the tumor is in the intracerebral location. When, however, a different drug is examined, such as *N*-

TABLE 2. CIRCADIAN RHYTHMICITY OF 6-MERCAPTOPURINE (50 mg/kg, i.v.) IN SRAGUE–DAWLEY RATS

Time of injection	Peak serum level (μg/ml ± S. E.)	
	Males	Females
9:00 a.m.	81 ± 6	50 ± 5
9:00 p.m.	90 ± 1	99 ± 6*

*$P<0.05$.

TABLE 3. HYDROCORTISONE (1.54 mg/kg, i.v.) HALF-LIVES IN HUMAN PLASMA AFTER INJECTION IN THE MORNING OR AFTERNOON*

Time of injection	$T_{1/2}$ (min)
8:00 a.m.	107 ± 11
4:00 p.m.	73 ± 8.4

*Data are from reference 2.
†$P<0.05$.

TABLE 4. DRUG CONCENTRATION IN THE TUMOR AND RESPONSIVENESS OF EHRLICH CARCINOMA GROWING IN VARIOUS SITES *in vivo* AFTER ADMINISTRATION OF CYCLO-PHOSPHAMIDE (cyclo-P) OR *N*-METHYLNITROSOUREA (MNU)*

Site of tumor growth	Cyclo-P		MNU	
	Peak level	Responsiveness *in vivo*	Peak level	Responsiveness *in vivo*
i.p.	85 ± 2	++	9 ± 0.4	–
s.c.	67 ± 7	+	3 ± 0.4	–
i.c.	25 ± 2	±	25 ± 1	++

*Cyclo-P (85 mg/kg) or MNU (20 mg/kg) was injected i.v. at various times after tumor transplantation, i.e. 12 days after 10^5 tumor cell injection intracerebrally (i.c.); 13 days after 10^6 cell injection i.p., and 16 days after 5×10^6 cell transplantation s.c. Levels of cyclo-P metabolites are expressed as nmoles HN_2-equiv./g and those of MNU as μg/g of tumor tissue (± S. E.).

methylnitrosourea (MNU), the opposite type of picture can be observed, and in fact MNU markedly accumulates in the brain. The possible therapeutic implication of these drug distribution data can be appreciated by observing that the drug responsiveness of the tumor *in vivo* in different sites correlates very well with the tissue distribution results.

A major factor that determines the body levels, and consequently the activity *in vivo*, of many therapeutic agents, is the capacity of the liver to metabolize the drug with the formation of other chemical species that may be more or less active than the parent compound. The system which is recognized as the most important for these biotransformation processes of foreign as well as many endogenous substances, is the liver microsomal fraction, which contains an array of enzymes, collectively referred to as mixed oxygenases, capable of carrying out several types of biochemical transformations.[3–5]

A simple experimental model that can be used to investigate the importance of the liver microsomes is schematically illustrated in Fig. 2. In principle, the system employs growing cancer cells *in vitro*, in order to measure (by the degree of cell growth inhibition) the antitumoral activity of the products originating from the drug of interest after interaction with isolated microsomes. In the "direct test," the drug is added to the growing cancer cells *in vitro*, whereas in the "indirect test" the medium includes the complete drug-metabolizing microsomal system. Details of this procedure are presented elsewhere.[6] Besides permitting the evaluation of the state of activity of the liver microsomes, an additional advantage of this method is that it may make possible the identification *in vitro* of active metabolites of anticancer agents; moreover, it may also be of some interest for screening purposes. A convenient model drug to illustrate this approach is cyclophosphamide; it is known[7,8] that this agent *per se* displays little or no cytotoxic activity, as is also shown by the fact that in the direct test no inhibition of cell growth is observed (Table 5). To exhibit cytotoxic activity, cyclo-P must be processed by the microsomal enzymes, which transform it into more active metabolites; the precise biochemistry of this process is under intense study in a number of laboratories.[9–15]

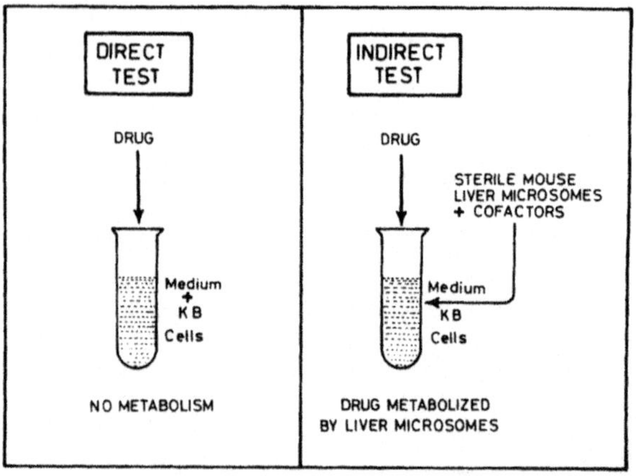

FIG. 2. A simple experimental model for evaluating the state of activity of liver microsomes. Details are given in the text.

The activation of cyclo-P by the microsomes is evidenced by the results obtained with the indirect test where the development of cytotoxic compound(s) is indicated by the reduction of growth of the test cells. Table 5 shows that in these experimental conditions, the cyctotoxicity produced is proportional to the amount of microsomes

TABLE 5. CYTOTOXIC ACTIVITY *in vitro* OF CYCLOPHOSPHAMIDE (1000 μg/ml) EXPOSED OR NOT EXPOSED TO 105,000 *g* MOUSE LIVER MICROSOMAL PREPARATIONS

Experimental group*	Growth inhibition (%)	Cell destruction (%)
Untreated	0	0
Cyclo-P	2	0
M 750 + CF	0	0
Cyclo-P + CF	1	0
M(25) + CF + cyclo-P†	42	0
M(50) + CF + cyclo-P†	82	0
M(100) + CF + cyclo-P†	100	25
M(250) + CF + cyclo-P†	100	72
M(500) + CF + cyclo-P†	100	91

*M = 105,000 *g* liver microsomal preparation; CF = cofactors; for details of experimental conditions see reference 6.

†The number in parentheses refers to the amount of microsomal preparation obtained from 25, 50, etc. mg liver.

TABLE 6. CELL DESTRUCTION *in vitro* BY DIMETHYLTRIAZENO-IMIDAZOLE CARBOXAMIDE (DIC) EXPOSED OR NOT EXPOSED TO MOUSE LIVER MICROSOMAL PREPARATIONS

Experimental group*	Cell destruction (%)
Controls	0
M + CF	0
DIC	88
DIC + CF	81
DIC + M	77
DIC + M + CF	0

*DIC = 170 μg/ml; M = 105,000 *g* liver microsomal fraction; CF = cofactors; see reference 6 for procedural details.

present. It should be recalled, however, that drugs may not only be activated through processing by the microsomes, but may also give rise to less active compounds. This latter event is illustrated (Table 6) by the pattern of results obtained in the direct and indirect tests when one investigates 5-(3,3-dimethyl-1-triazeno)imidazole-4-carboxamide (DIC), an agent which has lately received considerable attention for its activity on various types of human neoplasms.[16–18]

In view of the fact that a considerable number of substances may modify the activity of the liver microsomes in the sense of an increased capacity (the well known phenomenon of drug induction[19]) as well as in the direction of a decreased metabolizing activity, it is possible that drug interactions may be explained by such a mechanism. The aspect of drug interactions is of special interest in cancer chemotherapy where the use of combinations of agents is almost standard practice and it is common for most hospitalized patients to receive quite a large number of pharmacological agents.[20] We should be concerned not only with possible interactions of antineoplastic drugs, a topic examined by others in this meeting, but also with the possibility of interactions of anticancer and non-anticancer agents, since cancerous patients will frequently be given a whole range of other supportive treatments. It is, therefore, relevant to examine how these other treatments may affect the activity of antineoplastic drugs *in vivo*.

A model system that we have investigated is represented by the phenobarbital–cyclophosphamide interaction. The rationale behind these studies lies in the fact that phenobarbital (PB), like other barbiturates, is frequently employed clinically as an hypnotic-sedative agent; in addition, its capacity to "induce" the liver microsomal system has been amply documented.[3,5] If mice are pretreated with PB at actively inducing doses (80 mg/kg, i.p.) 48 and 24 hr before a single injection of cyclo-P, the activity of the latter *in vivo* is markedly diminished, as evidenced by reduction of the drug's antileukemic and immunosuppressant activities (Table 7). Immunosuppressant activity was estimated by counting the number of anti-sheep erythrocyte hemolytic plaque-forming cells (PFC) detectable in the spleen by the technique of Jerne and Nordin.[21] The diminished activity of cyclo-P *in vivo* in phenobarbital-pretreated mice is reflected in a striking reduction in the serum half-life of cyclo-P-derived alkylating activity measurable in these animals (Table 8). As regards the possible mechanism for such a result, the most likely explanation seems to be an "induction" of the liver microsomes by PB with consequent speeding up of the cyclo-P activation steps and, to a greater extent, of those leading to less active metabolites. A study by Field *et al.* [22] supports this reasoning and the effects of such drug combination in humans have been recently

TABLE 7. EFFECT OF PHENOBARBITAL (PB) (80 mg/kg, i.p.) PRETREATMENT ON THE IMMUNOSUPPRESSIVE AND ANTITUMORAL ACTIVITIES OF CYCLOPHOSPHAMIDE IN MICE*

Experimental group	PFC/10^6 spleen cells	No. leukemia cells ($\times 10^6$) in peritoneal cavity 5 days after transplant	Median survival time (days)
Controls	641	409	7.6
PB	683	476	8.2
Cyclo-P	8	34	18.7
PB + cyclo-P	225†	158†	14.4†

*For immunosuppression studies, mice were injected on day 0 with 4×10^8 sheep erythrocytes; PB was given on days 0 and 1, and cyclo-P (35 mg/kg, i.p.) was injected on day 2; antibody-producing cells were counted on day 4. CDF_1 mice were injected with 10^6 L1210 leukemia cells i.p. on day 0; PB was given on days 0 and 1, and cyclo-P (50 mg/kg, i.p.) was injected on day 2. PFC = plaque-forming cells.

†P<0.01.

TABLE 8. EFFECT OF PHENOBARBITAL (PB) (80 mg/kg, i.p. × 2) PRETREATMENT ON SERUM ALKYLATING ACTIVITY AFTER INJECTION OF CYCLOPHOSPHAMIDE (50 mg/kg, i.v.) IN MICE

Experimental group	Alkylating activity (mμmoles HN_2 equiv./ml)					$T_{1/2}$ (min)
	10 min	15 min	20 min	40 min	60 min	
Cyclo-P	116	119	115	48	24	18.6
PB + cyclo-P	129	125	77*	27*	9*	10.4

*$P<0.05$.

examined.[23] The same type of treatment with PB described above is capable of modifying, in either direction, the activity *in vivo* of a number of other frequently employed antitumoral and immunosuppressive agents, as summarized in Table 9. Of special interest, in view of its wide use, is the very marked reduction in activity of hydrocortisone after treatment with PB; studies in humans[24] have shown, for instance, that a sharply reduced plasma half-life of corticosteroids can be found even 3 weeks after discontinuation of PB treatment.

The possible importance of the schedule of treatment in influencing the final response *in vivo* should also be emphasized. This can be illustrated by the data of Table 10 which show that if, instead of short courses of PB followed by a single dose of cyclo-P, mice are given more prolonged treatment with both agents concomitantly, the interaction changes direction from what was described earlier, and a

TABLE 9. EFFECT OF PHENOBARBITAL (PB) (80 mg/kg, i.p. × 2) PRETREATMENT ON THE IMMUNOSUPPRESSIVE ACTIVITY OF VARIOUS COMPOUNDS IN MICE*

Increase	No change	Decrease
6-MP†	Methotrexate	Hydrocortisone†
PCZ‡	5-FU	cyclophosphamide†
BCNU§	HN_2	
TEM§	Daunomycin	
	ALS	

*PCZ = procarbazine; BCNU = 1,3-bis(2-chloroethyl)-1-nitrosourea; TEM = triethylenmelamine; 5-FU = 5-fluorouracil; HN_2 = mechlorethamine; ALS = antilymphocytic serum; 6-MP = 6-mercaptopurine.

†Modification of response compared to that of mice not pretreated with PB>50%.

‡Increase was 10–25% compared to response of mice not pretreated with PB.

§Increase was 25–50% compared to response of mice not pretreated with PB.

TABLE 10. IMMUNOSUPPRESSIVE ACTIVITY IN MICE GIVEN A SERIES OF CONCOMITANT INJECTIONS OF PHENOBARBITAL (PB) AND CYCLOPHOSPHAMIDE (cyclo-P)*

Experimental group	Dose (mg/kg, i.p.)	PFC/spleen
Controls		68,120
PB	40 × 4	61,530
Cyclo-P	35 × 4	6,080
PB + Cyclo-P	40 × 4 35 × 4	1,875†

*Mice were injected on day 0 with 4 × 10^8 sheep erythrocytes; PB and cyclo-P were given from day −4 to day −1; immune responsiveness was assessed on day 4. PFC = plaque-forming cells.

†$P<0.05$.

significant increase in the cytotoxic activity of cyclo-P is now observed in comparison to animals receiving only the cytotoxic agent. A further example of the possible importance of the schedule of treatment is presented in Table 11, which contains data on the combination of prednisone with cyclo-P. It is evident from these data that seemingly minor changes in a chemotherapeutic protocol can have profound effects on the ultimate results *in vivo*.

In addition to the influence of non-anticancer agents on the activity of antitumoral drugs, the reverse possibility should also be borne in mind, since it has been repeatedly demonstrated that treatment with cytotoxic agents may affect the liver drug-metabolizing capacity. An example of this type of interaction with cyclo-P and

TABLE 11. IMMUNOSUPPRESSIVE ACTIVITY OF THE PREDNISONE–CYCLOPHOSPHAMIDE DRUG COMBINATION ACCORDING TO THE RESPECTIVE TIME OF INJECTION*

Treatment (mg/kg, i.p.)	Day of injection	PFC/spleen (% of controls)
Prednisone (50)	1 or 2	100
Cyclo-P (25)	2	2.3
Prednisone + cyclo-P	1 2	7.4†
Cyclo-P + prednisone	2 2	0.5†

*Mice were injected on day 0 with 4 × 10^8 sheep erythrocytes; immune response was assessed by counting the number of anti-sheep erythrocyte plaque-forming cells (PFC) by the technique of Jerne and Nordin[21] on day 4.

†$P<0.05$.

pentobarbital (PT) is shown in Table 12. To close the circle, Table 13 shows the effect of previous administration of cyclo-P on circulating levels of 6-mercaptopurine (6-MP) administered 7 days later. The mechanism(s) of this effect, which may have an important bearing on the practice of sequential antitumoral chemotherapy, has not yet been fully elucidated.

TABLE 12. EFFECT OF A PREVIOUS INJECTION OF CYCLOPHOSPHAMIDE (120 mg/kg, i.p.) ON THE METABOLISM AND ACTIVITY *in vivo* OF PENTOBARBITAL (35 mg/kg, i.p.) IN RATS

Time after cyclo-P injection (hr)	Sleeping time (min)	Brain pentobarbital $T_{1/2}$ (min)	Liver microsomal activity (%)
0	30	31	100
1	50*		
4	46*		
14	55*		
24	56*		
96	86*	45*	56*

*$P<0.05$.

TABLE 13. EFFECT OF CYCLOPHOSPHAMIDE GIVEN 7 DAYS BEFORE ON THE KINETIC PARAMETERS OF 6-MERCAPTOPURINE (50 mg/kg, i.v.) IN SARCOMA 180 BEARING MICE

Parameter	Controls	Cyclo-P-treated*
Serum peak level (μg/ml)	52 ± 3	66 ± 3†
Serum $T_{1/2}$ (min)	5 (4–6)	11 (8–14)†
Serum Vd (l/kg)	0.8(0.6–1.0)	0.9(0.8–1.1)

*Mice were injected with 1×10^6 S180 cells i.p. on day 0; cyclo-P (300 mg/kg, i.p.) was given on day 6.
†$P<0.05$.

In still other cases, a metabolite may have an influence on the effectiveness *in vivo* of the active compound from which it was derived. An unexpected example of this type of interaction emerged during a study on the comparative activity of 6-MP and its derivative, azathioprine (AZA), the latter being at the present time the most widely used chemical immunosuppressant. When equimolar doses of 6-MP and AZA are given to mice by the i.v. route (the same result is observed with any parenteral route of administration), 6-MP is consistently found (Table 14) to be a more active immunosuppressant than AZA, the difference in activity being approximately a factor of 3. Since AZA is believed to act through its liberation of 6-MP,[25,26] the levels of the latter, i.e. the active compound, were measured in the serum and spleen after injections of AZA or of 6-MP as such. Full details of these results are presented in

TABLE 14. COMPARATIVE IMMUNOSUPPRESSIVE ACTIVITY OF EQUIMOLAR DOSES OF 6-MERCAPTOPURINE (6-MP) AND AZATHIOPRINE (AZA) GIVEN i.v. TO MICE*

Experimental group	Dose (mg/kg)	Response (%)
Controls		100
6-MP	50	31.2
AZA	81	67.7
6-MP	100	18.4
AZA	163	56.8
6-MP	150	9.9
AZA	244	32.6

*Mice were injected on day 0 with 4 × 10^8 sheep erythrocytes; drugs were administered 2 days later and the immune response was assessed on day 4.

another publication.[27] In summary, it was found that the total quantity of 6-MP present in the blood or in the spleen (the main target organ in our experimental conditions) was equal, over the time period investigated, after injections of 6-MP or of AZA, despite the marked differences in the activity of the two drugs *in vivo*.

The major mechanism responsible for the splitting of AZA *in vivo* is believed[26] to be through a nucleophilic attack by SH groups, mainly glutathione, which gives rise to 6-MP and to 5-thio-1-methyl-4-nitroimidazole (MIZ), as indicated in Fig. 3. We thus investigated whether this mercaptoimidazole moiety exerts some influence on the activity of 6-MP *in vivo*. As shown in Table 15, when MIZ, by itself inactive as an immunosuppressant, is injected together with 6-MP, the latter's activity is markedly reduced and levels of immunosuppression are obtained which are practically indistinguishable from those found in mice given AZA. Even low amounts of MIZ (the

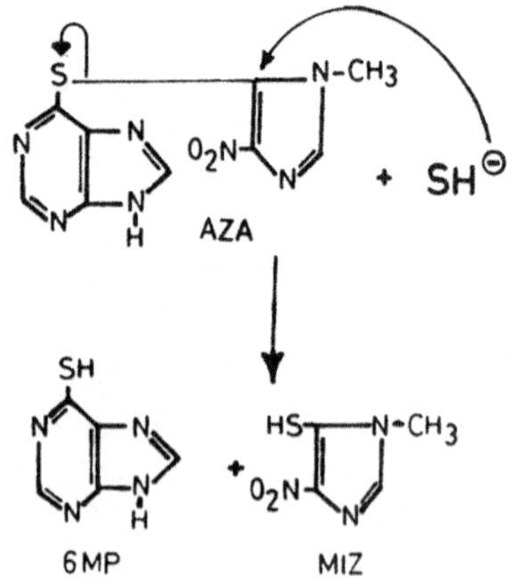

FIG. 3. Diagram of the mechanism by which azathiopurine (AZA) hydrolyzed, yielding 6-mercaptopurine (6-MP) and 5-thio-1-methyl-4-nitroimidazole (MIZ).

lowest quantity shown in Table 15 corresponds to the amount expected from a 33 per cent splitting of AZA by SH groups) are capable of antagonizing 6-MP, through mechanisms which still remain to be elucidated. Nevertheless, we thought it might be of some interest to present this cast of "inbuilt interaction" not only to show an additional factor that may exert an influence on the effectiveness of antitumor agents *in vivo*, but also to indicate some of the limitations as well as possible heuristic benefits of studies of correlations between activity *in vivo* and body concentrations of a drug. Results from the same study may also be usefully exploited to illustrate the importance of another obvious factor, i.e. the route of administration, in affecting the potency of drugs *in vivo*. In fact, when the comparative immunosuppressive activity of 6-MP and AZA was measured, employing the oral route of drug administration, AZA was found to be more effective than 6-MP, i.e. the results obtained were the opposite of those observed with parenteral routes (Table 16). This finding is attributable to the greater intestinal absorption of AZA in comparison to 6-MP, which produces significantly higher levels of AZA in the circulation.

Discussion has so far been devoted to consideration of several factors which may affect the metabolism, and hence the activity, of antitumor agents. However, the picture is rendered more complicated by the fact that the presence of a tumor *per se* can influence in several ways the distribution and metabolism of foreign compounds, including antineoplastic agents. This is a factor which should be kept in mind in extrapolating information obtained in normal subjects directly to patients with malignancies. A tumor may influence the excretion of drugs by affecting renal elimination or, for instance, by blocking biliary flow; because of the reduction of adipose tissue, it may affect the storage of drugs in this important body compartment.

TABLE 15. EFFECT OF 5-THIO-1-METHYL-4-NITROIMIDAZOLE (MIZ) ON THE IMMUNOSUPPRESSIVE ACTIVITY OF 6-MERCAPTOPURINE (6-MP) IN MICE*

Experimental group	Dose (mg/kg, i.p.)	PFC/spleen
Controls		100,580
6-MP	100	10,525
AZA	193	51,400
MIZ	93	106,320
6-MP + MIZ	100+ 93	47,300
6-MP + MIZ	100+ 62	48,000
6-MP + MIZ	100+ 31	46,100

*CD_1 mice were injected on day 0 with 4×10^8 sheep erythrocytes; 6-MP, AZA or MIZ was injected on day 2; plaque-forming cells (PFC) were counted on day 4.

TABLE 16. IMMUNOSUPPRESSIVE ACTIVITY OF EQUIMOLAR AMOUNTS OF 6-MERCAPTOPURINE AND AZATHIOPRINE (AZA) GIVEN ORALLY TO MICE*

Experimental group	Dose (mg/kg)	Response (%)
Controls		100
6-MP	150	91.4
AZA	244	65.3†
6-MP	300	55.8
AZA	489	24.3†
6-MP	600	21.5
AZA	978	9.6†

*CD_1 mice were given the drugs 2 days after antigenic stimulation with sheep erythrocytes; the immune response was assessed on day 4 by the technique of Jerne and Nordin.[21]

†$P<0.01$ relative to AZA group.

TABLE 17. ACTIVITY AND METABOLISM *in vivo* OF ZOXAZOLAMINE (50 mg/kg, i.v.) IN NORMAL AND WALKER CARCINOMA-BEARING RATS*

Experimental group	Paralysis (min)	Brain peak level (μg/g)	Plasma peak level (μg/ml)	Amount metabolized (nmoles/g liver)
Normal	160	3.8	3.3	803
Walker	330†	12.5†	6.4†	160†

*Rats were transplanted with 150 mg of Walker carcinoma s.c.; zoxazolamine was injected 16 days after tumor transplantation. Data are from reference 29.

†$P<0.05$.

Tumors may influence transport of drugs through modifications in plasma protein concentration and, therefore, protein binding of drugs. Furthermore, a tumor may change the activity of the liver microsomal enzymes (see Fig. 1). In Table 17 is shown the effect of the presence of Walker carcinoma on the metabolism of zoxazolamine, a useful model drug for these studies because of its metabolism through the microsomes. It can be seen that the tumor impairs the biotransformation of the drug, resulting in increased plasma and tissue levels with a consequent enhancement of the paralyzing activity of zoxazolamine in tumor-bearing rats. Studies conducted with the isolated perfused liver model[28] seem to indicate that such an impairment of liver metabolism is due to the presence of an as yet unidentified toxic factor (or factors) released by the tumor into the circulation.

The data presented indicate some of the complexities we must face in trying to make rational use of chemotherapeutic agents in the pursuit of more effective treatments of cancer. It is also clear that the surface has just been scratched in this field. In spite of the difficulties of the task ahead, it seems obvious that considerably more attention should be paid to these crucial subjects.

Acknowledgement – The experimental work summarized in this paper was supported by Grant EURATOM No. 088-72-1-BIAC and by Contracts NIH-NCI-C-72-3242 and CNR 72-.00207-.04.

REFERENCES

1. O. H. FRIEDMAN and E. BOGER, *Analyt. Chem.* **33**, 906 (1961).
2. P. L. MORSELLI, V. MARC, S. GARATTINI and M. ZACCALA, *Biochem. Pharmac.* **19**, 1643 (1970).
3. A. H. CONNEY, *Pharmac. Rev.* **19**, 317 (1967).
4. J. R. GILLETTE, *Adv. Pharmac.* **4**, 219 (1967).
5. R. KUNTZMAN, *A. Rev. Pharmac.* **9**, 21 (1969).
6. E. DOLFINI, A. MARTINI, M. G. DONELLI, L. MORASCA and S. GARATTINI, *Eur. J. Cancer* **9**, 375 (1973).
7. N. BROCK and H. J. HOHORST, *Cancer, Philad.* **20**, 900 (1967).
8. G. E. FOLEY, O. M. FRIEDMAN and B. P. DROLET, *Cancer Res.* **21**, 57 (1961).
9. R. A. ALARCON, J. MEIENHOFER and E. ATHERTON, *Cancer Res.* **32**, 2519 (1972).
10. J. H. COHEN and J. Y. JAO, *J. Pharmac. exp. Ther.* **174**, 206 (1970).
11. T. A. CONNORS, P. L. GROVER and A. M. MCLOUGHLIN, *Biochem. Pharmac.* **19**, 1533 (1970).
12. D. L. HILL, M. C. KIRK and R. F. STRUCK, *J. Am. chem. Soc.* **92**, 3207 (1970).
13. D. L. HILL, W. R. LASTER and R. F. STRUCK, *Cancer Res.* **32**, 658 (1972).
14. H. J. HOHORST, A. ZIEMAN and N. BROCK, *Arzneimittel-Forsch.* **21**, 1254 (1971).
15. N. E. SLADEK, *Cancer Res.* **32**, 535 (1972).
16. J. Z. FINKLESTEIN, V. ALBO, I. ERTEL, M. KARON and D. HAMMOND, *Cancer Chemother. Rep.* **56**, 523 (1972).
17. E. FREI, J. K. LUCE, R. W. TALLEY, V. K. VAITKEVICIUS and H. E. WILSON, *Cancer Chemother. Rep.* **56**, 667 (1972).
18. J. A. GOTTLIEB and A. A. SERPICK, *Oncology* **25**, 225 (1971).
19. G. J. MANNERING, in *Selected Pharmacological Testing Methods* (Ed. A. BURGER), p. 51. Dekker, New York (1968).
20. D. P. RALL, *Cancer Res.* **27**, 2650 (1967).
21. N. K. JERNE and A. A. NORDIN, *Science, N.Y.* **140**, 405 (1963).
22. R. B. FIELD, M. GANG, I. KLINE and J. M. VENDITTI, *J. Pharmac. exp. Ther.* **180**, 475 (1972).
23. J. Y. JAO, W. J. JUSKO and J. L. COHEN, *Cancer Res.* **32**, 2761 (1972).
24. P. L. MORSELLI, V. MARC, S. GARATTINI and M. ZACCALA, *Revue Ètud. clin. biol.* **15**, 195 (1970).
25. G. B. ELION, *Fedn Proc.* **26**, 898 (1967).
26. G. B. ELION, *Proc. R. Soc. Med.* **65**, 257 (1972).
27. F. SPREAFICO, M. G. DONNELLI, A. BOSSI, A. VECCHI, S. STANDEN and S. GARATTINI, *Transplantation* **16**, 269 (1973).
28. I. BARTOSEK, A. GUAITANI and M. G. DONELLI, *Biochem. Pharmac.* **21**, 2359 (1972).
29. R. ROSSO, M. G. DONELLI, G. FRANCHI and S. GARATTINI, *Eur. J. Cancer* **7**, 565 (1971).

Pp. 35–45, Supplement Number 2, 1974.
Biochemical Pharmacology. Printed in the U.S.A.

THE PRODUCT OF CONCENTRATION AND TIME*

LAWRENCE B. MELLETT

Kettering–Meyer Laboratories, Southern Research Institute
Birmingham, Ala., U.S.A.

MANY attempts have been made to formulate a relation between the quantity of a substance causing a physiological effect and the time necessary to produce this effect. Clark[1,2] published his remarkable monographs on the action of drugs on cells and general pharmacology approximately 35 years ago. In these works he reviewed the attempts to establish a formulation for these relationships. In numerous instances the relationship could be expressed by the formula $C \times T$ = a constant. Stated in words, the formula indicated that to obtain a given biological effect when concentration (C) of the drug is changed, the time of exposure (T) must be suitably modified so that their product yields a constant value. This is obviously an oversimplification which does not account for removal of drug from the system or for changes in the rate of removal during exposure. Clark was aware of the shortcomings of this formula and made suitable modifications which have been discussed elsewhere.[3]

The extensive studies by Skipper *et al.*[4–7] demonstrated, among other things, that for a given dose of an antitumor agent the per cent kill, or fractional reduction, of leukemic cell populations of various sizes is reasonably constant. He further pointed out that, similar to the effect of a disinfectant on bacterial cells, the $C \times T$ requirement for killing a given percentage of the leukemic cell population was constant within substantial variations of C and T. A mathematical formulation relating $C \times T$ to cell kill has been developed by Loo.[8]

Relationship of C × T *to cytotoxicity* in vitro. The techniques of tissue culture studies lend themselves effectively for demonstrating the relationships between biological response, concentration of the drug, and the time required to produce the biological effect. In many instances the relationships are simplified because the drug is not metabolized to any significant degree in the tissue culture system. Thus, the concentration of the drug and time of exposure may be manipulated within wide ranges and related to the biological effect, e.g. total cell kill in the system.

Himmelfarb *et al.*[9] have devised a spin-filter culture technique which allows the investigator to manipulate drug exposures *in vitro* under conditions paralleling the situation *in vivo*. Regulation of flow rates and drug concentrations in the apparatus may be varied to yield drug half-times ($T_{1/2}$) observed *in vivo*. Subsequently, Thayer *et al.*,[10] using the spin-culture apparatus, demonstrated that continuous perfusion of amethopterin at varying rates to provide the same daily integrated $C \times T$ value resulted in an equivalent cell-killing effect over a 2-day period. The $C \times T$ value they obtained

*Supported by Contract PH43-65-654 with the Division of Cancer Treatment, National Cancer Institute.

for equal cell-killing effects was the same as that obtained by Wilkoff *et al.*,[11] where concentrations of amethopterin were held constant for 24 hr.

Skipper *et al.* [12] presented data from tissue culture studies which indicated that the rate of cell kill for L1210 leukemic cells with arabinosyl cytosine (ara-C) was concentration-dependent up to approximately 5.0 μg of drug/ml of medium. They also demonstrated that the minimum cytotoxic concentration of the drug was approximately 0.1 μg/ml of medium for a 24-hr exposure. Thayer and Martin,[13] utilizing the spin-culture technique, pulsed doses of ara-C every 3 hr and controlled flow rates through the system to produce drug-disappearance rates with a $T_{1/2}$ (20–30 min) equal to those observed *in vivo* in the mouse. The results of these studies were compared with results obtained in studies where the concentration of the drug was held constant. In both instances, the cumulative $C \times T$ values were identical for equal cell-killing effects. Skipper *et al.*[12] further demonstrated that pulsed doses of ara-C every 3 hr for 24 hr in BDF_1 mice bearing L1210 leukemic cells were necessary to maintain continuous critical levels of the drug and to provide a $C \times T$ value *in vivo* sufficient to produce cures in the animals.

Relationship of C × T, *dose and toxicity in various species.* A variety of factors must be considered in the design of optimal therapeutic schedules for the chemotherapy of tumors. Among these are: (1) site of action of different drugs at the molecular level; (2) knowledge of cell-cycle parameters, the proliferative state and rate of growth of the tumor cell population; (3) maximum body fluid concentration of various drugs after maximum tolerated doses for different schedules; (4) the rate of fall in drug concentrations; (5) minimum cytotoxic concentrations of various drugs for tumor cells; (6) the influence of drug concentration *per se* and of concentration with time on the rate of tumor cell kill; (7) the influence of drug concentration *per se* and of concentration with time on the destruction of normal hematopoietic stem cells and on lethal toxicity to the host. In the following discussion, I shall be touching principally on items 3, 4, 5, 6 and 7 listed above.

In what practical way may a knowledge of dose, drug metabolism and elimination rates, drug plasma or tissue levels and pharmacological response be related within a species and between various species? Even among closely related species (man and monkey), differences in drug metabolism and drug elimination rates may arise simply from differences in the size of the subjects. "A man could not be reduced to the size of a rhesus monkey without important physiological alterations that might be expected to affect the disposition of drugs. If the pattern of distribution of a drug in the tissues is the same in different species, the concentration of the drug at the site of action will be approximately proportional to the total amount of drug in the body divided by the body weight, regardless of the size of the animal or species. However, the processes removing the drug from the body are likely to be correlated not with the body weight itself, but with the body weight raised to a power less than unity."[14] Many functions and physiological properties in different species of animals of diverse size are approximately proportional to powers of the body weight less than one. These are all functions and properties that in proportion to body weight are generally greater in small animals than in large. Details of these concepts have been discussed elsewhere.[3,15]

Pinkel[16] first suggested the applicability of body surface area as a criterion for relating drug dosages in laboratory and clinical studies. He reasoned that smaller animals had relatively larger surface areas (relative to body weight) than larger animals and, therefore, various functions and properties such as basal metabolic rate, blood volume, cardiac output and renal function would be proportionately greater in smaller animals. To the extent that mammalian species are broadly similar and have corresponding organs and tissues, it is true that any body surface area will increase approximately with the two-thirds power of body weight. Pinkel presented data which indicated that when doses of antitumor drugs were expressed in mg/m^2 of body surface area, more meaningful correlations could be made between animal and human studies than when doses were expressed in mg/kg of body weight. (Modern scaling concepts indicate that an exponent between 0.70 and 0.75 provides more precise correlation than the exponent 0.67.)

The most telling argument for the use of body surface area as a criterion for relating animal and human drug doses was presented by Freireich *et al.*[17] They made a quantitative comparison of toxicity of 18 different anticancer agents in the mouse, rat, hamster, dog, monkey and man. The compounds examined included antimetabolites and alkylating agents as well as other types of antitumor drugs. The authors concluded that relationships among various animal species and man are simpler and more direct when dosage is expressed on a mg/m^2 basis, and that experimental test systems used to evaluate the toxicities of potential anticancer drugs correlate remarkably closely with results in man. Their results are summarized in Fig. 1.

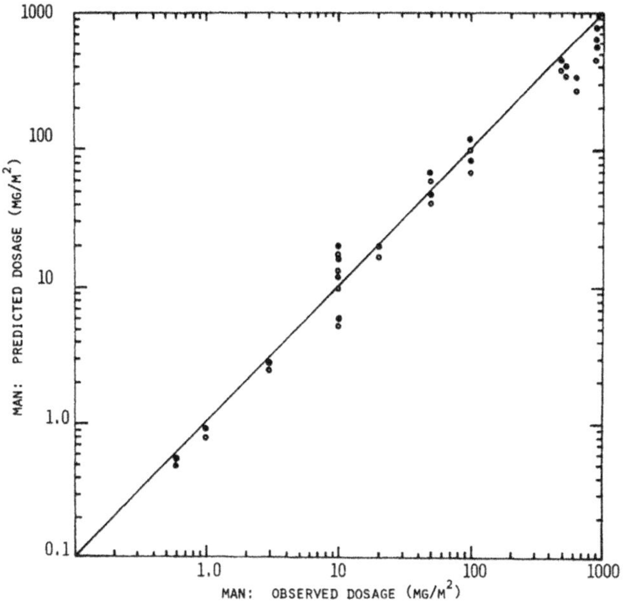

FIG. 1. Observed and predicted dosages (mg/m^2) in man using all animal systems. Data are from Freireich *et al.*[17]

In an extension of these concepts, we[15] examined the relationship between the dose (on a mg/m^2 basis) and serum levels of cyclophosphamide and amethopterin in animals and humans. The cyclophosphamide toxicologic data from animals[17] indicated that the maximum tolerated dose for man should be 362 mg/m^2 on a 1–5 day schedule (Table 1). The maximum tolerated dose determined from clinical data was 370 mg/m^2 for cyclophosphamide. In the case of amethopterin (Table 2), the predicted toxic dose for man from animal studies was 15.7 mg/m^2 *q.d.* 1–5 days, while the dose determined from clinical data was 15.0 mg/m^2 on the same schedule. Plasma levels *per se* are difficult to compare in various species because of differences in

TABLE 1. QUANTITATIVE COMPARISON OF CYCLOPHOSPHAMIDE TOXICITY IN MICE, HAMSTERS, RATS, DOGS, MONKEYS AND MAN*

Species	LD_{10} *q.d.* 1–5 days (mg/kg)	(mg/m^2)	Predicted maximum tolerated dose for man (mg/m^2)
Swiss mouse	93	280	388
BDF_1 mouse	110	340	439
Hamster	80	320	424
Rat	12	64	133
	Maximum tolerated dose, *q.d.* 1–5 days		
Dog	12	234	246
Monkey	54	621	711
Weighted over-all estimate for man based on all animal data			362
Man	Maximum tolerated dose, *q.d.* 1–5 days, determined from clinical data		370

*Data are from Freireich *et al.*[17]

TABLE 2. QUANTITATIVE COMPARISON OF AMETHOPTERIN TOXICITY IN MICE, HAMSTERS, RATS, DOGS, MONKEYS AND MAN*

Species	LD_{10} *q.d.* 1–5 days (mg/kg)	(mg/m^2)	Predicted maximum tolerated dose for man (mg/m^2)
Swiss mouse	3.2	10	13.2
BDF_1 mouse	5.2	16	20.6
Hamster	25.7	103	116.0
Rat	0.58	3.1	6.4
	Maximum tolerated dose, *q.d.* 1–5 days		
Dog	0.12	2.0	2.5
Monkey	3.0	35.0	40.2
Weighted over-all estimate for man based on all animal data			15.7
Man	Maximum tolerated dose, *q.d.* 1–5 days, determined from clinical data		15.0

*Data are from Freireich *et al.*[17]

time relationships with respect to peak levels and rates of disappearance of the drug. Therefore, the area under the serum curve, represented by the product of drug concentration x time, $C \times T$ (μg/ml x min), was employed as an arithmetical measure of exposure for inter-species comparisons. The area under the serum curve at varying doses in various species was plotted against the dose expressed in mg/m^2 for both drugs. The results for cyclophosphamide are shown in Fig. 2; the results for amethopterin are shown in Fig. 3.

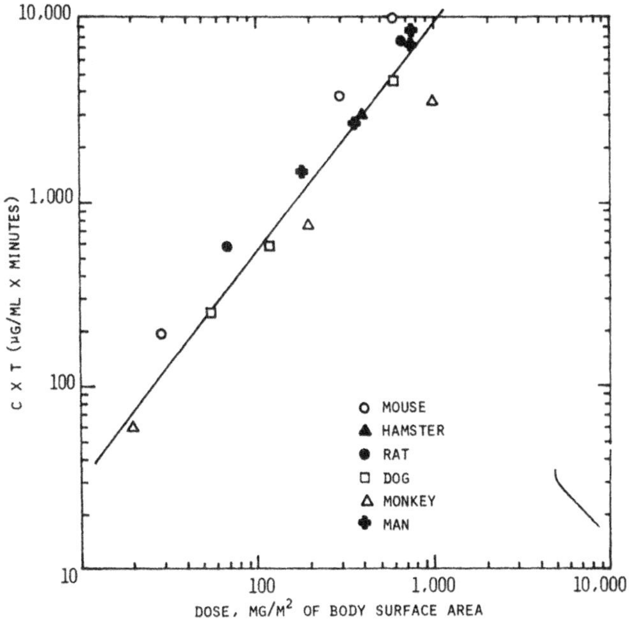

FIG. 2. Area under the serum curve ($C \times T$) versus dose of cyclophosphamide in mg/m^2 of body surface area in various species. Data are from Mellett.[15]

Not all of the correlations showed such precision. In the case of 6-mercaptopurine (6-MP), the animal toxicity data underpredicted the toxic dose for the human. This is shown in Table 3. The pooled animal data predicted a toxic dose for man of 444 mg/m^2, *q.d.* 1–5, whereas the clinically determined toxic dose was 1000 mg/m^2. In terms of $C \times T$ values, this is partially explained by the data in Fig. 4.[18*] When equal doses on a mg/m^2 basis were administered to animals and humans, man consistently gave $C \times T$ values lower than anticipated. The lower $C \times T$ values in man are the result of a relatively short serum half-life of the drug (average, 57 min), which was not substantially different from the serum half-life in the experimental animals (35–60 min).

Similar though less extensive data have been obtained for *N,N′,N″*-triethylenethiophosphoramide (thio-TEPA), daunomycin and 6-methylmercaptopurine riboside and show similar correlations. These relationships are shown for daunomycin in Fig. 5.[19–22,*]

*J. Finkel and L. B. Mellett, unpublished data.

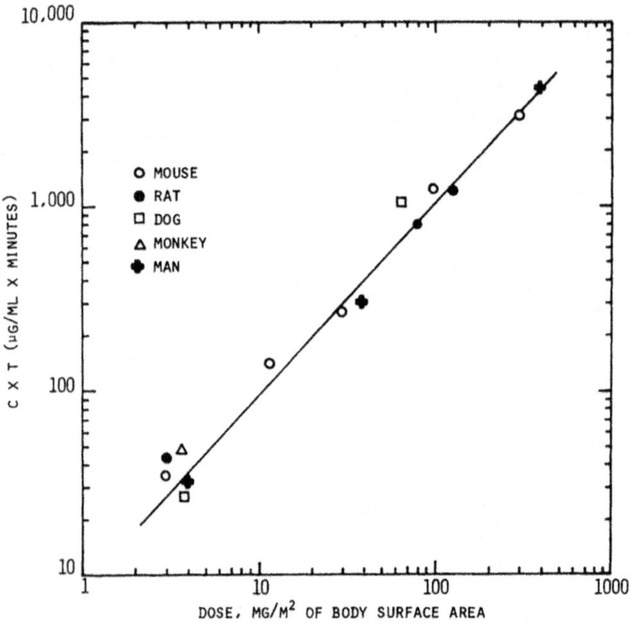

FIG. 3. Area under the serum curve ($C \times T$) versus dose of amethopterin in mg/m² of body surface area in various species. Data are from Mellett.[15]

TABLE 3. QUANTITATIVE COMPARISON OF 6-MP TOXICITY IN MICE, HAMSTERS, RATS, DOGS, MONKEYS AND MAN*

Species	LD_{10} *q.d.* 1–5 days (mg/kg)	(mg/m²)	Predicted maximum tolerated dose for man (mg/m²)
Swiss mouse	86	257	357
BDF_1 mouse	62	186	240
Hamster	80	320	424
Rat	51	266	554
	Maximum tolerated dose, *q.d.* 1–5 days		
Dog	22	434	457
Monkey	56	644	740
Weighted over-all estimate for man based on all animal data			444
Man	Maximum tolerated dose, *q.d.* 1–5 days, determined from clinical data		1000

*Data are from Freireich *et al.*[17]

With regard to these particular drugs, several conclusions may be drawn from the data. (a) When doses are expressed on a mg/m² basis for various species, then equal doses give equivalent $C \times T$ values in the different species. (b) Equivalent $C \times T$ values in various species give equivalent toxicological (or pharmacological) responses in

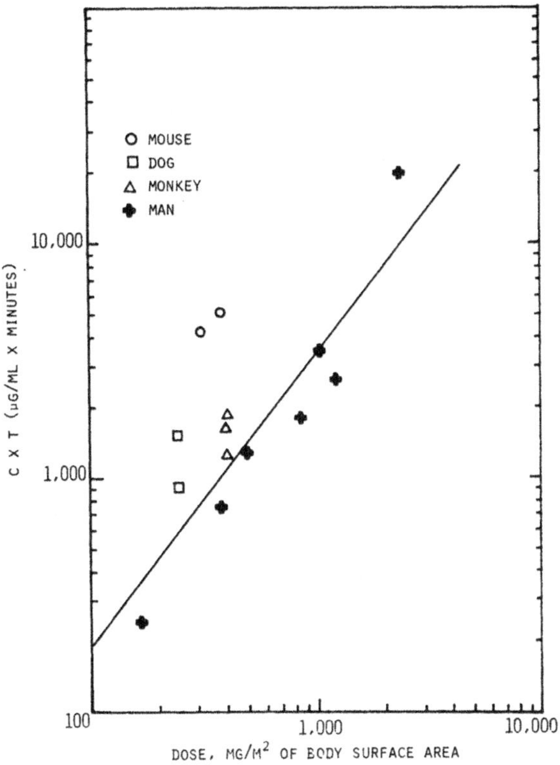

FIG. 4. Area under the serum curve ($C \times T$) versus dose of 6-mercaptopurine in mg/m² of body surface area in various species.

different species. (c) The serum half-life of the drugs tends to be shorter in animals and longest in humans, and is a prime determinant of the total $C \times T$ value attained in the various species. In general, our experience with drugs which are slowly, incompletely or erratically absorbed after oral administration indicates that these relationships held less well than after parenteral administration.

The comparative rates of metabolism of arabinosyl cytosine (ara-C) in various species have been studied by a number of investigators.[23–25] After administration of a standard dose to animals and humans, drug serum levels are depleted in an apparently haphazard fashion in relation to body size. The serum half-life of the drug was 95, 60, 30, 30 and 4 min for the dog, rat, mouse, hamster and monkey respectively. In man, an initial half-life of 10–12 min was noted, followed by a slower rate of disappearance, with a half-life of 90–150 min. This lack of correlation of the rate of drug disappearance with body surface area is explainable on the basis of the unique distribution of cytidine aminohydrolase, the enzyme which deaminates and inactivates ara-C, in various tissues and various animal species. Despite this lack of relationship of serum levels to body size or surface area, some interesting relationships between $C \times T$ serum values and biological response were observed in animals under a variety of conditions of drug administration. These relationships are summarized in Table 4. In general, the $C \times T$ values attained in the various species after single large doses or constant infusions over a 24-hr period for similar toxicological endpoints were

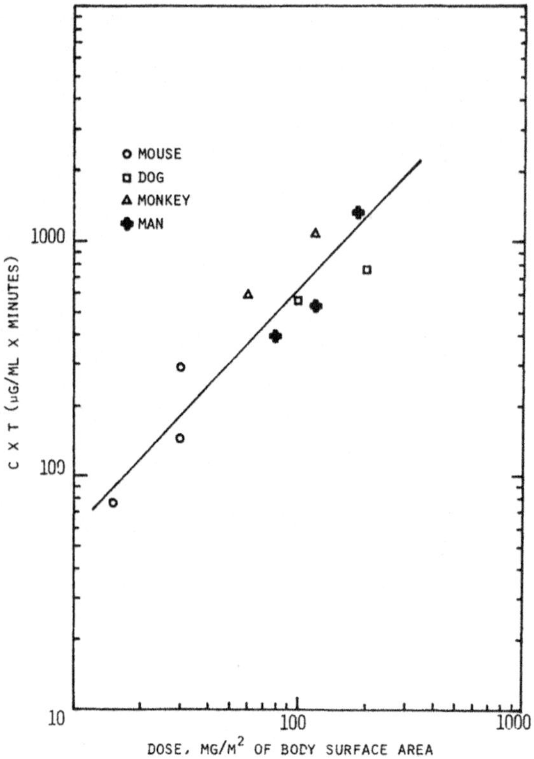

FIG. 5. Area under the serum curve ($C \times T$) versus dose of daunomycin in mg/m² of body surface area in various species. Data are from several sources.

TABLE 4. SOME RELATIONSHIPS OF AREA UNDER THE ARA-C SERUM CURVE ($C \times T$), DOSE AND TOXICITY IN VARIOUS SPECIES

Species	Route	Dose (mg/kg)	Dose (mg/m²)	$C \times T$ (μg/ml) × min)	Toxicity comments
Mouse	i.p.	3,000	9,000	115,000	LD_{10}
	i.p. continuous infusion (24 hr)	3,000	9,000	144,000	LD_{50}
Rat	i.p.	2,000	12,000	125,000	LD_{50}
Dog	i.v.	2,000	40,000	170,000	LD
	i.v. continuous infusion (24 hr)	298	5,600	105,000	MTD* re: hematopoietic toxicity
Monkey	i.v.	2,000	24,000	12,000	No toxicity
	i.v. continuous infusion (24 hr)	300	3,600	1,680	No toxicity

*MTD = maximum tolerated dose.

similar. The effects of dose and scheduling on the toxicity and therapeutic response to ara-C have been discussed by Skipper *et al.*[12]

Some relationships of C X T *to clinical responses.* We have examined retrospectively various successful and unsuccessful clinical regimens with ara-C that have been employed in the treatment of acute myelogenous leukemia (AML) in man. To implement these studies, a formula was developed which would allow a computer calculation of simulated serum levels of ara-C in humans after various treatment schedules. The computer simulations were challenged with experimental serum level data obtained in animals and man and showed good agreement. The details of these studies have been reported elsewhere.[26]

I have selected four simulations of ara-C serum levels after different doses and schedules in man. Three of these are shown in Fig. 6 and are based upon studies by Huguley[27] and Bickers and Freireich.[28] In these studies the complete remission rates ranged from 0 to 32 per cent. In all three schedules, the rate of infusion was 200 mg/m² for 24 hr and showed simulated serum levels of ara-C of 0.064 μg/ml. When this level was maintained for 5 days every 2 weeks (schedule 3), the remission rate was 32 per cent and the *C* X *T* serum value for 1 week was 467 μg/ml x min. When this level was maintained for 24 hr, twice a week, the remission rate dropped to 17 per cent (schedule 2) and the serum *C* X *T* value was 188 μg/ml x min. When this level was maintained for 24 hr, once a week, the remission rate dropped to 0 per cent and the serum *C* X *T* value was 94 μg/ml x min.

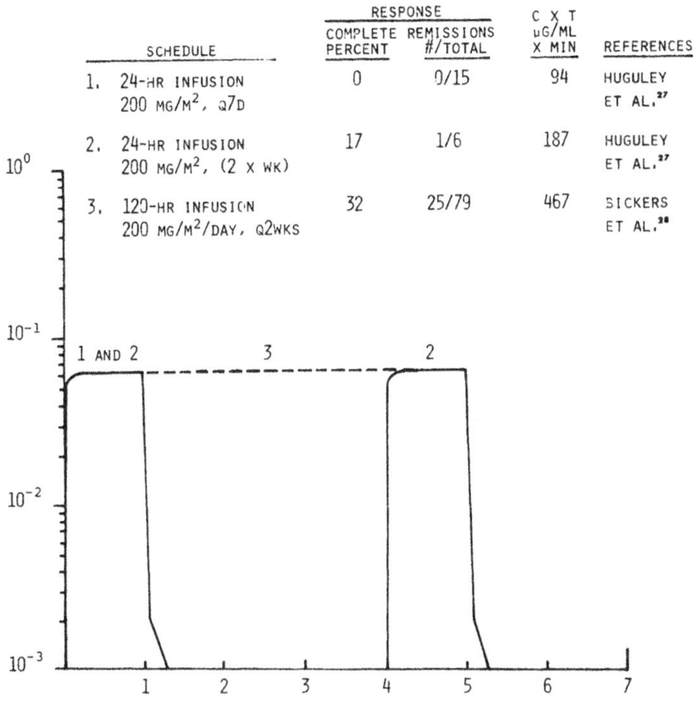

FIG. 6. Simulated serum levels and therapeutic responses in adult patients with acute myelogenous leukemia.

The fourth simulation (Fig. 7) is based upon the studies of Bodey *et al.*,[29] which employed a schedule of 1.8 mg/kg, *q.* 8 hr (x 15) every 2 weeks. This schedule produced remission rates of 38 per cent and the serum $C \times T$ value was 584 μg/ml x min. It should be noted that the two more successful schedules provided similar exposures in terms of $C \times T$ values.

From these and other studies,[26] we have concluded that a minimal effective serum concentration of ara-C for adult AML lies between 0.01 and 0.1 μg/ml, and that concentrations of drug in this range or at higher levels must be maintained for a sufficiently long period to prevent any significant number of leukemic cells from passing through S-phase unexposed. Furthermore, an effective exposure must be repeated at an interval which does not allow a significant net repopulation of leukemic cells between courses.

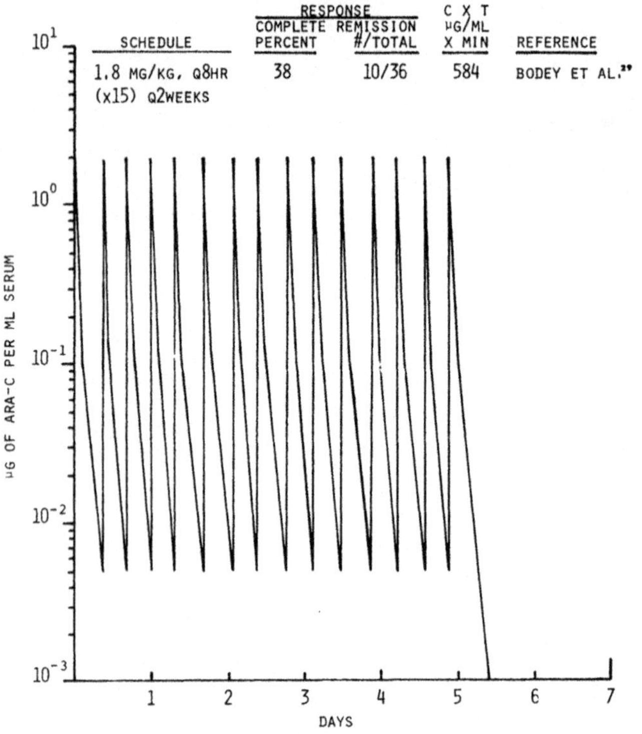

FIG. 7. Simulated serum levels and therapeutic responses in adult patients with acute myelogenous leukemia.

REFERENCES

1. A. J. CLARK, *The Mode of Action of Drugs on Cells,* 1st edn, p. 163. Arnold, London (1933).
2. A. J. CLARK, *General Pharmacology.* 1st edn, p. 105. Springer, Berlin (1937).
3. L. B. MELLETT, in *Antineoplastic and Immunosuppressive Agents,* (Eds. A. C. SARTORELLI and D. G. JOHNS), *Handbook of Experimental Pharmacology,* Springer, Berlin, in press.
4. H. E. SKIPPER, *Cancer Res.* **25**, 1544 (1965).
5. H. E. SKIPPER, F. M. SCHABEL, JR. and W. S. WILCOX, *Cancer Chemother. Rep.* **45**, 5 (1965).

6. R. F. PITTILLO, F. M. SCHABEL, JR., W. S. WILCOX and H. E. SKIPPER, *Cancer Chemother. Rep.* **47**, 1 (1965).
7. W. S. WILCOX, D. P. GRISWOLD, W. R. LASTER, F. M. SCHABEL, JR., and H. E. SKIPPER, *Cancer Chemother. Rep.* **47**, 27 (1965).
8. T. L. LOO, *Cancer Chemother. Rep.* **50**, 296 (1966).
9. P. HIMMELFARB, P. S. THAYER and H. E. MARTIN, *Science, N.Y.* **164**, 555 (1969).
10. P. S. THAYER, P. HIMMELFARB and D. ROBERTS, *Cancer Res.* **30**, 1709 (1970).
11. L. J. WILKOFF, W. S. WILCOX, J. A. BURDESHAW, G. J. DIXON and E. A. DULMADGE, *J. National Cancer Institute* **39**, 965 (1967).
12. H. E. SKIPPER, F. M. SCHABEL, JR., L. B. MELLETT, J. A. MONTGOMERY, L. J. WILKOFF, H. H. LLOYD and R. W. BROCKMAN, *Cancer Chemother. Rep.* **54**, 431 (1970).
13. P. S. THAYER and H. M. MARTIN, *Proc. Am. Ass. Cancer Res.* **13**, 18 (1972).
14. T. C. BUTLER, *Conference on Nonhuman Primate Toxicology* (Ed. C. O. MILLER), pp. 68–69. Dept. Health, Education and Welfare, Washington, D.C. (1966).
15. L. B. MELLETT, in *Progress in Drug Research*, Vol. 13, pp. 136–139, Birkaüser, Basel (1969).
16. D. PINKEL, *Cancer Res.* **18**, 853 (1958).
17. E. J. FREIREICH, E. A. GEHAN, D. P. RALL, L. H. SCHMIDT and H. E. SKIPPER, *Cancer Chemother. Rep.* **50**, 219 (1966).
18. T. L. LOO, J. K. LUCE, M. P. SULLIVAN and E. FREI, III, *Clin. Pharmac. Ther.* **9**, 180 (1968).
19. J. M. FINKEL, K. T. KNAPP and L. T. MULLIGAN, *Cancer Chemother. Rep.* **53**, 159 (1969).
20. D. W. YESAIR, E. SCHWARTZBACH, D. SHUCK, E. P. DENINE and M. A. ASBELL, *Cancer Res.* **32**, 1177 (1972).
21. D. S. ALBERTS, N. R. BACHUR and J. L. HOLTZMAN, *Clin. Pharmac. Ther.* **12**, 96 (1971).
22. D. H. HUFFMAN, R. S. BENJAMIN and N. R. BACHUR, *Clin. Pharmac. Ther.* **13**, 895 (1972).
23. L. T. MULLIGAN and L. B. MELLETT, *Pharmacologist* **10**, 167 (1968).
24. G. W. CAMIENER and C. G. SMITH, *Biochem. Pharmac.* **14**, 1405 (1965).
25. D. H. HO and E. FREI, III, *Clin. Pharmac. Ther.* **12**, 944 (1971).
26. L. B. MELLET, in *Proc. Fifth Int. Pharmacology Congr.* San Francisco, 1972, Vol. 3, p. 332 (Karger, Basel 1973).
27. C. HUGULEY, in *Minutes of the Meeting of the Southeastern Chemotherapy Group*, July, 1967.
28. J. BICKERS and E. J. FREIREICH, in *Proc. Chemotherapy Conference on Ara-C* (Eds. S. K. CARTER and R. B. LIVINGSTON), p. 59. National Cancer Institute, Washington, D.C. (1969).
29. G. P. BODEY, E. J. FREIREICH, R. W. MONTO and J. S. HEWLETT, *Cancer Chemother. Rep.* **53**, 59 (1969).

Pp. 47—50, Supplement Number 2, 1974.
Biochemical Pharmacology. Printed in the U.S.A.

TRANSPORT OF TUMOR-INHIBITORY AGENTS ACROSS CELL MEMBRANES

DAVID KESSEL*

Department of Pharmacology and Toxicology, The University of Rochester School of Medicine and Dentistry, Rochester, N.Y., U.S.A.

A TUMOR-INHIBITORY agent is, by definition, a compound (anti-metabolite, natural product, hormone, enzyme, alkylating agents, etc.) capable of interfering with some vital process necessary to the continued growth of certain neoplastic cells. Although most such agents also inhibit growth of "normal" mammalian cells, the use of the term "tumor-inhibitory" is generally taken to mean that an agent with some degree of selective toxicity is being considered.

The toxic effect of a tumor-inhibitory agent could be exerted via a variety of mechanisms, some of which require that the drug actually cross the cell membrane and interfere with intracellular processes. But such penetration is not necessarily a requisite for antitumor activity. The enzyme L-asparaginase is thought to act by depleting the extracellular environment of an amino acid essential for the growth of certain cells.[1] There are compounds like dimethylsulfoxide[2] and persantin[3] which inhibit the growth of cells by processes which involve action at the cell membrane, thereby preventing uptake of essential metabolites.

The majority of clinically useful tumor-inhibitory agents do, however, appear to act within the cell, and the transport of such agents across cell membranes, therefore, becomes an important pharmacologic parameter. When the rate of cross-membrane transport becomes a determinant of drug responsiveness, then one must consider this factor in the design of a chemotherapeutic program.

A considerable body of work has been accumulated concerning the role of transport processes in the biology of the cell; the early work was mainly concerned with bacterial cells, but later studies extended these early insights to the mammalian cell population. Pioneering studies in bacterial transport showed a multiplicity of transport systems involved in the accumulation of amino acids and sugars.

Meanwhile, Christensen[4] (and others) were carrying out similar work with the Ehrlich ascites tumor and other readily accessible mammalian cell types. The human blood cell was also extensively utilized for transport studies.[5,6] From all of this work, it became clear that certain substances were essentially excluded by cells; other materials entered by processes with characteristics of simple diffusion, while yet other substrates required rather complex, and often quite specific, access mechanisms to gain entry to a cell. The latter were divided into two categories: facilitated diffusion, being taken to mean that an access process mediated nonconcentrative uptake of a substrate, while active transport meant that net concentration against a gradient had occurred. In either case, saturability of the uptake process and evidence of structural specificity were generally found. The theories of transport processes, together with extensive discussions of evidence involved, have been reviewed.[7–9]

*Present address: Michigan Cancer Foundation, Detroit, Michigan, USA.

With regard to the commonly employed antitumor agents, some of the earliest transport studies were carried out with the antifol methotrexate using animal tumor models. Fischer,[10] in 1962, reported that a resistant clone of the L5178Y murine leukemia was apparently defective in its capacity to accumulate the drug. Hitherto, elevated levels of the target enzyme dihydrofolate reductase had been implicated in development of resistance to methotrexate.[11,12] In a survey of a large number of animal tumors, Roberts *et al.*[13] found no correlation between natural or inherent methotrexate responsiveness and levels of this target enzyme. Later, in our laboratory, we were able to establish a strong correlation between the rate of methotrexate uptake and drug responsiveness in all of the murine leukemias examined.[14] This work was later extended to provide a useful means for assessing probable responsiveness of human leukemias to methotrexate by studying the relative rate of uptake of radioactive drug by freshly isolated leukemic cells *in vitro.*[15] A detailed study of the methotrexate transport process was carried out by Goldman *et al.*,[16] who found evidence to suggest that a system normally functioning as a carrier for folinic acid and related molecules was responsible for methotrexate uptake.

The major importance of the studies with methotrexate was that a clear case had been made for considering transport phenomena, along with other pharmacologic parameters, as a potentially important determinant of drug responsiveness. Furthermore, development of agents which might modify transport rates might be a useful field for future exploration. The prototype study here was the work of Leive,[17] who found that treatment with EDTA removed a surface component which greatly increased the capacity of *Escherichia coli* cells to accumulate actinomycin D; the growth of such cells was thereby inhibited.

Another group of drugs for which transport rates appear to play some role in determining effectiveness is the alkylating agents. At first, it seemed that accumulation of nitrogen mustard and cytoxan by resistant vs sensitive animal tumors was not different.[18] But, in a series of papers, Wolpert, Goldenberg and Rutman *et al.*[19–23] established that development of resistance to nitrogen mustard in L5178Y and Ehrlich tumors was, in part, attributable to decreased uptake. Furthermore, the transport process involved seemed to be via a process normally responsible for uptake of choline.[23]

Sensitivity to actinomycin D also appeared to depend on the rate of transport of this drug across cell membranes.[24,25] Furthermore, the generally observed cross-resistance[26] between the group of agents including the vinca alkaloids, daunomycin, adriamycin and terephthalanilides and related agents suggests that all of these drugs are poorly accumulated by resistant cell types. In the case of actinomycin D, resistance has been found associated with well defined alterations in the cell membrane;[27,28] the resistant cell contains higher levels of cell-surface glycoportein, higher levels of enzymes involved in glycoprotein synthesis, and lower levels of enzymes involved in glycoprotein degradation. It is interesting to note that uptake of neither actinomycin D nor daunomycin was found impaired when drug-resistant cells were studied under non-growing conditions,[27,29] but that use of growing cells was required to demonstrate drug exclusion by the resistant cell population. Danø *et al.*,[30] using different cell types, concluded that impaired uptake of daunomycin, demonstrable *in vitro,* was a partial explanation for drug resistance.

Studies of the role played by transport of the purine, pyrimidine and nucleoside analogs are generally complicated by the very rapid intracellular metabolism of such compounds to nondiffusible products. The kinetics of uptake, therefore, suggest that a concentrative and temperature-sensitive process is involved. But when mutants incapable of further metabolism of such compounds are employed,[31,32] it becomes clear that only facilitated diffusion is actually involved in uptake of such compounds. Jacquez[33,34] had come to a similar conclusion without the use of mutant cell lines. The implications of these data are that resistance to the nucleic acid analogs does not involve transport barriers, but instead, results from defects in conversion of these drugs to the pharmacologically active nucleotide forms,[35–39] enhanced destruction of a drug by intracellular enzymes,[40] or by extracellular systems (e.g. the inactivation of cytosine arabinoside by a deaminase[41]).

This finding has not been without practical value. Since the free purine, pyrimidine or nucleoside analogs diffuse freely into and out of cells, washing of cells incubated with radioactive compounds will remove everything but intracellular nucleotides. Therefore, the rate of conversion of such compounds to "bound" radioactivity has proved useful in assessing probable responses in animal leukemias to fluorouracil,[42] cytosine arabinoside,[43] 6-mercaptopurine,[44] fluorouridine[32] and, in the case of the human leukemias, for 6-mercaptopurine[44] and cytosine arabinoside.[45]

As our knowledge of the determinants of drug responsiveness of newer antitumor agents increases, it is clear that the role of cross-membrane transport must be assessed before the optimal use of these drugs will be possible. If a transport system plays a rate-limiting role in drug entry, it may be possible to predict in advance, from studies *in vitro*, the potential usefulness of a drug in the clinical situation. It may be possible to design drugs to take advantage of existing transport systems and thereby gain entry to cells. Agents that are active in cell-free systems certainly must be evaluated to determine whether they are indeed taken up by mammalian cells before any clinical trials should be explored. Possible means for increasing permeability of membranes toward antitumor agents is another potential area in which useful work might be done.

Perhaps one of the most interesting aspects of the permeability problem consists of the role played by the development of drug resistance in the tumor-producing capacity of the cell. It is well known that many drug-resistant cells are less lethal to the host than are the drug-sensitive parent cells.[46] When cells become resistant to high levels of, for example, actinomycin D, they are no longer malignant,* and this is associated with significant alterations in the cell surface.[28] We often hear it said that there may be no essential difference between normal and malignant cells, but all workers in the field know of one essential difference: malignant cells have the potential for mutation to drug-resistant lines. Perhaps the proper direction of such mutations, i.e. toward development of cells with appropriately altered surfaces, may ultimately yield a drug-resistant cell much less able to survive in the environment of the host.

*J. Biedler, personal communication.

REFERENCES

1. D. A. COONEY and R. E. HANDSCHUMACHER, *A. Rev. Pharmac.* **10**, 421 (1970).
2. R. F. HAGEMANN and T. C. EVANS, *Nature, Lond.* **218**, 583 (1968).
3. C. SCHOLTISSEK, *Biochim. biophys. Acta* **158**, 435 (1968).
4. H. N. CHRISTENSEN, *Adv. Protein Chem.* **15**, 239 (1960).

5. A. YUNIS, G. ARRAMURA and D. KIPNIS, *J. Lab. clin. Med.* **62**, 465 (1963).
6. L. ROSENBERG and S. DOWNING, *J. clin. Invest.* **44**, 1382 (1965).
7. J. F. DANIELLI, *Symp. Soc. exp. Biol.* **8**, 502 (1954).
8. N. F. H. HO, J. TURI, C. SHIPMAN, JR. and W. I. HIGUCHI, *J. theoret. Biol.* **34**, 451 (1972).
9. W. D. STEIN, *The Movement of Molecules Across Cell Membranes*, Academic Press, New York (1967).
10. G. A. FISCHER, *Biochem. Pharmac.* **11**, 1233 (1962).
11. M. FRIEDKIN, E. CRAWFORD, S. R. HUMPHREYS and A. GOLDIN, *Cancer Res.* **22**, 600 (1962).
12. M. T. HAKALA, S. R. ZAKRZEWSKI and C. A. NICHOL, *J. biol. Chem.* **236**, 952 (1961).
13. D. ROBERTS, D. KESSEL and T. C. HALL, *Cancer Res.* **25**, 1899 (1965).
14. D. KESSEL, T. C. HALL and D. ROBERTS, *Science, N.Y.* **150**, 752 (1965).
15. D. KESSEL, T. C. HALL and D. ROBERTS, *Cancer Res.* **28**, 564 (1968).
16. I. D. GOLDMAN, N. S. LICHTENSTEIN and V. T. OLIVERIO, *J. biol. Chem.* **243**, 5007 (1968).
17. L. LEIVE, *Proc. Natn. Acad. Sci. U.S.A.* **53**, 745 (1965).
18. G. P. WHEELER and J. A. ALEXANDER, *Cancer Res.* **24**, 1331 (1964).
19. M. K. WOLPERT and R. W. RUDDON, *Cancer Res.* **29**, 873 (1969).
20. G. J. GOLDENBERG, C. L. VANSTONE, L. G. ISRAELS, D. ILSE and I. BIHLER, *Cancer Res.* **30**, 2285 (1970).
21. G. J. GOLDENBERG, R. M. LYONS, J. A. LEPP and C. L. VANSTONE, *Cancer Res.* **31**, 1616 (1971).
22. R. J. RUTMAN, E. H. L. CHUN and F. S. LEWIS, *Biochem. biophys. Res. Commun.* **32**, 650 (1968).
23. G. J. GOLDENBERG, C. L. VANSTONE and I. BIHLER, *Science, N.Y.* **172**, 1148 (1971).
24. M. N. GOLDSTEIN, K. HAMM and E. AMROD, *Science, N.Y.* **151**, 1555 (1966).
25. D. KESSEL and I. WODINSKY, *Biochem. Pharmac.* **17**, 161 (1968).
26. H. E. SKIPPER, D. J. HUTCHISON, F. M. SCHABEL, JR., L. H. SCHMIDT, A. GOLDIN, R. W. BROCKMAN, J. M. VENDITTI and I. WODINSKY, *Cancer Chemother. Rep.* **56**, 493 (1972).
27. D. KESSEL and H. B. BOSMANN, *Cancer Res.* **30**, 2695 (1970).
28. H. B. BOSMANN, *Nature, Lond.* **233**, 566 (1971).
29. D. KESSEL, V. BOTTERILL and I. WODINSKY, *Cancer Res.* **28**, 938 (1968).
30. K. DANØ, S. FREDERIKSEN and P. HELLUNG-LARSEN, *Cancer Res.* **32**, 1307 (1972).
31. D. KESSEL and S. B. SHURIN, *Biochim. biophys. Acta* **163**, 179 (1968).
32. D. KESSEL, R. BRUNS and T. C. HALL, *Molec. Pharmac.* **7**, 117 (1971).
33. J. A. JACQUEZ, *Proc. Soc. exp. Biol. Med.* **109**, 133 (1962).
34. J. A. JACQUEZ, *Biochim. biophys. Acta* **61**, 265 (1962).
35. M. Y. CHU and G. A. FISCHER, *Biochem. Pharmac.* **14**, 333 (1965).
36. P. REICHARD, O. SKÖLD, G. KLEIN, L. RÉVÉSZ and P. MAGNUSSON, *Cancer Res.* **22**, 235 (1962).
37. R. J. ALBERTINI, *Science, N. Y.* **169**, 482 (1970).
38. J. VESELÝ, A. ČIHÁK and F. ŠORM, *Cancer Res.* **30**, 2180 (1970).
39. R. W. BROCKMAN, *Adv. Cancer Res.* **7**, 129 (1963).
40. M. WOLPERT, S. P. DAMLE, J. E. BROWN, E. SZNYCER, K. AGRAWAL and A. SARTORELLI, *Cancer Res.* **31**, 1620 (1971).
41. G. W. CAMIENER and C. G. SMITH, *Biochem. Pharmac.* **14**, 1405 (1965).
42. D. KESSEL, T. C. HALL and I. WODINSKY, *Science, N.Y.* **154**, 911 (1966).
43. D. KESSEL, T. C. HALL and I. WODINSKY, *Science, N.Y.* **156**, 1240 (1967).
44. D. KESSEL and T. C. HALL, *Cancer Res.* **29**, 2116 (1969).
45. D. KESSEL, T. C. HALL and D. ROSENTHAL, *Cancer Res.* **29**, 459 (1969).
46. A. NICOLIN, S. VALAMAUDI, E. BONMASSAR and A. GOLDIN, *Proc. Am. Ass. Cancer Res.* **12**, 13 (1971).

Pp. 51—56, Supplement Number 2, 1974.
Biochemical Pharmacology. Printed in the U.S.A.

PHARMACOLOGICAL CONSIDERATIONS IN THE CHEMOTHERAPY OF CENTRAL NERVOUS SYSTEM TUMORS

JOSEPH D. FENSTERMACHER and RONALD G. BLASBERG

Membrane Transport Section, Office of the Associate Scientific Director
for Experimental Therapeutics, Division of Cancer Treatment
National Cancer Institute, National Institutes of Health
Bethesda, Md. 20014, U.S.A.

IN THE search for drugs which will be effective against tumors, the chemotherapist must seek compounds which not only can eliminate the malignant cells but also can be delivered successfully to the target site. As reported in several recent reviews, the chemotherapeutic treatment of central nervous system (CNS) and meningeal tumors has met with only limited success.[1,2] Much evidence suggests that the permeability of the capillaries of both normal and neoplastic CNS tissue severely limits the delivery of many compounds, including antineoplastic agents, to the brain and surrounding cerebrospinal fluid (CSF) and meninges. For example, Shapiro *et al.*[3] have pointed out that leukemic cells in both experimental and human meningeal leukemia are resistant to systemic chemotherapy even though the drugs used were effective against leukemic cells when located peripherally. Many clinicians, being aware of this apparent capillary permeability problem (the blood–brain barrier phenomena), have tried to improve CNS and meningeal uptake of antitumor agents by administering them directly into the lumbar or ventricular cerebrospinal fluid rather than into the vascular system. Nervous system leukemia has been fairly successfully treated by intrathecal methotrexate,[1,2] in some cases in combination with cranial radiation,[4] suggesting that better delivery of drug to intracranial tumor sites can be obtained with this route of administration.

The uptake of drug by normal and malignant cells is dependent upon a basic sequence of transport steps regardless of the route of injection or infusion. Each of these steps in the drug distribution process is a function of the physicochemical and pharmacological properties of the compound and the physiological properties of the organ systems involved. Since different routes of administration involve different systems with different physiological properties, factors which enhance drug uptake in one situation may lead to little or no tissue accumulation in another and vice versa. The purpose of this presentation is to consider the various components of blood–brain–CSF exchange and to suggest guidelines for choosing drug and route combinations which will yield more effective drug delivery to CNS tumors.

Components of drug distribution

In general, the movement of a drug from the point of entry to the various tissues of the body, including the target site, is accomplished by local inclusion and subsequent bulk distribution of the compound in one of the systemic fluids, e.g. the plasma. This fluid then becomes the source solution for tissue drug uptake. Inclusion in and bulk delivery by the source fluid plus the remaining components of drug distribution are listed below in Table 1. The site and the manner of administration contribute to the kinetics of the appearance of the drug in the source fluid. In addition, the absorption and solubility of the pharmacological material and its vehicle also affect the concentration of drug in the source fluid at the point of introduction into the body. Once the material has entered the source fluid, it is carried throughout this compartment by bulk flow or circulation. The speed of distribution depends on the rate of flow of the source fluid and the amount of mixing which occurs within the source fluid compartment.

For the actual exchange from the source fluid to the tissue extracellular fluid (ECF), two components – the driving force and the resistance – control the flow of drug. The driving force is the effective concentration (activity) gradient from source fluid to tissue ECF and depends on the concentration of free and exchangeable drug throughout the duration of the presence of the compound in both of these fluids. The source fluid–tissue interface, either a simple or complex membrane structure, provides the resistance to the flow of drug between these two fluid compartments.

Once the compound has crossed the interface and entered the ECF, it diffuses throughout the extracellular space (ECS) of the tissue. As the material diffuses through the ECS, it will enter the cells, provided the cell membrane is appropriately permeable, and the other circulating fluids, such as the lymph, of the tissue. For chemotherapy to succeed, all of these transport or distributive steps must interact to provide a compromising or lethal amount of the drug to the malignant cells.

TABLE 1. COMPONENTS OF DRUG DISTRIBUTION FROM SOURCE FLUID TO CELLS*

1. Inclusion in source fluid
2. Bulk flow of source fluid with entrained drug to tissue
3. Drug activity in source fluid at fluid-tissue interface
4. Source fluid-tissue interface permeability
5. Movement of drug through the extracellular space
6. Drug exchange between extracellular fluid and other tissue fluids

*Possible source fluids for brain tumor chemotherapy are the blood and cerebrospinal fluid.

Brain drug distribution and routes of administration

Based on the components of tissue distribution listed in Table 1, a useful comparison can be made of the entry and accumulation of drugs in the central nervous system from the two source fluids, plasma and CSF, which are commonly employed in brain tumor chemotherapy. This consideration of the distribution components will emphasize points of marked difference between these two delivery situations and suggest certain guidelines for improving drug delivery to normal and, hopefully, neoplastic brain and meningeal tissue.

Inclusion in source fluid. The inclusion of drug into the source fluid is dependent on both the input function, i.e. the time course of the appearance of drug in the source fluid at the site of introduction, and the capacity of the source fluid to hold the drug. When blood is the source fluid, the input function depends on the site (intravascular, intramuscular or oral) and the manner (quick injection or slow infusion) of administration. The solubility, plasma protein binding and cellular uptake of the drug, plus the blood flow to the input region, contribute to the capacity. Except for arterial infusions, the specific location of the input site relative to the lesion is comparatively unimportant. Because the flow of blood past the site of introduction is much larger than the volume and rate of administration, the subsequent circulation and mixing of drug is virtually independent of the input volume parameters.

Materials are only put directly into the CSF, and the input function is that of the injection or infusion procedure, *per se*. The capacity of the fluid depends primarily on the solubility of the drug in the fluid. Since the flow of cerebrospinal fluid is relatively slow, the variables of the administration – the speed, the volume and the site – are very important. In contrast to intravascular administration, the input volume and rate can significantly affect the subsequent bulk delivery of drug to the target site. More effective distribution of drug will be obtained with larger volumes, more dynamic injections or infusions, and closer proximity between administration and target sites.

Bulk flow of source fluid to tissue. The principal role of the circulatory system is the rapid delivery and removal of materials to and from the tissue, and thus, the bulk distribution of a drug from the point of vascular introduction to most tissue capillaries, the exchange sites, is quick and efficient. For drugs which readily cross capillary and cellular membranes, the tissue uptake may be partially limited by the rate of blood flow; nevertheless, only in a few cases, e.g. poorly perfused normal or malignant tissue, does this component of drug distribution present a major problem in delivery. Good mixing of the administered material is achieved throughout the source fluid compartment as the blood mixes in the heart and pulmonary circulation before flowing to the tissues.

On the other hand, bulk distribution of drug throughout the CSF compartment is slow and presents significant limitations in drug delivery. Very little mixing occurs in this source fluid and great regional variation in concentration is found.[5] As previously mentioned, better delivery throughout the CSF compartment is achieved by augmenting bulk flow and mixing with aggressive administration, e.g. barbotage.[6] However, even when such maneuvers are employed, a sizable fraction of the CSF system and adjacent CNS tissue may receive little or no drug because of slow fluid turnover. In addition, the presence of protruding tumor masses or tissue adhesions would reduce the flow of the source fluid to these areas and the delivery of CSF-entrained drug to the tissue sites needing chemotherapy.

Drug activity in source fluid at interface. The driving force for the unidirectional flux of drug from the source fluid to brain tissue is provided by the activity or effective concentration of the drug in the source fluid from the time the material first appears at the fluid–tissue interface until it disappears. For the blood, the exchange of material with the tissue occurs only at the capillaries; therefore, only the intracapillary activity must be considered. The time course of drug activity in the brain capillaries can be divided into two phases, the initial and the recirculation. The intracapillary activity during the initial phase depends on the factors previously mentioned – the input function, the capacity and the blood flow. The recirculation phase for the CNS depends on what all of the tissues, including the brain and spinal cord, do to the drug presented to them during their respective initial phases. It is important to emphasize that the time course of drug activity within most capillaries of the CNS will be fairly similar, that only small regional variations in this component of tissue distribution will be found when blood is the source fluid.

The blood-to-tissue exchange of material occurs only across the capillary portion of the vascular network; the exchange between the cerebrospinal fluid and the CNS and meninges, on the other hand, occurs throughout the CSF system. Marked local variations in the time course of drug activity will be found in the CSF all along the source fluid–tissue interface as a result of uneven bulk flow and poor mixing within the ventricular and subarachnoid spaces and of molecular loss of material to adjacent neural and meningeal tissue and blood. Compounds which readily enter CNS cells and/or circulating blood may be completely or nearly completely cleared from the CSF before reaching the necessary portion of the system unless the distance between the infusion and target sites is very small. For rapidly exchanging materials, this distance may be on the order of 10–20 cm. Thus, not only poor mixing but also molecular loss or exchange may severely compromise the bulk delivery of drug to the CSF–tissue interfaces of the brain, spinal cord and meninges.

Source fluid–tissue interface permeability. The respective interfaces for blood and CSF are formed by the capillary endothelium and the ependymal and pia-glial membranes. The exchange of material across the capillaries of normal brain and spinal cord is markedly different than that across most other capillaries. Lipid-soluble, nonpolar compounds readily move from blood to brain ECF, whereas polar, water-soluble materials enter CNS tissue from the blood very slowly.[7–10] When blood is the source fluid, the uptake of lipid-insoluble drugs to normal (and probably also neoplastic) neural tissue may be severely restricted by the permeability of the capillary complex, the so-called blood–brain barrier.

The ependymal and pia-glial membranes appear to offer little or no restriction to the CSF–CNS exchange of most molecules. Work from the laboratory of Rall indicates that compounds with molecular weights of 5000 or less readily exchange across these membranes and that even larger molecules, e.g. albumin, move at reasonable diffusional rates from CSF into brain tissue.[11–13]

Movement through the extracellular space. Regardless of the source fluid, movement of a drug through the extracellular space will occur by the same mechanism (diffusion) and at the same rate. However, because of the dissimilarity in the distances involved, a marked difference in the efficacy of drug delivery throughout the tissue ECS does exist between the two potential source fluids, blood and CSF. Blood capillaries are fairly uniformly distributed throughout the CNS parenchyma; estimates of the intracapillary distance range from 15 to 50 μm.[14] Diffusion over distances of this magnitude would lead to rapid distribution of most drugs within the ECS.[15] On the other hand, the distances between the CSF–tissue interfaces, i.e. the ependymal and pia-glial borders, and parenchymal tissue sites may range up to many millimeters in the human brain. Diffusional delivery of drugs to cells more than 1 or 2 mm into the tissue would be slow in time and limited in quantity. The penetration of drug, therefore, to deep tissues sites via the brain ECS would be significantly restricted by the effective diffusional distances when CSF is the source fluid.

Exchange between ECF and other tissue fluids. Once the drug has been transported from either the blood or the CSF into the extracellular fluid of the CNS, it may remain within the ECF, enter the cells, or diffuse into the CSF and blood. The course followed depends on the permeability of the cellular and interfacial membranes to the drug and the intracellular–extracellular fluid, plasma–extracellular fluid, and CSF–extracellular fluid activity gradients over the duration of the presence of the drug within the system. The importance of ECF–CSF exchange, the so-called sink action of the CSF,[16] in the over-all kinetics of brain uptake of drugs from the blood has only emerged in the last decade. This hypothesis suggests that the activity of various compounds in the tissue adjacent to the CSF will be maintained at a low level if the activity of drug in the CSF remains very low and significant ECF to CSF diffusional exchange occurs. Pollay and Kaplan[17] have demonstrated that the CSF does, indeed, act as a sink and creates diffusional gradients within the brain for the organic nonelectrolyte sucrose. The effects of the sink action of the CSF on the net uptake of specific antitumor agents by normal and neoplastic brain tissue have not been evaluated. This action, however, may be quite important for certain drugs and should be considered.

The reverse situation may hold, i.e. a sink action by the blood, when the drug has been infused or injected into the CSF. Drug loss from the tissue to the circulating blood will occur if the activity of drug in the blood is appreciably lower than that in the CSF and ECF, and the CNS capillaries are permeable to the compound. If the capillary permeability is high enough, as is the case for *N, N', N''*-triethylenethiophosphoramide (thio-TEPA) (Blasberg and Fenstermacher, unpublished observations), the drug will be cleared from the tissue nearly as rapidly as it enters from the CSF, and very little drug will penetrate into the parenchyma. Such transcapillary loss not only diminishes the depth of drug penetration and tissue accumulation but also augments the clearance of drug from the CSF. Such clearance reduces the amount of drug delivered to the more distal parts of the CSF system and adjacent CNS and meningeal tissue, as mentioned in the section on "Drug Activity in Source Fluid at Interface."

CONCLUSIONS

To obtain the most uniform and widespread distribution of drug to central nervous tissue, cerebrospinal fluid and meninges, the drug should be introduced into the bloodstream. However, for this route of delivery to provide adequate uptake, the drug must be lipid soluble enough to cross the capillaries of the brain and spinal cord readily. Lipid-insoluble drugs, unless transported by special processes, enter brain tissue from the blood very slowly and are generally ineffective against CNS and meningeal tumors when injected or infused into the vascular system.

Compounds which do not cross the blood–brain barrier may be effectively delivered to the brain, spinal cord and meninges by way of the CSF. There are, however, significant problems, such as adequate mixing throughout the CSF compartment and depth of tissue penetration, in drug distribution to CNS tissue when this route is used. Before administering the drug into the CSF, consideration must be given to the site and manner of infusion, the location of the tumor mass, and the transport properties of the drug. Drugs which readily penetrate the capillaries of the brain will have limited CNS distribution and effectiveness because of rapid clearance from the CSF and adjacent neural tissue.

The dynamics of blood–brain–CSF exchange may be considerably altered in and around CNS tumors. The pathophysiology of such lesions has only been examined in a few clinical studies.[18–20] Until an adequate brain tumor model has been developed and studied and more extensive clinical research has been done on patients, all suggestions for improving drug delivery to CNS and meningeal lesions must be based on our basic knowledge of normal blood–brain–CSF transport. Hopefully, we will not be greatly misled by this approach in efforts directed at the chemotherapeutic treatment of brain tumors.

REFERENCES

1. W. R. SHAPIRO and J. I. AUSMAN, in *Recent Advances in Neurology* (Ed. F. PLUM) pp. 149–235. F. A. Davis, Philadelphia (1969).
2. L. E. BRODER and D. P. RALL, in *Progress in Experimental Tumor Research* (Ed. W. G. BINGHAM, JR.) Vol. 17, pp. 373–99. Karger, Basle (1972).
3. W. R. SHAPIRO, J. I. AUSMAN and D. P. RALL, *Cancer Res.* **30,** 2401 (1970).
4. R. J. A. AUR, J. SIMONE, H. O. HUSTU, T. WALTERS, C. PRATT and D. PINKEL, *Blood* **37,** 272 (1971).
5. R. K. KOROBKIN, A. V. LORENZO and R. W. P. CUTLER, *J. Pharmac. exp. Ther.* **165,** 412 (1968).
6. R. E. RIESELBACH, G. DICHIRO, E. J. FREIREICH and D. P. RALL, *New Engl. J. Med.* **267,** 1273 (1962).
7. S. MAYER, R. P. MAICKEL and B. B. BRODIE, *J. Pharmac. exp. Ther.* **127,** 205 (1959).
8. D. P. RALL and C. G. ZUBROD, *A. Rev. Pharmac.* **2,** 109 (1962).
9. L. S. SCHANKER, in *Advances in Drug Research* (Eds. N. J. HARPER and A. B. SIMMONDS), pp. 71–106. Academic Press, London (1964).
10. H. DAVSON, *Physiology of the Cerebrospinal Fluid,* pp. 82–103. J. & A. Churchill, London (1967).
11. D. P. RALL, in *Progress in Brain Research* (Eds. A. LAJTHA and D. H. FORD), pp. 159–67. Elsevier, New York (1968).
12. V. A. LEVIN, J. D. FENSTERMACHER and C. S. PATLAK, *Am. J. Physiol.* **219,** 1528 (1970).
13. R. E. CURRAN, M. B. MOSHER, E. S. OWENS and J. D. FENSTERMACHER, *Expl Neurol.* **29,** 546 (1970).
14. S. S. KETY, *Pharmac. Rev.* **3,** 1 (1951).
15. A. L. COWLES and J. D. FENSTERMACHER, in *Handbook of Experimental Pharmacology* (Eds. A. C. SARTORELLI and D. G. JOHNS), Vol. 7, Springer, Berlin (1974).
16. H. DAVSON, C. R. KLEEMAN and E. LEVIN, *J. Physiol., Lond.* **159,** 67 (1961).
17. M. POLLAY and R. J. KAPLAN, *Expl Neurol.* **30,** 54 (1971).
18. L. BAKAY, *Brain* **93,** 693 (1970).
19. L. BAKAY, *Brain* **93,** 699 (1970).
20. D. M. LONG, *J. Neurosurg.* **32,** 127 (1970).

Pp. 57–69, Supplement Number 2, 1974.
Biochemical Pharmacology. Printed in the U.S.A.

DESCRIPTIVE AND OPERATIONAL CYTOKINETICS

G. GORDON STEEL

Department of Biophysics, Institute of Cancer Research, Belmont, Sutton, Surrey, England

IN SEEKING drugs and drug schedules that have maximum selectivity of action against tumor cells, it is necessary to examine and exploit any relevant differences in the biology of neoplastic and normal tissues. The reason for discussing cell population kinetics in a meeting such as this is that many of the chemotherapeutic drugs now in use which, when they were discovered were hoped to be tumor-specific, have in fact been found to be largely proliferation-specific and, insofar as this is so, their success must depend on differences in proliferative state between tumor cells and cells in critical normal tissues. The exploited differences may either exist before the start of treatment or may appear when both the normal and tumor tissues have been damaged and begin to repair. In this paper, I wish to review some aspects of cytokinetics which appear to be relevant to chemotherapy. I will do this by attempting to draw a distinction between two main classes of cytokinetic investigation. The difference between them is not always clear-cut, but I believe it to be a distinction that helps in the evaluation of the widely different experimental approaches that are now being made.

There are two general types of approach to the identification of exploitable differences in cytokinetics between tissues. One of these begins with the microscope, and, for want of a better label, I will call this the "descriptive approach" to cell population kinetics. Through the microscope one can see dividing and nondividing cells, and one can relate their proliferation to cell morphology and to the tissue architecture. By autoradiography, it is possible to measure the times that cells take to migrate or to undergo various cellular processes. By quantitative optical methods, it is possible to count how many cells exist in defined categories and thus to obtain further information on the proliferative state of a tissue. All of these methods centre upon the microscope, though in the case of radioactive labeling techniques the autoradiographic work can sometimes be supplemented by studies of the turnover of radioactivity in tissue homogenates. The aim of these methods is to describe in detailed terms the cytokinetic structure of tissues and hopefully to reveal differences that are therapeutically exploitable.

The alternative approach is based on assays of tissue function. The internal structure of the tissue is ignored in favour of a measurement of some overall property of the system. In relation to the cytokinetics of chemotherapy, one property is of special interest – the ability of a tissue to grow. The assays used are therefore assays of growth capacity and the line of reasoning is as follows. An assay is selected which is technically feasible and which can give an estimate of growth capacity in a tissue before and after experimental therapeutic treatment. The ratio of these estimates is taken as an indication of response, which can then be compared with the response of a different tissue that is subjected to a similar treatment. I will call this the "operational approach" to the cytokinetics of chemotherapy. Operational is a word that carries the idea of "assessment of performance," in mathematics the idea of "subjecting a quantity to a process that changes its value," in military terminology the idea of "assessment of performance under combat conditions." The distinction that I wish to draw is between the attempt to take a cell population apart in order to see how it works (the descriptive approach) and the attempt to study it in terms of some chosen measure of overall performance (the operational approach). In the four sections that follow, I will try to indicate briefly some of the types of information relevant to chemotherapy which have been obtained by each of these approaches in the study of normal tissues and tumors.

Descriptive cytokinetics of bone marrow and intestinal epithelium

The descriptive cytokinetics of small intestine and bone marrow has been studied in some detail in experimental animals, and it is convenient that these are two of the principal limiting normal tissues in chemotherapy. The intestinal epithelium consists of a highly convoluted but continuous sheet of epithelial cells which covers the villi that project into the lumen of the gut and also the associated crypts of Lieberkühn. Cell proliferation is normally restricted to the lower ¾ of the crypts, and the rest of the epithelium consists of nonproliferating cells which have probably lost the ability to divide (although this has not been finally proved). Most of the proliferating cells within the crypt have a very short intermitotic time. In the rat, the average is approximately 11 hr, with about 8 hr spent in DNA synthesis.[1] If all proliferating cells in the crypt had a cycle time of 11 hr and an 8-hr S period, one would predict that two doses of an S-phase specific cytotoxic agent given say 6 hr apart would eradicate the proliferating cell population. That this does not happen may be attributed to the existence of a small number of cells at the base of each crypt which have been shown to proliferate much more slowly.[1,2] The greater part of the intestinal epithelium is in a state of rapid turnover in which cell production within the crypts is normally balanced by an equivalent loss of differentiated cells from the tips of the villi into the intestinal lumen. The turnover time of the whole epithelium in the rat is about 36–48 hr. Cells on the villi thus have a very short lifespan. For an individual cell in the crypt, we may ask how many of its descendants will still be found in the epithelium after, say 5 days. For most crypt cells, the answer will be none, for the unidirectional flow of cells towards the villi will have carried all their descendants away. Only a few cells at the base of the crypts will produce large families of descendants and among these may be true stem cells, cells whose descendants continue for a long time to give rise to new epithelial cells. It will be noted that the stem cells are not actually identified through the microscope; their existence is inferred. Cytotoxic agents often produce severe damage to the intestinal epithelium in which crypt cells die *in situ* and the villi collapse, presumably due to continued exfoliation. When regeneration occurs from sublethal toxicity, it is often difficult to know which cells were responsible for the recovery. One would presume that the surivors were close to the base of the crypts at the time of treatment, but it cannot be ruled out that cells further up the crypts might have the capacity to revert to become new stem cells.

The architecture of bone marrow is much more difficult to identify than that of the intestine, although recent studies have shown some progress in this direction.[3]

However, between the three main lines of cells that make up the marrow there are marked differences in morphology and in staining properties, and within each line it is possible fairly reliably to place cells into a series of morphological categories that are known to be sequential. It is this morphological structure that provides the opportunity for detailed kinetic studies. It is possible to estimate the transit time and number of divisions of cells in each of the morphological stages and to investigate the stage at which cells lose their proliferative activity and become mature, functional cells.[4] Most of the recognisable cells in the erythroid system are normally in a state of rapid proliferation, with intermitotic times that are even shorter than those found in intestinal epithelium. Granulocyte precursors normally proliferate more slowly, but under stress a shortening of intermitotic time can occur in both systems to a value of 9 hr or less.[5,6] As might be expected, such cells are highly sensitive to many cytotoxic agents and, as with the small intestine, survival from sublethal toxicity often depends on the survival of a few of the most primitive cells. Microscopic techniques do not, however, allow the marrow stem cells to be studied, or even identified with great certainty.

Operational cytokinetics of bone marrow and intestine

As indicated above, the term "operational" is being used here to denote investigations that ignore the internal structure of a tissue but concentrate on assays of its overall growth performance. The bone marrow has readily lent itself to the development of assays because of the ease with which known numbers of cells can be withdrawn from a donor and transplanted into a recipient whose own marrow has been completely destroyed by radiation or drugs. Various properties of the growth of the transplant can be measured, yielding various possible assays of the growth potential of the transplanted marrow. For instance, if the dose of transplanted marrow cells is suitably chosen, discrete colonies, each of which arises from a single marrow stem cell, can subsequently be found in the spleen. The count of colonies per recipient spleen is thus a measure of the stem cell content of the implanted marrow.[7] A somewhat different approach is to measure the subsequent functional state of the transplanted marrow. A measurement of the rate of incorporation of radioactive iron into the peripheral blood of marrow recipients provides an assay of the erythroid repopulating ability of the original donor marrow.[8] An injection of bacterial endotoxin into animals that have received a marrow graft mobilises mature granulocytes from the marrow and the maximum concentration that they achieve in the peripheral blood provides a further assay of the growth potential of the donor marrow, in this case of its granulocyte repopulating ability.[9] In recent years, techniques have been developed that allow bone marrow cells to be grown *in vitro* in such a way that colonies develop, also apparently from single cells. This provides yet another assay of stem cell content of the marrow under test.[10]

Any of the assays just mentioned may be employed to examine the survival and regrowth characteristics of those cells in the bone marrow that can regenerate marrow in a lethally irradiated recipient or produce growth *in vitro*. The proliferative state of such cells in the donor may be examined by studying their survival under treatment with phase-specific cytotoxic agents. The most reliable agent for this purpose is ^{3}H-thymidine, which reaches maximum cytotoxicity at a dose of about 5 mCi in the mouse. This so-called "thymidine-suicide" technique has shown that marrow stem cells behave as though they have a much lower labeling index than the recognisable proliferating cells in the marrow and their turnover time has been estimated to be approximately 30 hr in the mouse. In marrow that is recovering from damage by acute irradiation or certain chemotherapeutic agents, the stem cells appear to increase their rate of proliferation.[11]

Techniques for measuring the regenerative capacity of the intestinal epithelium are much more difficult than for the bone marrow, and also less precise. Hornsey and Vatistas[12] used the 4-day survival of mice following X-irradiation as a measure of the survival of a minimal number of crypt cells and were able in split-dose experiments to show that the dose–response curve in intestinal epithelium appeared to have a very large shoulder (extrapolation number greater than 28). Withers and Elkind[13,14] confirmed this finding using a method in which colony regeneration could be assessed *in situ.* The conclusion was that the cells which limited the survival of intestinal epithelium to X-irradiation had a high capacity for repair of sublethal damage.

Descriptive cytokinetics of tumors

Bone marrow and intestinal epithelium maintain relatively uniform kinetic properties among animals of any one species. There are minor variations with age and strain, and interspecies differences have been clearly demonstrated. In contrast, neoplastic tissues display a wide variety of morphological and kinetic properties and defy simple generalisation. The bulk of available cytokinetic information is on transplanted tumors that have undergone many passages, and numerous investigations have shown that these differ considerably in kinetic properties from the initial autochonous tumors.[15,16] Perhaps the simplest cytokinetic parameter is volume doubling time. The doubling times of primary tumors appear to be species dependent, increasing as one moves from the mouse, through the rat, to tumors in larger animals and man. In small laboratory animals, tumor growth is invariably far from exponential, the doubling time increasing continuously with tumor size. The most detailed studies of the growth rate of human tumors have shown little evidence of growth rate dependence on tumor size. It thus appears that tumors have an initial growth rate (when first seen microscopically) that is species dependent and a retardation that is in part determined by the ratio of tumor weight to the host body weight.

Studies in primary tumors by the technique of labeled mitoses have shown that the average intermitotic time is always much shorter than the volume doubling time. Furthermore, there appears invariably to be a considerable variation among the intermitotic times of different cells within the same tumor,[17] probably reflecting the considerable morphological and vascular heterogeneity of most primary tumors. It is difficult to gain information on tumor cells whose intermitotic times are much longer than the average and to distinguish them from cells that are truly nondividing. However, thymidine studies have shown that in primary tumors there appear to be many cells that are slowly or noproliferating.[18] Studies by Refsum and Berdal[19] have shown that in human tumors the mitotic indices are often much higher than would be expected in view of the estimated tumor growth rate, and Steel[20,21] has shown that thymidine labeling indices are similarly high. From this we may conclude that extensive cell loss occurs in primary tumors and that the observed growth rate is often the result of a high rate of cell production competing with a high rate of cell loss.

The greatest difficulty in the descriptive approach to the cytokinetics of tumors is their morphological heterogeneity. The amount of detail gained in studies on normal tissues has depended on the ease with which a stable spatial or morphological structure can be defined. In tumors, such a structure is usually impossible to discern and most investigators are led to the unsatisfactory policy of producing results that are averages for the whole tumor. Since in many therapeutic situations tumor regrowth comes from a small minority of survivors, such a policy is probably incapable of contributing to our understanding of failure to cure.

The small amount of work that has been done on cell proliferation in relation to tumor structure has led to two general observations. First, in experimental tumors the rate of cell proliferation usually decreases from the tumor periphery to its centre.[22] This is not surprising in view of the hydrodynamics of tumor blood supply and the phenomenon of central necrosis. Second, in special types of experimental tumor, it has been shown by Tannock[23] that some patent blood vessels are surrounded by a cord of viable tumor cells whose cord radius is limited to about 100 μm. Within such cords, proliferation is fastest in cells that are close to the axial blood vessel, cells appear to be pushed outward as a result of this proliferation, and in less than one volume doubling time of the tumor as a whole, cells move from close to the blood vessel to the outer edge of the cord where they die at the boundary with necrosis. This spatially related process of cell turnover has so far only been clearly observed in one experimental tumor. It does, however, form the basis of a hypothesis about the structural cytokinetics of tumors, namely that the cellular proliferation rate is greatest close to blood vessels and that the extensive cell loss that can be demonstrated is mainly of cells that are distant from blood vessels. The examination of this hypothesis is a central problem in the descriptive cytokinetics of tumors. If it is valid, then under circumstances of unimpeded growth the stem cells of a tumor would be expected to be close to blood vessels, though if the tumor is damaged by an agent that selectively hits cells that are close to blood vessels, regrowth may then come from cells that were destined to be lost in the normal process of cell turnover. A therapeutically important question is to what extent the normal processes of cell loss continue after the start of cytotoxic therapy. It may be that, both for radiotherapy and chemotherapy, tumor cell survival is dominated by resistant cells that are not close to blood vessels. If this is so, then on the basis of the hypothesis outlined above, the resistant subpopulation may consist of cells that normally have a short lifespan. Their fate after the start of therapy will thus depend greatly on the normal processes of cell destruction. If, as the work of Sylvén and Holmberg[24] implies, advancing necrosis is partly due to cytotoxic materials diffusing out of a necrotic area, then this may not be stopped by an interruption of cell proliferation. This general theory of the persistence of cell loss processes is supported by the work of Denekamp,[25] who has observed that an immediate drop in tumor volume occurs predominantly in tumors which on the basis of thymidine studies appear to have a high rate of cell loss.

The structural characteristics that have just been described are observed in highly anaplastic tumors. Tumors that show differentiation presumably retain some of the characteristics of the tissue of origin and, in particular, carcinomas may retain the sequential process of cell turnover that is found in many normal renewal tissues. This has two implications: first, that extensive cell loss from differentiated tumors may take place not only by necrosis but also by processes of normal cell differentiation; and second, that only a proportion of the parenchymal tumor cells may retain the capacity to proliferate, and perhaps an even smaller proportion may retain the capacity to act as stem cells for regrowth after cytotoxic treatment.

Few direct attempts have been made to relate parameters of descriptive cytokinetics to therapeutic response. Wolberg and Ansfield[26] studied response to the administration of 5-fluorouracil in a group of 148 cases in which they also recorded the pretreatment thymidine labeling index of the tumor. No relationship was found between thymidine labeling and clinical response. A further example of lack of agreement between therapeutic response and predictions on the basis of descriptive cytokinetics will be given below.

Operational cytokinetics of tumors

The amount of experimental work that has been performed on tumors using the operational approach is enormous, and only a brief outline can be given here. Interest has mainly centred on the extent of cell kill by various cytotoxic agents and this problem is only in part a kinetic one. However, there are two areas in which kinetic considerations are important in understanding response and in which (as a corollary) information that is useful to the field of cytokinetics is obtained.

The first area is the attempt to understand response to acute treatment with cytotoxic agents, the assays being performed immediately. The pretreatment kinetic state of the cell population is important here, and the greatest contribution to our understanding of the problem has probably come through the work of Bruce *et al.*[27] Chemotherapeutic agents may be placed in three main categories: class I contains agents that give exponential survival curves whose slope is largely unaffected by the proliferation rate of the target cells; class II contains agents whose cell survival curves show an initial fall followed by a plateau; class II contains agents whose cell survival curves are close to exponential but with sensitivities that depend on the proliferative state of the target cells. This work has formed the basis for the classification of drugs as "proliferation dependent" (class III) or "phase specific" (class II), but it should be noted that the therapeutic value of this classification does not lie in this interpretation but in the fact that dose–response curves have different shapes, depending on the choice of agent and the state of the target tissue. For example, a plateau in a dose–response curve has therapeutic implications that are largely independent of its kinetic interpretation. The influence of pretreatment kinetics on dose–response curves has also been studied *in vitro* in two principal ways. In synchronised cultures it has been possible to investigate directly the phase specificity of drugs and radiation.[28,29] By comparing survival curves in exponentially growing and plateau-phase cultures, conclusions have been drawn about the drug or radiation sensitivity of slowly proliferating cells.[30,31] Clear evidence that kinetic considerations can only partly explain differences in therapeutic response has come from the recent work of Ogawa *et al.*[32]

The second area in which kinetics impinges on tumor cell survival is when a tumor is left *in situ* for a period before applying an assay or delivering a second treatment. Studies of this type can be divided into those in which the time interval was short (a few hr or less) or in which it was longer. With short time intervals between primary and secondary treatments, important changes occur in dose–response curves which have been attributed[33] to three "R's": repair of sublethal damage; reoxygenation (of hypoxic cells, when the second treatment is with radiation); and reassortment (i.e.

progression of a partially synchronised population of cells surviving the primary treatment). It is often difficult to know which of these mechanisms is responsible for a change in survival with short intervals between doses. When longer intervals are allowed after the primary treatment, a fourth mechanism becomes possible – regeneration. Descriptive evidence has been adduced to show that in solid tumors there is a period of rapid proliferation shortly after a primary treatment.[34,35] From a therapeutic point of view, the important question is whether enhanced sensitivity to cytotoxic agents can be demonstrated at this time (i.e. whether there is operational evidence for an effect), as has been found in the two-treatment response of bone marrow.[8,36] When, instead of a second treatment, an assay is applied at intervals after a single cytotoxic treatment, information of considerable kinetic interest is obtained. In some cases, the number of surviving cells remains constant for a few days before the regeneration process sets in.[34] In other cases, a further fall in the number of survivors occurs before regeneration starts, which could be interpreted either as an artifact due to the survivors having an initially high sensitivity to damage by the assay procedure or to their difficulty in surviving within an almost obliterated region of tissue.

Assays that have been used to study the survival of growth capacity in treated tumors have included the endpoint dilution assay,[37,38] the spleen colony assay,[39] the lung colony assay,[40] a standardised regrowth assay[41] and assay *in vitro*.[34]

Comparison between the descriptive and operational approaches to cytokinetics

The previous four sections have reviewed briefly the use of what are here called the "descriptive" and "operational" approaches to the study of cytokinetics in normal tissues and tumors. The contrast between the types of information gained by these approaches is marked. The descriptive approach (based on the microscope) can reveal important details in the relationship between cell proliferation and tissue structure, although in tumors progress is often thwarted by structural heterogeneity. The main drawback of this approach lies in the difficulty of identifying under the microscope those cells that have the capacity to produce a large family of descendants (stem cells).

The operational approach (based on growth assays) ignores tumor structure and concentrates upon the capacity of cells for regrowth after treatment. From the point of view of trying to understand drug selectivity in chemotherapy, it might be thought that this is by far the more direct of the two approaches. It does, however, have one major drawback, namely that it depends on the availability of valid assays of cell growth capacity (i.e. assays that can truly reflect the performance *in vivo* of cells left viable after treatment has finished).[42] Most of the assays that are used at present start by tearing apart the organised structure of a tissue (normal or tumor), producing a single-cell suspension, and then testing the ability of the cells to grow. It would not be surprising if some cells under these artificial circumstances failed to grow, though they could repopulate the tissue if left *in vivo*, or if some cells grew which would not do so under the controls that continue to operate during regrowth *in vivo*. The cells of normal tissues and primary tumors may be strongly influenced in their growth characteristics by their contacts with adjacent cells, and their growth characteristics when isolated *in vitro* or in abnormal surroundings *in vivo* may be to some extent artificial.

If we accept, therefore, that each of these two experimental approaches has important (but contrasting) limitations, two questions present themselves. First, to what extent can we see agreement between descriptive and operational cytokinetics? Second, can either approach make useful predictions about therapeutic response? Each of these questions would require a complete paper for a full review, but the following brief comments will be made here. Probably the best answer to the first question has come from the experimental therapeutic work of Skipper *et al.*[43,44] With their permission, I am reproducing here their data together with some theoretical derivations that I have made from them. In a number of transplanted mouse tumors and in spontaneous AK mouse leukemia, thymidine studies have been performed by the technique of labeled mitoses and by repeated thymidine injection.[45] The results allow distributions of intermitotic time to be calculated that are consistent with the labeled mitoses data, similarly distributions of residence times in G_1, S and G_2. The method used for these analyses was that described by Steel *et al.*[46] as elaborated by Steel and Hanes.[47] It assumes that the phase durations are log-normally distributed within the population (the data are not sufficiently precise to confirm or reject this assumption) and the shape of the distribution of intermitotic times is therefore intermediate between normal and log-normal. The distributions of phase duration allow age density distributions to be calculated, provided that some assumption is made about the fate of nonproliferating cells. Three different assumptions have been made in the present work, yielding three versions of what we have called the SAB model:[46,47]

SAB 1. Cell loss is assumed to occur only from the oldest nonproliferating cells and the age at which loss occurs is well defined. After the start of thymidine administration, no loss of labeled cells will occur until this age is reached.

SAB 2. Cell loss is assumed to occur only at mitosis. By comparison with SAB 1, this is the other extreme, for cell loss is from the youngest cells in the population and the loss of labeled cells begins almost immediately after the start of thymidine administration.

SAB 3. Cell loss is assumed to occur randomly with respect to age and proliferative status. This is an intermediate situation between the other two models in regard to the age dependence of cell loss.

The reason for choosing these three models is that they allow three different continuous thymidine labeling curves to be calculated: SAB 1 and SAB 2 give two extreme curves and SAB 3 an intermediate one. These curves therefore show the range of forms that is possible in the continuous labeling curves, for different assumptions about the mode of cell loss. The curves are based on three basic items of data: the labeled mitoses curve, an initial labeling index, and a volume doubling time.

The approach of Skipper *et al.*[43,44] was to relate the results of such a study to studies of continuous thymidine labeling and to estimates of cell survival under a continuous infusion of cytosine arabinoside (Ara-C). This agent is thought to show a highly selective toxicity against cells undergoing DNA synthesis. In each of the four tumor types referred to here, comparisons have been made of the cytotoxic effects of Ara-C and high doses of ^{3}H-thymidine, and the agreement has been good[48–50] (and personal communication from H. E. Skipper). The experiments consisted of taking two comparable groups of tumors, one of which received repeated (effectively continuous) administration of ^{3}H-thymidine followed by autoradiography to determine the proportion of labeled cells, while the other received a similar administration of Ara-C followed by a bioassay (usually at 24 hr) to determine the proportion of surviving stem cells. What might be expected is that the proportion of cells surviving the Ara-C would correspond to the proportion of cells remaining unlabeled by ^{3}H-thymidine. This proportion should also correspond to the residual unlabeled fraction as indicated by the range of theoretical continuous labeling curves.

The results on four of the tumor types within this study are shown in Fig. 1. In others, the results were comparable. Each chart shows "survival" as a function of time of effectively continuous administration. "Survival" consists of the survival of cells with repopulating ability in the Ara-C study, and "survival" in the unlabeled state in

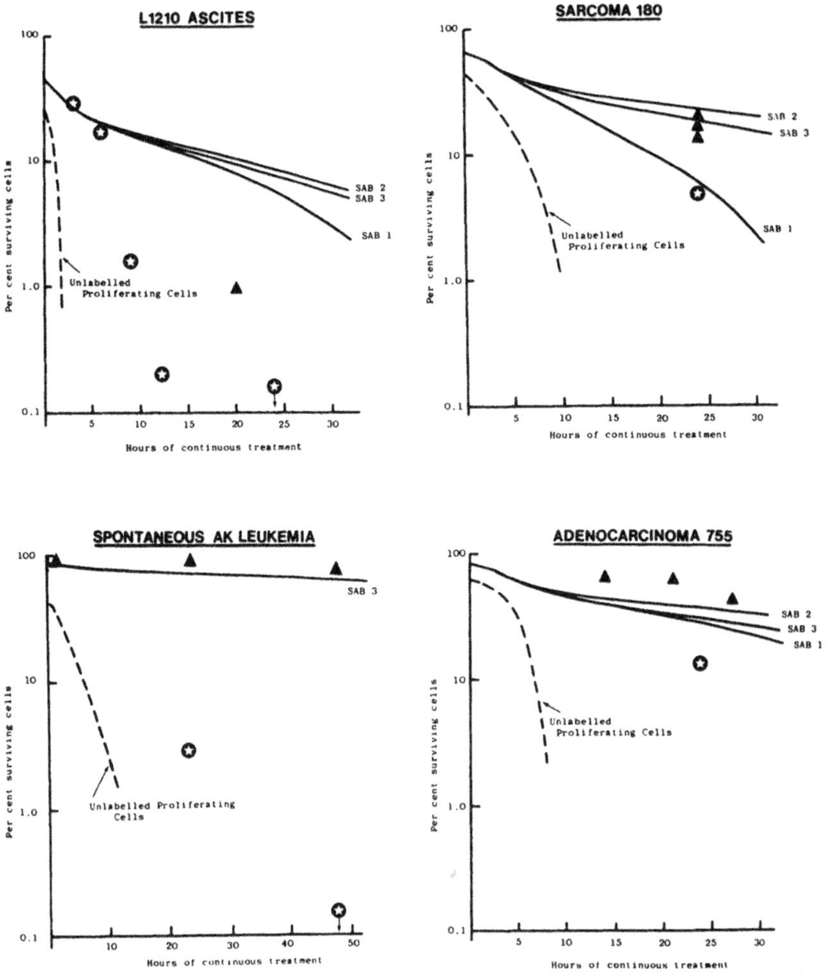

FIG. 1. Comparison for four experimental tumors between the results of semicontinuous labeling with ^{3}H-thymidine (as studied by autoradiography) and semicontinuous treatment with cytosine arabinoside (as studied by bioassay). The stars indicate estimated cell survival after treatment with Ara-C; the triangles represent the proportion of cells unlabeled by thymidine. The lines show predictions of the proportion of cells remaining unlabeled during continuous administration of ^{3}H-thymidine, on the basis of the initial labeling index and the labeled mitoses data. The solid lines apply to the whole cell population (using three different mathematical models); the broken lines apply to proliferating cells only.

the thymidine studies. The broken line shows the calculated survival of proliferating cells, i.e. the proportion that have not entered the S phase at various times. In each case, these curves predict rapid killing of the proliferating cell population and the fact that survival was always greater than this indicates that survival was dominated by cells that the thymidine studies classify as nonproliferating. The theoretical "thymidine survival" curves do not differ widely for these tumors, except in the case of Sarcoma 180 where SAB 1 predicts a considerably lower survival. The curve for SAB 3 agrees well with the continuous thymidine labeling data for this tumor; in Ca 755, all three theoretical curves overestimate the amount of labeling actually observed; in L1210 ascites, the curves underestimate the labeling. From this, one must conclude that the theoretical models used in this work are inadequate to simulate both the pulse-labeling and continuous thymidine labeling data.

The more important comparison, however, is between the thymidine survival and Ara-C survival data. In each tumor the survival point lies below the thymidine labeling points, indicating that the extent of kill was found to be greater than that predicted by thymidine labeling. In Sa 180 and Ca 755, the difference is a factor of 4 or 5; in L1210, the factor is difficult to estimate because all survivals are very low; in spontaneous AK leukemia, the factor is 2 decades at 24 hr and more than 3 decades at 48 hr. Again, one must conclude that thymidine labeling gives a poor indication of the extent of kill by Ara-C.

The conclusions of this study are of considerable interest and it would be valuable for these experiments to be repeated on other experimental tumors. Three possible explanations of the discrepancies could be given and it is not at this stage possible to decide among them: (1) that Ara-C is not purely S phase specific, but kills some cells that do not undergo DNA synthesis (studies with cytotoxic doses of ^{3}H-thymidine argue against this possibility); (2) that the bioassay for some reason overestimated the extent of kill of cells left *in situ*; and (3) that tumor stem cells were kinetically unrepresentative of the whole tumor cell population. The latter hypothesis implies that the tumor stem cells constitute a more rapidly proliferating subpopulation and that many of the nonproliferating cells in the tumor had lost their capacity to repopulate. A fourth possible explanation, that ^{3}H-thymidine failed to label some cells that were killed by Ara-C within the S phase, seems unlikely, although in the case of L1210 the discrepancy amounts to less than 1 per cent of residual unlabeled cells, and such an error in labeling index cannot be ruled out.

CONCLUSIONS

One general conclusion that follows from this attempt to make a direct comparison between descriptive and operational cytokinetics in tumors is that despite the possible sources of error in the assays available for the operational approach, the possible errors in trying to predict cell survival from thymidine studies are considerably greater. In the experiments referred to here, direct studies of thymidine labeling of the whole cell population were more reliable than predictions made from labeled mitoses curves (and theoretical models), but even these had two major drawbacks. First, estimates of the proportion of unlabeled cells become very inaccurate when more than 95 per cent of the population is labeled (a "survival" of 5 per cent or less), yet the successful treatment of tumors involves many decades of cell kill. Thymidine labeling might help in the understanding of palliative treatment (the first decade of kill), but it can make only rough predictions about high levels of cell kill. Second, any predictions about cell kill that are made on the basis of thymidine labeling assume that tumor stem cells are kinetically typical of the whole tumor. This does not seem to have been the case from the present studies, which show that while ultimate tumor survival is predominantly due to slowly or nonporliferating stem cells, such cells may form only a small proportion of all nonproliferating cells, most of which may be incapable of repopulation.

One of the main objects of this paper has been to show how concepts that have come from two very different experimental approaches interact. There is a tendency to take an idea that has come from survival curve studies and relate it to a phenomenon seen through the microscope, and *vice versa,* but such a link is often hard to prove. Some examples of analogies of this type are shown in Table 1. To enlarge on one example, consider the concept of resting cells. Autoradiographic work demonstrates that in tumors some cells must be proliferating very slowly, though it is hard to show that they are nonproliferating. Cell survival studies show that some stem cells are resistant to protracted treatment with proliferation-dependent cytotoxic agents, and it is sometimes concluded that the resistant survivors must be "G_0 cells." But the autoradiographic work cannot prove that the nonproliferating cells are stem cells and the cell survival work cannot show that the resistant minority are not in fact resistant by virtue of a property that is unconnected with proliferation. It is important, for clarity of thought, to beware of such conceptual terms as "G_0 cells", "cycle specific", "therapeutic synchronisation" and "cell cycle time",[17] but to relate them always to what the data directly show. At the present time the links between the descriptive and operational approaches cannot be seen clearly. In the development of rational chemotherapeutic schedules, it would seem that information gained by the descriptive approach is less directly useful than that gained by the operational approach (despite its own limitations), and the strategy proposed by Bruce and Lin[51] may be the way to achieve an early improvement in scheduling. The long-term future of cancer therapy

TABLE 1. ANALOGIES BETWEEN DESCRIPTIVE AND OPERATIONAL CONCEPTS*

Operational approach	Descriptive approach
Stem cells registered by their ability to produce a discrete number of descendants under test conditions	Stem cells postulated as a source of continued proliferation
Acute survival curve has a well defined plateau	Phase specificity
Short-term synergism or antagonism between treatments in the absence of known biochemical interactions	Treatment-induced synchrony (plus phase specificity)
Subpopulation resistant to protracted treatment with proliferation-dependent agents	Cells "out of cycle"
Sensitivity to proliferation-dependent agents increased by prior treatment	Mobilisation of nonproliferating cells

*A phenomenon that is observed by one approach may be thought to correspond to an analogous phenomenon detected by the other approach, but the correspondence may be largely hypothetical.

will, however, depend on a deeper understanding of the biology of tumors and the normal tissues that limit therapy, and for this an improvement in knowledge gained by many different experimental approaches will be necessary.

Acknowledgements – I acknowledge with gratitude the support and advice of Professor L. F. Lamerton and helpful discussions with Drs. N. M. Blackett and R. P. Hill. Dr. H. E. Skipper and his colleagues supplied the data shown in Fig. 1. I am also grateful to Dr. Skipper for much stimulating discussion.

REFERENCES

1. A. B. CAIRNIE, L. F. LAMERTON and G. G. STEEL, *Expl Cell Res.* **39**, 528 (1965).
2. N. WRIGHT, A. MORLEY and D. APPLETON, *Cell Tissue Kinet.* **5**, 351 (1972).
3. T. M. FLIEDNER, W. CALVO, R. HASS, J. FORTEZA and F. BOHNE, in *Hemopoietic Cellular Proliferation* (Ed. F. STOHLMAN, JR.), Grune & Stratton, New York (1970).
4. R. G. TARBUTT and N. M. BLACKETT, *Cell Tissue Kinet.* **1**, 65 (1968).
5. I. R. A. HANNA, R. G. TARBUTT and L. F. LAMERTON, *Br. J. Haemat.* **16**, 381 (1969).
6. C. J. F. SPRY, *Cell Tissue Kinet.* **4**, 351 (1971).
7. J. E. TILL and E. A. MCCULLOCH, *Radiat. Res.* **14**, 213 (1961).
8. N. M. BLACKETT, *J. natn. Cancer Inst.* **41**, 909 (1968).
9. S. HELLMAN and H. E. GRATE, *Blood,* **30**, 103 (1967).
10. T. R. BRADLEY and D. METCALF, *Aust. J. exp. Biol. med. Sci.* **44**, 287 (1966).
11. T. B. CONSTABLE and N. M. BLACKETT, *J. natn. Cancer Inst.* **48**, 941 (1972).
12. S. HORNSEY and S. VATISTAS, *Br. J. Radiol.* **36**, 795 (1963).
13. H. R. WITHERS and M. M. ELKIND, *Radiology* **91**, 998 (1968).
14. H. R. WITHERS and M. M. ELKIND, *Radiat. Res.* **38**, 598 (1969).
15. A. C. BEGG, *Cell Tissue Kinet.* **4**, 401 (1971).
16. G. G. STEEL, K. ADAMS, J. HODGETT and P. JANIK, *Br. J. Cancer* **25**, 802 (1971).
17. G. G. STEEL, *Cell Tissue Kinet.* **5**, 87 (1972).
18. M. L. MENDELSOHN, *J. natn. Cancer Inst.* **28**, 1015 (1962).
19. S. B. REFSUM and P. BERDAL, *Eur. J. Cancer* **3**. 235 (1967).
20. G. G. STEEL, *Eur. J. Cancer* **3**, 381 (1967).
21. G. G. STEEL, *Cell Tissue Kinet.* **1**, 193 (1968).
22. A. F. HERMENS and G. W. BARENDSEN, *Eur. J. Cancer* **3**, 361 (1967).
23. I. F. TANNOCK, *Br. J. Cancer* **22**, 258 (1968).
24. B. SYLVÉN and B. HOLMBERG, *Eur. J. Cancer* **1**, 199 (1965).
25. J. DENEKAMP, *Eur. J. Cancer* **8**, 335 (1972).
26. W. H. WOLBERG and F. J. ANSFIELD, *Cancer Res.* **31**, 448 (1971).
27. W. R. BRUCE, B. E. MEEKER and F. A. VALERIOTE, *J. natn. Cancer Inst.* **37**, 233 (1966).
28. W. K. SINCLAIR and R. A. MORTON, *Radiat. Res.* **29**, 450 (1966).
29. D. PETROVIC and A. H. W. NIAS, *Eur. J. Cancer* **3**, 321 (1967).
30. F. M. SCHABEL, JR, H. E. SKIPPER, M. W. TRADER and W. S. WILCOX, *Cancer Chemother. Rep.* **48**, 17 (1965).
31. G. M. HAHN, in *Time and Dose Relationships in Radiation Biology as Applied to Radiotherapy* (Eds. V. P. BOND, H. D. SUIT and V. MARCIAL), BNL 50203 (C-57). Brookhaven Laboratory (1970).
32. M. OGAWA, D. F. BERGSAGEL and E. A. MCCULLOCH, *Blood* **41**, 7 (1973).
33. H. R. WITHERS in *Time and Dose Relationships in Radiobiology as Applied to Radiotherapy* (Eds. V. P. BOND, H. D. SUIT and V. MARCIAL), BNL 50203 (C-57). Brookhaven National Laboratory (1970).
34. A. F. HERMENS and G. W. BARENDSEN, *Eur. J. Cancer* **5**, 173 (1969).
35. H. A. VAN PEPERZEEL, *Eur. J. Cancer* **8**, 665 (1972).
36. F. A. VALERIOTE and W. R. BRUCE, *J. natn. Cancer Inst.* **38**, 393 (1967).
37. H. B. HEWITT and C. W. WILSON, *Br. J. Cancer* **13**, 69 (1959).
38. R. F. KALLMAN in *Methods in Cancer Research* (Ed. H. BUSCH), Vol. 4, Academic Press, New York (1968).
39. W. R. BRUCE and H. VAN DER GAAG, *Nature, Lond.* **199**, 79 (1963).
40. R. P. HILL and R. S. BUSH, *Int. J. Radiat. Biol.* **15**, 435 (1969).
41. H. H. LLOYD, *Proc. Am. Ass. Cancer Res.* **12**, 6 (1971).
42. T. ALPER, *Br. med. Bull.* **29**, 3 (1973).
43. H. E. SKIPPER and S. PERRY, *Cancer Res.* **30**, 1883 (1970).

44. H. E. SKIPPER, F. M. SCHABEL, JR. and W. S. WILCOX, *Cancer Chemother. Rep.* **51**, 125 (1967).
45. L. SIMPSON-HERREN and H. H. LLOYD, *Cancer Chemother. Rep.* **54**, 143 (1970).
46. G. G. STEEL, K. ADAMS and J. C. BARRETT, *Br. J. Cancer* **20**, 784 (1966).
47. G. G. STEEL and S. HANES, *Cell Tissue Kinet.* **4**, 93 (1971).
48. W. R. BRUCE and B. E. MEEKER, *J. natn. Cancer Inst.* **34**, 849 (1965).
49. W. R. BRUCE, B. E. MEEKER, W. E. POWERS and F. A. VALERIOTE, *J. natn. Cancer Inst.* **42**, 1015 (1969).
50. L. J. WILKOFF, A. DULMADGE and H. H. LLOYD, *J. natn. Cancer Inst.* in press.
51. W. R. BRUCE and H. LIN, *Cancer Res.* **29**, 2308 (1969).

Pp. 71—82, Supplement Number 2, 1974.
Biochemical Pharmacology. Printed in the U.S.A.

ROLE OF ENZYMATIC ACTIVATION AND INACTIVATION IN DRUG SELECTIVITY

J. FRANK HENDERSON

University of Alberta Cancer Research Unit (McEachern Laboratory) and
Department of Biochemistry, Edmonton, Alberta, Canada T6G 2E1

THE BROAD problem of drug selectivity in cancer chemotherapy will be considered from three related but slightly different points of view. The first concerns the bases of selective toxicity itself: i.e., why can drugs in some cases selectively inhibit tumor growth in a patient? The second concerns the bases of variation in selective toxicity: i.e., why can only some types of tumors be inhibited in some patients some times? The third concerns the prediction of selective toxicity: i.e., how can the drug sensitivity of a particular tumor in a particular patient at any one time be predicted?

Selective toxicity in cancer chemotherapy, when it is achieved, is the sum result of a wide variety of biological,[1] pharmacological[2] and biochemical factors,[3] and in no one tumor–patient–drug system are these factors completely understood at the present time. One of these many factors is the metabolism of the drug used, both in the tumor and in the patient. In particular, the phenomenon of the conversion in the body of inactive drugs to active drugs and of active drugs to inactive drugs will be considered here.

With respect to activation and inactivation reactions, cancer chemotherapeutic agents may be divided into several general classes.

(1) A few antitumor drugs are not significantly metabolized at all; this group includes such compounds as methotrexate,[4,5] methylglyoxal-*bis*-guanylhydrazone,[6,7] guanazole,[8] aminocyclopentane carboxylic acid,[9] actinomycin D[10] and mithramycin.[11]

(2) A second group includes those that may be activated and inactivated in the body, but by nonenzymatic processes. Thus alkylating agents of the mustard class, for example, are activated by nonenzymatic conversion to aziridines,[12,13] and they may be inactivated by nonenzymatic reaction with various biological molecules, including sulfhydryl-containing compounds[7] and bicarbonate.[12–16] Certain of the methylhydrazine derivatives also are nonenzymatically activated,[17] and 1-(2-chloroethyl)-3-cyclohexyl-1-nitrosourea may be nonenzymatically metabolized, at least in part.[18] The highly reactive compounds of this group are also often subject to enzymatic inactivation, as will be mentioned below.

(3) Another important group of anticancer drugs includes compounds that are administered in pharmacologically inactive forms, which then are enzymatically converted to active agents. This group includes most (but not all) purine and pyrimidine antimetabolites, and such alkylating agents as cyclophosphamide and the triazinoimidazoles (See references.)

(4) Finally, the largest group includes all the drugs that are enzymatically inactivated. These really may be divided into two subclasses. One of these includes active compounds that undergo inactivation, such as hydroxyurea, daunomycin, streptonigrin, vinblastine, the heterocyclic thiosemicarbazones and activated forms of cyclophosphamide, triazenoimidazoles and many purine and pyrimidine antimetabolites. The second class includes inactive precursors of active agents, which are converted to compounds that cannot subsequently be activated; purine and pyrimidine antimetabolites are prominent members of this group. (See references.)

Having classified in this way many of our present growth-inhibitory drugs with respect to activation and inactivation reactions, the reactions themselves may be further classified according to their tissue distribution. For this purpose it is sufficient to divide all tissues into two groups. The first, which will be called "drug-sensitive" tissues, includes the neoplastic tissues and those growing normal tissues whose growth is frequently inhibited by antineoplastic drugs; intestinal mucosa, bone marrow, skin and lymphatic tissues may be placed in this category. The second group of tissues, termed "drug-insensitive," includes all other normal tissues, which may or may not metabolize the drugs in question but in general are not adversely affected by them. This classification is, of course, both oversimplified and relative, but is useful for the subsequent discussion.

Enzymatic activation and inactivation reactions may have the following types of tissue distributions. (a) Some drugs are not activated, but are inactivated both in sensitive and insensitive tissues; the methylhydrazines are an example. (b) Some drugs are not activated, and are inactivated only in insensitive tissues; hydroxyurea, mycophenolic acid and probably vinblastine are in this group. (c) Among the drugs which undergo enzymatic activation, some, such as cyclophosphamide and triazenoimidazoles, are activated only in insensitive tissues, in this case, the liver. (d) Drugs which have been activated can be inactivated both in sensitive and insensitive tissues, as is the case with the triazenoimidazoles. (e) Drugs which have been activated may also be inactivated mainly in insensitive tissues, as is the case with cyclophosphamide. (f) Most purine and pyrimidine antimetabolites may be activated both in sensitive and insensitive tissues. (g) Most purine and pyrimidine antimetabolites may also be inactivated both in sensitive and insensitive tissues.

With respect to drug selectivity, it is obvious that the relative rates of enzymatic activation and inactivation reactions in sensitive tissues are very important determinants of their drug sensitivity, but they affect only that portion of the administered drug that reaches and enters these tissues. Activation and inactivation in insensitive tissues, in contrast, affect mainly the amount of drug that reaches the sensitive tissues because their main effect now is on drug pharmacokinetics. Thus, depending on the tissue distribution of activating and inactivating enzymes, their effect on drug selectivity may be direct or indirect or both.

The implications of these general considerations regarding enzymatic activation and inactivation for the problem of drug selectivity may now be considered. Inasmuch as there is still much to learn in this regard, only selected examples can be given here.

Purine and pyrimidine antimetabolites

The activation of purine and pyrimidine antimetabolites in normal and neoplastic tissues will be considered first (reviews[19–22]). Activation of purine and pyrimidine analogs and derivatives may involve one or more of the following types of reactions: (a) conversion to nucleotides, (b) phosphorylation of these nucleotides, (c) further metabolism of the purine or pyrimidine portion of the nucleotide, (d) conversion of ribonucleotides to deoxyribonucleotides, and (d) incorporation into nucleic acids. These may be considered one at a time.

Purine and pyrimidine antimetabolites may be converted to nucleotides by three types of reactions. The first is the simple phosphorylation of a nucleoside by adenosine triphosphate to form the nucleoside monophosphate. With purine ribonucleosides such as 6-methylmercaptopurine ribonucleoside and 2-fluoroadenosine, this process is catalyzed by the enzyme adenosine kinase. With pyrimidine ribonucleosides such as 5-fluorouridine and 6-azauridine, the enzyme involved is uridine kinase.

The phosphorylation of purine and pyrimidine deoxyribonucleosides and arabinosides and those containing other sugars by adenosine triphosphate is a similar process, but requires different enzymes. Thus the phosphorylation of arabinosyl cytosine is catalyzed by deoxycytidine kinase, and that of fluorodeoxyuridine, iododeoxyuridine and bromodeoxyuridine is catalyzed by thymidine kinase. At the present time, the identity of the enzyme or enzymes that phosphorylate adenine arabinoside and the α- and β-deoxythioguanosines is not known.

The second type of nucleotide-forming process starts with purine and pyrimidine bases and, in one step, adds a phosphoribosyl moiety to form a ribonucleoside monophosphate. Purines such as 2,6-diaminopurine, 8-azaadenine and 2-fluoroadenine are converted to nucleotides by the enzyme adenine phosphoribosyltransferase, whereas a different enzyme, hypoxanthine-guanine phosphoribosyltransferase, converts 6-mercaptopurine, 6-thioguanine and 8-azaguanine to the nucleotide form. In some cells a uracil phosphoribosyltransferase is responsible for the conversion of 5-fluorouracil to the ribonucleotide.

A fourth process, applicable only to pyrimidine base antimetabolites, converts the pyrimidine to the ribonucleoside, using the enyzme uridine phosphorylase, and then phosphorylates this, using uridine kinase, as has already been described.

Some of the purine and pyrimidine antimetabolite nucleotides thus formed exert their growth-inhibitory activity in their monophosphate form; this is true of 6-methylmercaptopurine ribonucleoside, 6-azauridine and 5-fluorodeoxyuridine, for example. Others are further phosphorylated to their di- and triphosphate derivatives. Those compounds, for example, that are incorporated into DNA, have first to be converted to triphosphates; iododeoxyuridine, bromodeoxyuridine, 6-thioguanine and, in some cells, 6-mercaptopurine are examples of this class. Others, such as arabinosyl cytosine and arabinosyl adenine, also are solely or primarily active as triphosphates.

The third general type of activating reaction involves changes in the base portion of the nucleotide. This is not common, and is perhaps best exemplified by 6-mercaptopurine ribonucleotide, which may be methylated to form 6-methylmercaptopurine ribonucleotide, and may also be oxidized to 6-thioxanthine ribonucleotide and then converted to 6-thioguanine ribonucleotide.

A fourth type of activating reaction is conversion of purine and pyrimidine antimetabolite ribonucleotides into deoxyribonucleotides, which takes place at the diphosphate level of phosphorylation. Examples include the conversion of 6-thioguanine ribonucleoside diphosphate to the deoxyribonucleotide, and probably also the formation of 5-fluorouracil deoxyribonucleoside diphosphate from the ribonucleoside. Neither of these two reactions has been demonstrated directly, but their existence is inferred from other studies of the metabolism of 6-thioguanine and 5-fluorouracil.

Finally, some purine and pyrimidine analogs and derivatives are activated by incorporation into DNA, and the process of nucleic acid synthesis must therefore be considered a fifth class of activating reactions. As already mentioned, 6-thioguanine, 6-mercaptopurine, 5-iodouracil and 5-bromouracil are in this group. 8-Azaguanine is active only after incorporation into RNA and, at least in some systems, the incorporation of 5-fluorouracil into RNA is also pharmacologically important.

For the most part, only conversion to nucleotides has been considered in relation to the question of drug sensitivity, and in fact relatively little is known concerning possible differences in these activation reactions between tumors in general and sensitive normal tissues such as bone marrow, intestinal mucosa, skin, etc. However, normal human bone marrow does not phosphorylate α-deoxythioguanosine, whereas many tumors are able to convert it to the nucleotide.[23] In the mouse, phosphorylation of α-deoxythioguanosine in bone marrow did occur, but at low rates.[24]

More information, however, is available regarding activation of purine and pyrimidine antimetabolites, which helps to account for their differential toxicity to one or another normal tissue. Thus, different rodent,[25] monkey[26] and human[27] tissues vary widely in their purine phosphoribosyltransferase activities, and such differences are one basis for the observation that concentrations of 6-thioguanine nucleotides are higher in bone marrow than in intestinal mucosa.[28,29] Normal human bone marrow cells also converted 6-mercaptopurine to nucleotides more rapidly than did normal peripheral leukocytes.[30] The tissue distribution of deoxycytidine kinase also is related to the toxicity of arabinosyl cytosine in certain tissues.[31] In contrast, no correlation between sensitivity to 6-methylmercaptopurine ribonucleoside and adenosine kinase activity was noted in normal human and mouse tissues.[32]

Variation in selective toxicity includes differences in drug sensitivity of different histological types of neoplasms, differences among individual tumors of the same type, and the drug resistance which sometimes emerges during courses of chemotherapy. It must also be expected that individual variation, although perhaps of lesser magnitude, will occur in the non-neoplastic tissues of individual patients, and even in a single patient over a period of time. A good beginning has been made in relating variation in drug activation and inactivation reactions to these phenomena.

Numerous cases of resistance to purine and pyrimidine antimetabolites, at least in animal cells, are due to decreased activity of one or another of these activating enzymes (reviews[33,34]). Among the purine and purine nucleoside analogs, numerous cases of resistance to 6-mercaptopurine,[35,36] 6-thioguanine[37,38] and 8-azaguanine[39,40] have been attributed to complete or partial loss of hypoxanthine-guanine phosphoribosyltransferase activity. In other tumors, resistance to 2,6-diaminopurine[41,42] and 2-fluoroadenine[43] has been attributed to decreased adenine phosphoribosyltransferase activity, and resistance to 6-methylmercaptopurine ribonucleoside and related compounds[44,45] to decreased adenosine kinase activity.

Among the pyrimidine antimetabolites, resistance of animal tumors to 5-azacytidine[46] and 6-azauridine[47] has been attributed to decreased uridine kinase activity, resistance to cytosine arabinoside[48,49] and 2′-deoxy-5-azacytidine[46] to decreased deoxycytidine kinase activity, resistance to 5-fluorodeoxyuridine[50,51] and

5-bromodeoxyuridine[52] to decreased thymidine kinase activity; resistance to 5-fluorouracil in different cells has been attributed to decreased activities of uridine phosphorylase,[53] uridine kinase[54] and uracil phosphoribosyltransferase.[55–57]

Studies of a variety of animal tumors have shown good correlations between chemotherapeutic response to 6-methylmercaptopurine ribonucleoside,[32] 6-mercaptopurine,[30] arabinosyl cytosine[48,58] and 5-fluorouracil[59] and the ability of tumor cells or extracts to convert these compounds to nucleotides. In the case of 6-thioguanine, there is a correlation between chemotherapeutic sensitivity and incorporation of drug into DNA, but not with respect to nucleotide formation alone.[60,61] In apparent contrast to these observations, there was an inverse relationship between growth inhibition and ability of cell extracts to phosphorylate 5-fluorodeoxyuridine in several mouse tumors,[62] but drug metabolism in intact cells was not measured.

Wide variations have also been noted in the abilities of human neoplasms, even of the same histological type, to convert purine and pyrimidine antimetabolites to their active nucleotide derivatives. This has been observed, for example, in studies of the metabolism of 6-mercaptopurine[30] and arabinosyl cytosine[58,63] in human leukemic leukocytes, in studies of the metabolism of α- and β-deoxythioguanosine[23] and 6-methylmercaptopurine ribonucleoside[32] by extracts of solid tumors, and in measurements of the potential ability of solid tumor extracts to phosphorylate arabinosyl adenine.[64,65]

Thus far the discussion has been confined to activation reactions in drug-sensitive tissues only, in which they are important determinants both of pharmacological activity and of chemotherapeutic selectivity. However, activation in insensitive tissues may also be an important determinant of activity, as it will affect the amount of drug that reaches the sensitive tissues. Although drug activation in insensitive tissues is usually thought not to be a significant influence on drug pharmacokinetics, in several cases important effects have been noted. Thus high rates of phosphorylation of 6-methylmercaptopurine ribonucleoside[66] and tubercidin[67] by human erythrocytes (and low rates of dephosphorylation) lead to extensive drug accumulation in these cells. This in turn leads to a substantial decrease in the per cent of the administered dose that is available to sensitive tissues, and to drastic alterations in the pharmacokinetics of these drugs; the half-life of 6-methylmercaptopurine ribonucleoside is 4–6 days,[66] and that of tubercidin is 8 days.[67]

Information gained regarding bases of selective toxicity in general and of variation in selective toxicity should be applicable to the prediction of drug selectivity in individual patients with their own specific tumors. Thus, appropriate enzymes may be measured in tissue extracts, drug metabolites may be measured after incubation of intact cell preparations *in vitro*, and drug metabolites may be measured in cells removed from the patient after drug treatment *in vivo*.

For example, nucleotide formation from 6-mercaptopurine[30,68,69] and arabinosyl cytosine[63,68,69] has been studied in intact human leukemic leukocytes incubated *in vitro* with drug; in general, there was a correlation between the rate of this process and the response of the individual patient to treatment with these drugs. Similarly, human leukemias, which are generally unresponsive to treatment with 5-fluorouracil, showed only a low capacity to form nucleotides of this drug *in vitro*.[68] Measurements of adenosine kinase activity in extracts of human solid tumors have likewise been carried out in attempts to predict sensitivity to arabinosyl adenine and xylosyladenine.[64,65]

The inactivation of purine and pyrimidine antimetabolites may occur both before and after the activating reactions outlined above. That is, the administered pharmacologically inactive form of the drug, may be converted to derivatives that cannot be activated, and already activated forms may be converted back into pharmacologically inactive derivatives. The precise enzymatic reactions to which a particular compound will be subjected will depend on the structure of the particular purine or pyrimidine base that is involved, and on whether the drug is in the form of the base, nucleoside or nucleoside phosphate (reviews[19–22]). The range of enzymatic reactions which potentially take part in inactivation processes include: (a) dephosphorylation of nucleotides, (b) removal of sugar moieties, (c) deamination, (d) oxidation or reduction or both, and (e) cleavage of the purine or pyrimidine ring. Other reactions may also occur but are of lesser importance.

Inactivation of those purine and pyrimidine antimetabolites which are administered as bases may involve deamination, as, for example, the deamination by guanine deaminase of 6-thioguanine to 6-thioxanthine and of 8-azaguanine to 8-azaxanthine. 6-Thioxanthine may also be formed by oxidation of 6-mercaptopurine and, in either case, it may be further oxidized to 6-thiouric acid by xanthine oxidase. In some species this product may be further broken down, but in man this occurs at a low rate because of the absence of the enzyme urate oxidase.

The main route of catabolism of pyrimidine bases is reduction and cleavage of the pyrimidine ring. In the course of this process, the bromide and iodide of bromouracil and iodouracil are removed, whereas the fluoride of fluorouracil remains attached to the carbon chain.

If members of this class of drugs are administered in the form of nucleosides, they may undergo deamination and removal of the sugar moiety, if their structures are appropriate for the enzymes which carry out these reactions. Thus arabinosyl adenine, xyloxyl adenine, formycin and similar adenosine analogs are deaminated by adenosine deaminase, and arabinosyl cytosine and bromodeoxycytosine are deaminated by deoxycytidine deaminase. In these cases the sugars are not cleaved from the bases. Other compounds, such as 6-mercaptopurine ribonucleoside, 6-thioguanine ribonucleoside and 6-fluorouracil ribonucleoside, are phosphorolytically cleaved to the base and ribose 1-phosphate. The bases may then be metabolized as described above.

Finally, if the purine or pyrimidine antimetabolites have first been converted to active nucleotide derivatives, they are subject to enzymatic dephosphorylation to form nucleosides that may then be metabolized as described above. There are a number of enzymes which potentially may catalyze this dephosphorylation, but in most cases their relative importance is not known.

In a few cases the toxicity of some purine antimetabolites to certain normal tissues has been related inversely to their ability to inactivate the precursor form. Thus the toxicity of 8-azaguanine to skin has been attributed to the low level of guanine deaminase in this tissue.[70] It is also thought that the rapid deamination of 6-thioguanine by intestinal mucosa is one basis for its insensitivity to this drug,[29] whereas the lack of guanine deaminase in bone marrow contributes to drug toxicity in this tissue. In a similar manner, the lack of toxicity of xylosyl adenine and arabinosyl adenine in thymus, spleen and bone marrow may be due to the high adenosine deaminase activities of these tissues.[71,72] Phosphorolysis of 5-fluorodeoxyuridine[73] and catabolism of 5-fluorouracil[74–77] by intestinal mucosa may likewise protect this tissue from the toxicity of these drugs.

Several cases of resistance to purine antimetabolites appear to be due to accelerated catabolism of their activated nucleotide derivatives. Thus, several cases of resistance to 6-thioguanine,[78,79] 4-aminopyrazolopyrimidine[80] and 6-methylmercaptopurine ribonucleoside[81] have been attributed to increased rates of dephosphorylation of the corresponding nucleoside monophosphates. The exact enzyme involved was not identified. Recently, increased alkaline phosphatase activity was demonstrated in a tumor whose resistance to 6-mercaptopurine and 6-thioguanine was associated with accelerated dephosphorylation of drug nucleotides.[82]

Several other examples of resistance to purine antimetabolites in animal tumors are known to be due to inactivation of the inactive precursor form. Thus resistance to 8-azaguanine has been attributed to guanine deaminase activity,[83] and insensitivity to arabinosyl adenine and xylosyladenine has been attributed to increased adenosine deaminase activity.[72,84] In some human leukemias, resistance to cytosine arabinoside has been associated with an increased ability of the leukemic cells to deaminate the drug.[85]

Measurements of the ability of different human solid tumors (or of tumor extracts) and of different human leukemia cell populations to deaminate arabinosyl adenine[64,65,86] and cytosine arabinoside[85] have demonstrated the wide variations in this property which exist even among tumors of the same type.

In most cases, inactivation of precursor forms of purine and pyrimidine antimetabolites in insensitive tissues is quantitatively more important than their activation in insensitive tissues. The major site of deamination of cytosine arabinoside, for example, is the liver,[87] and although it is not normally catabolized by erythrocytes, it has recently been observed that erythrocytes made in response to stress are able to carry out this reaction.[88] The deamination of arabinosyl adenine,[72] 6-thioguanine,[89] the oxidation of 6-mercaptopurine,[90,91] the phosphorolysis of many purine and pyrimidine antimetabolites,[71,73,77] and the catabolism of 5-fluorouracil[74–77] also take place at substantial rates in various insensitive tissues. Enzyme activities in these tissues thus are important determinants of concentrations of many purine and pyrimidine antimetabolites in blood and hence of the amount of drug that reaches the tumor and sensitive normal tissues. Variations in the rates of these reactions in different patients, or in a single patient during a course of chemotherapy, have in general not been much studied with respect to the problem of drug selectivity.

The use of measurements of adenosine deaminase activity[21,64,65] and deoxycytidine deaminase activity[85] in human tumor cell extracts has been initiated in attempts to predict sensitivity of patients to treatment with arabinosyl adenine and arabinosyl cytosine respectively. In these cases, the ability of individual tumors to phosphorylate the drugs is also being measured, and prediction is being based on the ratio of phosphorylating and deaminating capacities.

Cyclophosphamide and dimethyl-triazeno-imidazole carboxamide

Cyclophosphamide and dimethyl-triazeno-imidazole carboxamide and drugs structurally related to them are activated solely or mainly in the liver; in particular, the activation is catalyzed by the same hepatic mixed-function oxidases that are functional in the oxidative metabolism of many other drugs (reviews[92–94]). In addition, both drugs, after activation, can be converted to inactive forms both nonenzymatically and enzymatically in the liver. The active forms which are produced in the liver must travel via the circulation to the sensitive tissues to exert their growth-inhibitory activity.

In liver, cyclophosphamide is activated by oxidation to aldophosphamide by microsomal oxidase[95,96] and inactivated by conversion to carboxyphosphamide, the latter reaction being catalyzed by aldehyde oxidase, a soluble enzyme.[96]

Dimethyl-triazeno-imidazole carboxamide was originally synthesized as a latent form of diazo-imidazole carboxamide, to be activated by enzymatic demethylation.[97–99] This does indeed occur, and is catalyzed by hepatic mixed-function oxidase.[99,100] It is not certain, however, whether diazo-imidazole carboxamide is formed, or whether the monomethyl intermediate is nonenzymatically cleaved (presumably in sensitive tissues) to diazomethane, which is known to be a potent alkylating agent. Certainly aminoimidazole carboxamide, a product of such a cleavage, is a major urinary metabolite.[101,102]

Because the enzymatic activations of cyclophosphamide and dimethyl-triazeno-imidazole carboxamide take place solely or mainly in a drug-insensitive tissue, these reactions cannot themselves be the bases of the tumor–host selectivity exhibited by these drugs. However, a number of experiments have been carried out in attempts to alter the activity or selectivity (or both) of these compounds by altering the activities of the hepatic microsomal enzymes that convert them to active forms. Thus the activation of cyclophosphamide *in vivo* has been both stimulated[92,103,104] and inhibited[92,93,105] by appropriate treatments, and similar alterations have been made in the metabolism of dimethyl-triazeno-imidazole carboxamide *in vivo.*[94] However, such treatments had no effect on inhibition of leukemia L1210[106] or Walker carcinoma 256[92,93] growth by cyclophosphamide, and had only small effects on leukopenia induced by cyclophosphamide treatments. However, the lethality of cyclophosphamide to mice could be altered by inhibition[106,107] and stimulation[106,108] of cyclophosphamide inhibition. Further studies are required to detail the possible effects of alteration of hepatic microsomal enzyme activity on the activity and selectivity of these drugs.

Other drugs inactivated in insensitive tissues

Most anticancer drugs do not require enzymatic activation, but can be enzymatically inactivated at least to some degree; frequently this occurs in the liver (review[109]).

Thus, mycophenolic acid,[110,111] streptonigrin,[112] and *p*-hydroxyaniline mustard[113,114] are converted at least in part to glucuronidated derivatives; hydroxyurea can be reduced to urea;[115,116] and dichloromethotrexate can be oxidized by hepatic aldehyde oxidase.[117,118] Both heterocyclic carboxaldehyde thiosemicarbazones[119] and vinblastine[120–122] are extensively metabolized, probably by the liver. Daunomycin is hydroxylated and the glycoside portion removed in the liver, but also in brain and heart.[123–127] Hepatic microsomal oxidases can dealkylate nitrogen mustard[128,129] and the methyl hydrazines.[130–134]

It should be pointed out that, although the metabolism of these drugs by liver and other insensitive tissues is very important, certain of these reactions may also be carried out by tumors. Thus several mouse tumors can demethylate methylhydrazines[135] and dimethyl-triazeno-imidazole carboxamide.[136] The pharmacological significance of these observations has not been evaluated.

As previously discussed, such enzymatic inactivation cannot directly affect drug selectivity, but indirectly may do so by affecting the concentration and amount of drug that reaches the sensitive tissues. Blood flow, tissue and tumor permeability, intracellular binding, and other factors that determine the effectiveness of the drug intracellularly are of primary importance in determining selectivity. However, the possibility that variation among patients, and variation in a given patient over a period of time, may be factors in variation in drug toxicity and selectivity, must also be considered. Little information is available on this point, however, and firm conclusions must await further evidence.

Inactivation followed by reactivation

Several cases of drug activation and inactivation do not fit exactly into the pattern which has been discussed above. Mycophenolic acid, for example, does not require activation and is rapidly and extensively inactivated in the liver by conjugation with glucuronic acid. However, the circulating glucuronide may be reactivated by tumors that have sufficient β-glucuronidase activity at their outer surface.[110,111,137]

A similar but slightly more complicated situation exists with respect to aniline mustard, a compound of relatively low toxicity. It is converted in the liver to the much more toxic *p*-hydroxy derivative which, however, is immediately completely inactivated – also in the liver – by conjugation with glucuronic acid. Tumors which have high β-glucuronidase activity can then reactivate the highly toxic *p*-hydroxyaniline mustard.[113,114]

CONCLUSIONS

Enzymatic activation, inactivation, or both, are important determinants of the toxicity of most anticancer agents. They play a role in the tissue selectivity of some drugs, are responsible for variation in the selectivity of some, and are almost certainly involved in the basic tumor–host selectivity of some drugs. Information on these points has made predictive tests possible in certain cases, but there is still much to be learned about enzymatic activation and inactivation and their application to the practical problems of selective cancer chemotherapy.

REFERENCES

1. H. E. SKIPPER, in *The Cell Cycle and Cancer* (Ed. R. BASERGA), pp. 355–387. Marcel Dekker, New York (1971).
2. F. S. PHILIPS, in *Handbuch der Experimentallen Pharmakologie: Antineoplastic and Immunosuppressive Agents* (Eds. A. C. SARTORELLI and D. JOHNS). Springer, Berlin, in press.
3. J. F. HENDERSON, in *Handbuch der Experimentallen Pharmakologie: Antineoplastic and Immunosuppressive Agents* (Eds. A. C. SARTORELLI and D. JOHNS). Springer, Berlin, in press.
4. E. S. HENDERSON, R. H. ADAMSON, C. DENHAM and V. T. OLIVERIO, *Cancer Res.* **25**, 1008 (1965).
5. E. S. HENDERSON, R. H. ADAMSON and V. T. OLIVERIO, *Cancer Res.* **25**, 1018 (1965).
6. V. T. OLIVERIO, R. H. ADAMSON, E. S. HENDERSON and J. D. DAVIDSON, *J. Pharmac. exp. Ther.* **141**, 149 (1963).
7. R. H. ADAMSON, C. DENHAM and V. T. OLIVERIO, *Archs int. Pharmacodyn Thér.* **161**, 364 (1966).
8. M. A. HAHN and R. H. ADAMSON, *Pharmacologist* **12**, 282 (1970).

9. W. R. STERLING, J. F. HENDERSON, H. G. MANDEL and P. K. SMITH, *Biochem. Pharmac.* **11**, 135 (1962).
10. H. WEISSBACH, B. REDFIELD, T. O'CONNOR and M. A. CHIRIGOS, *Cancer Res.* **26**, 1832 (1966).
11. B. J. KENNEDY, M. SANDBERG-WALLHEIM, M. LOKEN and J. W. YARBRO, *Cancer Res.* **27**, 1534 (1967).
12. W. C. J. ROSS, *Biological Alkylating Agents*, pp. 32–63. Butterworths, London (1962).
13. G. P. WARNICK, *Cancer Res.* **23**, 1315 (1963).
14. H. M. RAUEN, K. NORPATH and K. P. KRAMER, *Arzneimittel-Forsch.* **15**, 1048 (1965).
15. C. E. WILLIAMSON, J. G. KIRBY, J. I. MILLER, S. SASS, S. P. KRAMER, A. M. SELIGMAN and B. WITTEN, *Cancer Res.* **26**, 323 (1966).
16. H. MATSUDOIRA, T. SEKIGUCHI, H. ORII, F. SEKIGUCHI and H. NAGASAWA, *Gann* **58**, 415 (1967).
17. G. R. GALE, J. G. SIMPSON and A. B. SMITH, *Cancer Res.* **27**, 1186 (1967).
18. V. T. OLIVERIO, W. M. VIETZKE, M. K. WILLIAMS and R. H. ADAMSON, *Cancer Res.* **30**, 1330 (1970).
19. J. F. HENDERSON and A. R. P. PATERSON, *Nucleotide Metabolism*, Academic Press, New York (1973).
20. A. R. P. PATERSON and D. M. TIDD, in *Handbuch der Experimentellen Pharmakologie: Antineoplastic and Immunosuppressive Agents* (Eds. A. C. SARTORELLI and D. JOHNS). Springer, Berlin, in press.
21. G. A. LEPAGE, in *Handbuch der Experimentellen Pharmakologie: Antineoplastic and Immunosuppressive Agents* (Eds. A. C. SARTORELLI and D. JOHNS). Springer, Berlin, in press.
22. P. ROY-BURMAN, *Analogues of Nucleic Acid Components*, Springer, New York (1970).
23. A. PERRY and G. A. LEPAGE, *Cancer Res.* **29**, 617 (1969).
24. G. A. LEPAGE, I. G. JUNGA and B. BOWMAN, *Cancer Res.* **24**, 835 (1964).
25. A. W. MURRAY, *Biochem. J.* **100**, 664 (1966).
26. T. A. KRENITSKY, *Biochim. biophys. Acta* **179**,506 (1969).
27. F. M. ROSENBLOOM, W. N. KELLEY, J. MILLER, J. F. HENDERSON and J. E. SEEGMILLER, *J. Am. med. Ass.* **202**, 175 (1967).
28. E. C. MOORE and G. A. LEPAGE, *Cancer Res.* **18**, 1075 (1958).
29. S. L. MARCHESI and A. C. SARTORELLI, *Cancer Res.* **23**, 1769 (1963).
30. D. KESSEL and T. C. HALL, *Cancer Res.* **29**, 2116 (1969).
31. J. P. DURHAM and D. H. IVES, *Molec. Pharmac.* **5**, 358 (1969).
32. D. H. W. HO, J. K. LUCE and E. FREI, *Biochem. Pharmac.* **17**, 1025 (1968).
33. R. W. BROCKMAN, *Adv. Cancer Res.* **7**, 129 (1963).
34. J. F. HENDERSON, *Proc. Fifth Int. Congr. Pharmac.* **3**, 365 (1972).
35. R. W. BROCKMAN, *Cancer Res.* **20**, 643 (1960).
36. J. D. DAVIDSON, *Cancer Res.* **20**, 225 (1960).
37. D. B. ELLIS and G. A. LEPAGE, *Cancer Res.* **23**, 436 (1963).
38. P. STUTTS and R. W. BROCKMAN, *Biochem. Pharmac.* **12**, 97 (1963).
39. R. W. BROCKMAN, L. L. BENNETT, JR., M. S. SIMPSON, A. R. WILSON, J. R. THOMSON and H. E. SKIPPER, *Cancer Res.* **19**, 856 (1959).
40. J. MORROW, *Genetics* **65**, 279 (1970).
41. J. H. ATKINS and S. M. GARTLER, *Genetics* **60**, 781 (1968).
42. D. G. R. BLAIR and A. D. HALL, *Can. J. Biochem.* **43**, 1857 (1965).
43. L. L. BENNETT, JR., M. H. VAIL, S. CHUMLEY and J. A. MONTGOMERY, *Biochem. Pharmac.* **15**, 1719 (1966).
44. L. L. BENNETT, JR., H. P. SCHNEIBLI, M. H. VAIL, P. W. ALLAN and J. A. MONTGOMERY, *Molec. Pharmac.* **2**, 432 (1966).
45. I. C. CALDWELL, J. F. HENDERSON and A. R. P. PATERSON, *Can. J. Biochem.* **45**, 735 (1967).
46. J. VESELY, A. CIHAK and F. SORM, *Cancer Res.* **30**, 2180 (1970).
47. C. A. PASTERNAK, G. A. FISCHER and R. E. HANDSCHUMACHER, *Cancer Res.* **21**, 110 (1961).
48. W. KREIS, D. DRAHOVSKY and H. BORBERG, *Cancer Res.* **32**, 696 (1972).
49. A. R. SCHRECKER, *Cancer Res.* **30**, 632 (1970).
50. N. R. MORRIS and G. A. FISCHER, *Biochim. biophys. Acta* **68**, 84 (1963).
51. P. A. MORSE and V. R. POTTER, *Cancer Res.* **25**, 499 (1965).
52. S. KIT, D. R. DUBBS, L. J. PICKARSKI and T. C. HSU, *Expl Cell Res.* **31**, 297 (1963).
53. P. REICHARD, D. SKÖLD and G. KLEIN, *Nature, Lond.* **183**, 939 (1959).

54. O. SKÖLD, P.-H. MAGNUSSON and L. REVESZ, *Cancer Res.* **22**, 1226 (1962).
55. R. W. BROCKMAN, J. M. DAVIS and P. STUTTS, *Biochim. biophys. Acta* **40**, 22 (1960).
56. D. KESSEL, J. DEACON, B. COFFEY and A. BAKAMJIAN, *Molec. Pharmac.* **8**, 731 (1972).
57. P. REYES and T. C. HALL, *Biochem. Pharmac.* **18**, 2587 (1969).
58. D. KESSEL, T. C. HALL and I. WODINSKY, *Science, N.Y.* **156**, 1240 (1967).
59. D. KESSEL, T. C. HALL and I. WODINSKY, *Science, N.Y.* **154**, 911 (1966).
60. G. A. LEPAGE, *Cancer Res.* **20**, 403 (1960).
61. G. A. LEPAGE and M. JONES, *Cancer Res.* **21**, 1590 (1961).
62. D. KESSEL and I. WODINSKY, *Molec. Pharmac.* **6**, 251 (1970).
63. D. KESSEL, T. C. HALL and D. ROSENTHAL, *Cancer Res.* **29**, 459 (1969).
64. G. A. LEPAGE, *Adv. Enzyme Regulat.* **8**, 323 (1970).
65. G. A. LEPAGE, *Natn. Cancer Inst. Monogr.* **34**, 184 (1971).
66. T. L. LOO, J. K. LUCE, H. P. SULLIVAN and E. FREI, *Clin. Pharmac. Ther.* **9**, 180 (1968).
67. C. G. SMITH, L. M. REINEKE, M. R. BURCH, A. M. SHEFNER and E. E. MUIRHEAD, *Cancer Res.* **30**, 69 (1970).
68. D. KESSEL, *Natn. Cancer Inst. Monogr.* **34**, 138 (1971).
69. T. C. HALL, *Natn. Cancer Inst. Monogr.* **34**, 145 (1971).
70. A. GELLHORN, *Cancer* **6**, 1030 (1953).
71. G. A. LEPAGE and I. G. JUNGA, *Cancer Res.* **25**, 46 (1965).
72. J. J. BRINK and G. A. LEPAGE, *Cancer Res.* **24**, 1042 (1964).
73. G. D. BIRNIE, H. KROEGER and C. HEIDELBERGER, *Biochemistry, N.Y.* **2**, 566 (1963).
74. K. L. MUKHERJEE and C. HEIDELBERGER, *J. biol. Chem.* **235**, 433 (1960).
75. K. L. MUKHERJEE, J. BOOJAR, D. WENTLAND, F. J. ANSFIELD and C. HEIDELBERGER, *Cancer Res.* **23**, 49 (1963).
76. K. L. MUKHERJEE, A. R. CURRERI, M. JAVID and C. HEIDELBERGER, *Cancer Res.* **23**, 67 (1963).
77. C. HEIDELBERGER and F. J. ANSFIELD, *Cancer Res.* **23**, 1226 (1963).
78. A. L. BIEBER and A. C. SARTORELLI, *Cancer Res.* **24**, 1210 (1964).
79. A. C. SAROTRELLI, G. A. LEPAGE and E. C. MOORE, *Cancer Res.* **18**, 1232 (1958).
80. L. L. BENNETT, JR., P. W. ALLAN, D. SMITHERS and M. H. VAIL, *Biochem. Pharmac.* **18**, 725 (1969).
81. J. F. HENDERSON, I. C. CALDWELL and A. R. P. PATERSON, *Cancer Res.* **27**, 1773 (1967).
82. M. K. WOLPERT, S. P. DAMLE, J. E. BROWN, E. SZNYCER, K. C. AGRAWAL and A. C. SARTORELLI, *Cancer Res.* **31**, 1620 (1971).
83. E. HIRSCHBERG, J. KREAM and A. GELLHORN, *Cancer Res.* **12**, 524 (1952).
84. J. J. BRINK and G. A. LEPAGE, *Cancer Res.* **24**, 312 (1964).
85. C. D. STEUART and P. J. BURKE, *Nature New Biol.* **233**, 109 (1971).
86. R. KOSHUIRA and G. A. LEPAGE, *Cancer Res.* **28**, 1014 (1968).
87. G. W. CAMIENER and C. G. SMITH, *Biochem. Pharmac.* **14**, 1405 (1965).
88. I. K. ROTHMAN, *J. clin. Invest.* **49**, 2051 (1970).
89. E. C. MOORE and G. A. LEPAGE, *Cancer Res.* **18**, 1075 (1958).
90. H. R. SILBERMAN and J. B. WYNGAARDEN, *Biochim. biophys. Acta* **47**, 178 (1961).
91. G. B. ELION, S. CALLAHAN, R. W. RUNDLES and G. H. HITCHINGS, *Cancer Res.* **23**, 1207 (1963).
92. N. E. SLADEK, *Cancer Res.* **32**, 535 (1972).
93. N. E. SLADEK, *Cancer Res.* **32**, 1848 (1972).
94. J. L. SKIBBA, D. D. BEAL, G. RAMIREZ and G. T. BRYAN, *Cancer Res.* **30**, 147 (1970).
95. N. E. SLADEK, *Cancer Res.* **31**, 901 (1971).
96. D. L. HILL, W. R. LASTER, JR. and R. J. STRUCK, *Cancer Res.* **32**, 658 (1972).
97. Y. F. SHEALEY, I. A. MONTGOMERY and W. R. LASTER, JR., *Biochem. Pharmac.* **11**, 674 (1962).
98. K. HANO, A. AKASKI, I. YAMAMOTO, S. NARUMI and H. IWATA, *Gann* **59**, 207 (1968).
99. I. YAMAMOTO, *Biochem. Pharmac.* **18**, 1463 (1969).
100. J. L. SKIBBA, G. RAMIREZ, D. D. BEAL and G. T. BRYAN, *Biochem. Pharmac.* **19**, 2043 (1970).
101. G. E. HOUSEHOLDER and T. L. LOO, *Life Sci.* **8**, 533 (1969).
102. C. L. VOGEL, V. T. DEVITA, C. DENHAM, H. T. FOLEY, R. B. FIELD and P. P. CARBONE, *Cancer Chemother. Rep.* **55**, 159 (1971).
103. H. M. RAUEN and K. P. KRAMER, *Arzneimittel-Forsch.* **14**, 1066 (1964).
104. N. BROCK, *Cancer Chemother. Rep.* **51**, 315 (1967).
105. N. BROCK and H. J. HOHORST, *Arzneimettel-Forsch.* **13**, 1021 (1963).

106. L. G. HART and R. H. ADAMSON, *Archs int. Pharmocodyn. Thér.* **180**, 391 (1969).
107. R. L. DIXON, *Proc. Soc. exp. Biol. Med.* **127**, 1151 (1968).
108. J. L. COHEN and J. Y. JAO, *J. Pharmac. exp. Ther.* **174**, 206 (1970).
109. R. H. ADAMSON, *Ann. N.Y. Acad. Sci.* **179**, 432 (1971).
110. M. J. SWEENEY, D. H. HOFFMAN and M. A. ESTERMAN, *Cancer Res.* **32**, 1803 (1972).
111. J. LINTRUP, P. HYLTOFT-PETERSON, S. KNUDTZON and N. I. NISSEN, *Cancer Chemother. Rep.* **56**, 229 (1972).
112. N. S. MIZUNO and E. W. HUMPHREY, *Cancer Chemother. Rep.* **41**, 23 (1964).
113. T. A. CONNORS and M. E. WHISSON, *Nature, Lond.* **210**, 866 (1966).
114. T. A. CONNORS, *Cancer Res.* **29**, 2443 (1969).
115. R. H. ADAMSON, S. L. AGUE, S. M. HESS and J. D. DAVIDSON, *J. Pharmac. exp. Ther.* **150**, 322 (1965).
116. M. COLVIN and V. H. BONO, JR., *Cancer Res.* **30**, 1516 (1970).
117. T. L. LOO and R. H. ADAMSON, *J. med. Chem.* **8**, 513 (1965).
118. J. D. DAVIDSON and V. T. OLIVERIO, *Clin. Pharmac. Ther.* **6**, 321 (1965).
119. W. A. CREASEY, K. C. AGRAWAL, R. L. CAPIZZI, K. K. STINSON and A. C. SARTORELLI, *Cancer Res.* **32**, 565 (1972).
120. C. T. BEER and J. F. RICHARDS, *Lloydia* **27**, 352 (1964).
121. H. F. GREENIUS, R. W. MCINTYRE and C. T. BEER, *J. med. Chem.* **11**, 252 (1968).
122. J. F. HEBDEN, J. R. HADFIELD and C. T. BEER, *Cancer Res.* **30**, 1417 (1970).
123. N. R. BACHUR and J. C. CRADOCK, *J. Pharmac. exp. Ther.* **175**, 331 (1970).
124. N. R. BACHUR and M. GEE, *J. Pharmac. exp. Ther.* **177**, 567 (1971).
125. N. R. BACHUR, *J. Pharmac. exp. Ther.* **177**, 573 (1971).
126. D. H. HUFFMAN and N. R. BACHUR, *Cancer Res.* **32**, 600 (1972).
127. M. A. ASBELL, E. SCHWARTZBACH, I. WODINSKY and D. W. YESAIR, *Cancer Chemother. Rep.* **56**, 315 (1972).
128. E. G. TRAMS and C. T. KLOPP, *Cancer Res.* **15**, 617 (1955).
129. E. G. TRAMS and M. V. NADKARNI, *Cancer Res.* **16**, 1069 (1956).
130. M. BAGGIOLINE, M. H. BICKEL and F. M. MESSIHA, *Experientia* **21**, 334 (1965).
131. W. KREIS, S. B. PIEPHO and H. V. BERNHARD, *Experientia* **22**, 431 (1966).
132. D. E. SCHWARTZ, *Experientia* **22**, 212 (1966).
133. B. DEWALD, M. BAGGIOLINE and H. AEBI, *Biochem. Pharmac.* **18**, 2179 (1969).
134. M. BAGGLIOLINI, B. DEWALD and H. AEBI, *Biochem. Pharmac.* **18**, 2187 (1969).
135. W. KREIS, *Cancer Res.* **30**, 82 (1970).
136. N. S. MIZUNO and E. W. HUMPHREY, *Cancer Chemother. Rep.* **56**, 465 (1972).
137. M. J. SWEENEY, D. H. HOFFMAN and G. A. POORE, *Cancer Res.* **31**, 477 (1971).

Pp. 83—88, Supplement Number 2, 1974.
Biochemical Pharmacology. Printed in the U.S.A.

GENERAL MECHANISMS OF CLINICAL RESISTANCE TO CANCER CHEMOTHERAPY

MONTAGUE LANE

Sadie Darsky Laboratory for Clinical Cancer Research
Division of Clinical Oncology, Department of Pharmacology
Baylor College of Medicine, Houston, Tex., 77025, U.S.A.

THE MAJORITY of patients treated with cancer chemotherapeutic agents fail to demonstrate an objective response. When response does occur, it is generally of limited duration and the patient relapses despite continued drug therapy. Only a very small number of responding patients remain free of evident disease sufficiently long to be considered "cured" and these "cures" occur with only a few types of tumor such as choriocarcinoma of women, Burkitt's lymphoma, Wilms' tumor, acute leukemia, testicular tumors and perhaps Hodgkin's disease. Thus, in one sense or another, resistance to drugs remains a central problem in clinical cancer chemotherapy. As implied by these introductory remarks, resistance falls into two categories. Natural or inherent resistance is the failure of a drug to inhibit the progressive growth of a neoplasm in a patient who has not previously received the drug or its congeners, although dosage is sufficient to inflict severe toxicity upon the patient. In one sense, natural toxicity is a reflection of the lack of selective toxicity of the drug for the neoplasm. Resistance is defined as acquired if, after initial response to drug therapy, the tumor grows progressively despite the continued administration of the previously successful drug regimen, often with doses increased until toxicity to the patient is severe. To set the stage for the ensuing detailed discussions of clinical resistance to specific drugs, I shall present briefly some general considerations of the subject.

Some general biochemical mechanisms of resistance to drugs that have been demonstrated in microbial and neoplastic cells are as follows: (1) deletion of activating enzymes; (2) induction or activation of drug-catabolizing enzymes; (3) inhibition of transport; (4) conformational change in target enzyme; (5) increase in concentration of inhibited enzyme or an isoenzyme; (6) decreased requirement for product of inhibited reaction; (7) development of or increased utilization of alternate pathway; and (8) induction or activation of repair mechanisms. The first three mechanisms protect the cell by limiting the intracellular concentration of active drug. Mechanisms 4 and 5 limit the action of the drug by minimizing its direct effect upon target enzymes. Mechanisms 6 and 7 permit the cell to skirt the direct action of the drug, and by mechanism 8 the cell survives by repairing the damage done by the drug. It may be seen that mechanisms of resistance can be elucidated from knowledge of some of the pharmacological determinants of a drug's action without a precise knowledge of its molecular mechanism of action.

Tables 1 and 2 illustrate some of the biochemical mechanisms of resistance that have been reported for some anticancer drugs in animal tumor systems. (The references cited are intended to be illustrative rather than comprehensive.) It will be seen that for some drugs many different mechanisms have been found, depending upon the resistant tumor line that has been examined. Table 1 illustrates that for several purine analogs tumors may develop resistance through loss of hypoxanthine:guanine phosphoribosyltransferase, which converts these analogs by "lethal synthesis" to their active mononucleotides. Other resistant lines have increased enzymatic activities either for inactivating the analog via deamination or by hydrolysis of the nucleotide that is synthesized. Thioguanine, unlike the others, is converted to deoxynucleotides which are incorporated into DNA. The degree of its incorporation has been correlated with cell toxicity. One mechanism of resistance to thioguanine is decreased activity of ribonucleotide reductase, the enzyme that converts its ribonucleotide to deoxynucleotide.

TABLE 1. BIOCHEMICAL MECHANISMS OF RESISTANCE IN ANIMAL TUMORS TO PURINES AND PYRIMIDINES

Drug	Mechanism	Reference No.
Purines		
8-Azaguanine	↑ Guanine deaminase	1
	↓ Hypoxanthine-guanine phosphoribosyltransferase	2,3
6-Mercaptopurine	↓ Hypoxanthine-guanine phosphoribosyltransferase	4
	↑ Alkaline phosphohydrolase	5
6-Thioguanine	↓ Hypoxanthine-guanine phosphoribosyltransferase	6,7
	↑ Guanine deaminase	8,9
	↓ Ribonucleotide reductase	10
	↑ Alkaline phosphohydrolase	5
Pyrimidines		
5-Fluorouracil	↓ Uridine phosphorylase	11
	↓ Uridine kinase	12
	↓ Pyrimidine phosphoribosyltransferase	13
	Altered thymidylate synthetase	14
	↓ Thymidine kinase	15,16
	↑ Thymidine kinase	17
	↑ Degradation of nucleosides and deoxynucleosides	18,19
Cytarabine	↓ Deoxycytidine kinase	20
	↑ Pyrimidine nucleoside deaminase	21

Table 1 also illustrates many of the mechanisms of resistance to fluorouracil and/or its nucleosides. Several of these are due to decreased activity of enzymes required for various steps in the anabolism of the drug to 5-fluoro-2′-deoxyuridine-5′-monophosphate (FdUMP), the fraudulent nucleotide that competitively inhibits thymidylate synthetase with resultant inhibition of DNA synthesis. Another mechanism is rapid degradation of nucleosides and deoxynucleosides to fluorouracil. Alteration of the target enzyme, thymidylate synthetase, so that it is not inhibited by FdUMP and changes in activity of the salvage pathway enzyme, thymidine kinase, have also been described.

In the case of cytarabine, two major mechanisms for resistance have been noted: decreased enzymatic conversion of the nucleoside to the active nucleotide, and increased catabolism of the drug to the inactive arabinosyluracil.

Table 2 illustrates mechanisms that have been described for resistance to methotrexate. These include an increased concentration of the target enzyme, dihydrofolate reductase, two forms of the enzyme with differing affinities for methotrexate resulting in a net increase in cellular catalytic activity, increases in thymidylate synthetase activity (this enzyme having been proposed as another site of action of the drug) and impaired transport of the drug into the cell.

TABLE 2. BIOCHEMICAL MECHANISMS OF RESISTANCE TO VARIOUS CANCER CHEMOTHERAPEUTIC AGENTS

Drug	Mechanism	Reference No.
Methotrexate	↑ Dihydrofolate reductase	22–24
	↑ Dihydrofolate reductase isozymes	25
	↓ Transport into cell	26,27
Actinomycin D	↓ Transport into cell *in vitro*, change in membrane glycoprotein	28,29
	↓ Intracellular retention, ↓ Drug–DNA interaction	30
Daunomycin	↓ Drug–DNA interaction	29,31
Vincristine, vinblastine	Cross-resistant with actinomycin D and daunomycin; ? related mechanism in some mouse tumor cells	29
Terephthalanilide	Cross-resistant with actinomycin D and daunomycin; ? related mechanism in some mouse tumor cells; increased efflux of drug–lipid complexes	32
Alkylating agents	↑ Repair of DNA	33,34
	↓ Transport into cell	35–37
L-Asparaginase	↑ Asparagine synthetase	38,39
	↑ Immune clearance	40,41

Inhibition of intracellular transport of actinomycin D has been found in resistant cells *in vitro* and was associated with changes in cell membrane glycoprotein and the activities of membrane glycosidases and glycoprotein transferases. In addition, normal drug uptake by resistant cells *in vivo*, but increased subsequent release of both actinomycin D and daunomycin, suggested interference with the interaction of these antibiotics and DNA. A similar mechanism has been suggested for vinca alkaloids and terephthalanilides in cross-resistant cell lines. In the case of the latter drugs, marked cellular efflux of drug–lipid complexes occurs *in vitro.*

Mechanisms of resistance to the alkylating agents have been difficult to demonstrate and have included enhanced ability of the cell to excise monoalkylated and cross-linked guanine moieties with repair of DNA and the inhibition of intracellular transport of these drugs.

Resistance to the enzyme L-asparaginase has been related to increased activity of asparagine synthetase as a result of gene derepression, which then relieves the cell of the need for an exogenous supply of asparagine. Other proposed resistance mechanisms appear less likely.

In examining the mechanisms of drug resistance by human tumors, one must bear in mind that mechanisms of resistance to the same drug may differ in tumors that have inherent and those that have acquired resistance, that the most common mechanism in animal tumors may not be prevalent in human tumors, and that the mechanisms of resistance to a drug in different patients with the same tumor type may be different. Care must be taken also in interpreting results of studies of cells *in vitro,* since they may not reflect events *in vivo.*

The definitions of natural and acquired resistance which were offered at the beginning of this discussion were oversimplified. The concept that resistance occurs when the tumor progresses despite severe host toxicity is valid only if the schedule of drug administration is relatively optimal, or the "resistance" observed may be more apparent than real. Some of the determinants of an optimal dose schedule are listed below.

(1) Pharmacology of drug:
absorption, transport, distribution, concentration at and in targets, half-life, metabolism, mechanism of action, storage, detoxification, excretion.

(2) Action with respect to events of cell cycle.

(3) Inherent sensitivity of tumor and host target cells.

(4) Kinetics of tumor cell populations, for each tumor type.

(5) Kinetics of host target cell populations.

(6) Recovery and repair of host versus tumor cells.

(7) Effects of drug on host – tumor immunology.

Often many of these determinants are unknown. Nevertheless, schedule sensitivity can be shown in animal models and tolerated doses for various schedules can be determined and compared for efficacy in patients with cancer.

Possible causes for apparent natural resistance to drugs are: (1) inadequate duration of therapy; (2) inadequate dosage; (3) improper schedule of therapy; (4) excessive dosage, i.e. toxicity, which precludes proper trial; and (5) inadequate sample size for a tumor type. These may be "booby traps" in a "phase II" study. Table 3 lists several possible explanations for apparent acquired resistance to drugs when, in fact, tumors may still be sensitive.

The foregoing comments illustrate some of the difficulties involved in studying mechanisms of resistance to cancer chemotherapy in man. The investigator must be certain that reasonably optimal dose regimens are used in evaluating biochemical

TABLE 3. APPARENT ACQUIRED RESISTANCE

1. Inadequate exposure of tumor to drug – "pharmacological hide-outs"

2. Population kinetics:

   (a) Tumor recovers before host; small log-kill
   (b) Increased host toxicity with retreatment due to changes in host target cell populations

3. Cumulative drug toxicity to host results in dose reduction

mechanisms in patients with "natural resistance," and these regimens may be different for various tumor types treated with the same drug. This trap may be avoided in studies of acquired resistance by performing experiments prior to initial therapy and again when the patient relapses. The investigator should evaluate the several mechanisms of resistance to a drug that have been revealed with animal tumor models, since any of these may occur in human tumors and he may have to search for new mechanisms if none of these applies. Finally, he will have to select his patients carefully in order that adequate quantities of tumor tissue may be obtained for study of "solid tumors." On occasion, it may be possible to establish mechanisms of resistance with reasonable certainty and ease, as when activating enzymes are deleted or catabolic enzymes are greatly increased in activity. Other mechanisms of action must be interpreted with caution if tumor cells are studied only *in vitro*.

REFERENCES

1. E. HIRSCHBERG, J. KREAM and A. GELLHORN, *Cancer Res.* **12**, 524 (1952).
2. R. W. BROCKMAN, M. C. SPARKS and M. S. SIMPSON, *Biochim. biophys. Acta* **26**, 671, (1957).
3. R. W. BROCKMAN, L. L. BENNETT, JR., M. S. SIMPSON, A. R. WILSON, J. R. THOMPSON and H. E. SKIPPER, *Cancer Res.* **19**, 856, (1959).
4. R. W. BROCKMAN, *Cancer Res.* **20**, 643 (1960).
5. M. K. WOLPERT, S. P. DAMLE, J. E. BROWN, E. SZNYCER, K. C. AGRAWAL and A. C. SARTORELLI, *Cancer Res.* **31**, 1620 (1971).
6. D. B. ELLIS and G. A. LE PAGE, *Cancer Res.* **23**, 436, (1963).
7. P. STUTTS and R. W. BROCKMAN, *Biochem. Pharmac.* **12**, 97 (1963).
8. A. C. SARTORELLI, G. A. LE PAGE and G. C. MOORE, *Cancer Res.* **18**, 1232 (1958).
9. E. C. MOORE and G. A. LE PAGE, *Cancer Res.* **21**, 257 (1958).
10. G. A. LE PAGE, *Adv. Enzyme Regulat.* **8**, 323 (1969).
11. P. REICHARD, O. SKÖLD and G. KLEIN, *Nature, Lond.* **183**, 939 (1959).
12. P. REICHARD, O. SKÖLD, G. KLEIN, L. RÉVÉSZ and P. -H. MAGNUSSON, *Cancer Res.* **22**, 235 (1962).
13. P. REYES and T. C. HALL, *Biochem. Pharmac.* **18**, 2587 (1969).
14. C. HEIDELBERGER, G. KALDOR, K. L. MUKHERJEE and P. B. DANNEBERG, *Cancer Res.* **20**, 903 (1960).
15. N. R. MORRIS and G. A. FISCHER, *Fedn Proc.* **20**, 358 (1961).
16. M. UMEDA and C. HEIDELBERGER, *Cancer Res.* **28**, 2529 (1968).
17. D. KESSEL and I. WODINSKY, *Molec. Pharmac.* **6**, 251 (1970).
18. C. HEIDELBERGER, H. KROEGER and G. D. BIRNIE, *Fedn Proc.* **21**, 378 (1962).
19. J. A. JACQUEZ, *Biochim. biophys. Acta* **61**, 265 (1962).
20. M. Y. CHU and G. A. FISCHER, *Biochem Pharmac.* **13**, 333 (1965).
21. W. A. CREASEY, *J. biol. Chem.* **238**, 1772 (1963).
22. G. A. FISCHER, *Biochem. Pharmac.* **7**, 75 (1961).

23. M. T. HAKALA, S. F. ZAKRZEWSKI and C. A. NICHOL, *J. biol. Chem.* **236**, 952 (1961).
24. D. K. MISRA, S. R. HUMPHREYS, M. FRIEDKIN, A. GOLDIN and E. J. CRAWFORD, *Nature, Lond.* **189**, 39 (1961).
25. F. OTTING, R. JACKSON, D. NIETHAMMER, M. BAUGHAN and F. M. HUENNEKENS, *Am. Soc. Hemat. Fourteenth Meeting,* San Francisco, Calif., abstr. 117, p. 67.
26. G. A. FISCHER, *Biochem. Pharmac.* **11**, 1233 (1962).
27. W. C. WERKHEISER, L. W. LAW, R. A. ROOSA and C. A. NICHOL, *Proc. Am. Ass. Cancer Res.* **4**, 71 (1963).
28. M. N. GOLDSTEIN, K. HAMM and E. AMROD, *Science, N. Y.* **151**, 1555 (1966).
29. D. KESSEL, in *Prediction of Response in Cancer Therapy* (Ed. T. C. HALL), pp. 134-139. U.S. Government Printing Office, Washington, D. C. (1971).
30. D. KESSEL and I. WODINSKY, *Biochem. Pharmac.* **17**, 161 (1968).
31. D. KESSEL, V. BOTTERILL and I. WODINSKY, *Cancer Res.* **28**, 938 (1968).
32. D. W. YESAIR and C. HOFOOK, *Cancer Res.* **28**, 314 (1968).
33. B. PAPIRMEISTER and C. L. DAVISON, *Biochem. biophys. Res. Commun.* **17**, 608 (1964).
34. K. W. KOHN, N. M. STEIGBIGEL and C. L. SPEARS, *Proc. natn. Acad. Sci. U.S.A.* **53**, 1154 (1965).
35. R. J. RUTMAN, E. H. L. CHUN and F. S. LEWIS, *Biochem. biophys. Res. Commun.* **32**, 650 (1968).
36. E. H. L. CHUN, L. GONZALES, F. S. LEWIS, J. JONES and R. J. RUTMAN, *Cancer Res.* **29**, 1184 (1969).
37. G. J. GOLDENBERG, C. L. VANSTONE, L. G. ISRAELS, D. ILSE and I. BIHLER, *Cancer Res.* **30**, 2285 (1970).
38. B. HOROWITZ, B. K. MADRAS, A. MEISTER, L. J. OLD, E. A. BOYSE and E. STOCKERT, *Science, N. Y.* **160**, 533 (1968).
39. R. H. ADAMSON and S. FABRO, *Cancer Chemother. Rep.* **52**, 617 (1968).
40. J. ROBERTS, M. D. PRAGER and N. BACHYNSKY, *Cancer Res.* **26**, 2213 (1966).
41. S. VADLAMUDI, M. PADARATHSINGH, V. S. WARAVDEKAR and A. GOLDIN, *Proc. Am. Ass. Cancer Res.* **10**, 95 (1969).

ACKNOWLEDGEMENT

Supported by grants from the National Cancer Institute, CA 10893 and CA 3392.

Pp. 89—100, Supplement Number 2, 1974.
Biochemical Pharmacology. Printed in the U.S.A.

MECHANISMS OF CLINICAL DRUG RESISTANCE TO ALKYLATING AGENTS

THOMAS A. CONNORS

Chester Beatty Research Institute, Institute of Cancer Research
Royal Cancer Hospital, Fulham Road, London, SW3 6JB, England

CLASSES OF ALKYLATING AGENT AND MECHANISM OF ACTION

SIX alkylating agents are in general clinical use, the nitrogen mustards, HN2, cyclophosphamide, melphan and chlorambucil, the aziridine, *N, N', N''*-triethylenethiophosphoramide (thio-TEPA), and the sulphonoxyalkane busulphan (Myleran). Although their chemical structures are quite varied, they can all form reactive compounds in body fluids. In Fig. 1 these reactive entities are shown as positively charged carbonium ions formed by loss of chloride ion from nitrogen mustards, by loss of the methanesulphonyl ion in the case of busulphan and by ring opening in the case of thio-TEPA. In

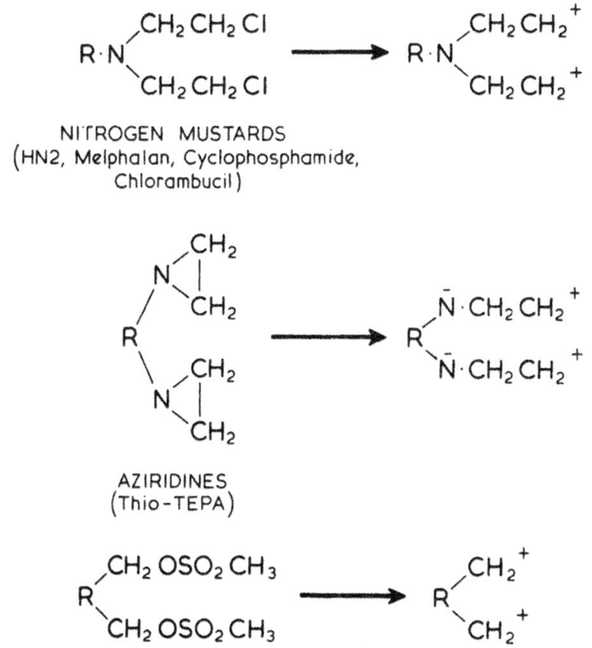

FIG. 1. Types of alkylating agent used in the clinic, showing the reactive intermediates formed in body fluids.

fact, the reactive carbonium ions may never exist as separate entities, but they are written this way to make clear their mechanism of action. A further similarity of the antitumour alkylating agents is that they are at least difunctional, that is they can form at least two reactive centres in each molecule.

Once a positively charged carbonium ion has formed, the compound will be very reactive to, and bind covalently to, molecules which are negatively charged or have areas of high electron density. Amino acids containing ionised carboxyl groups and uncharged amino groups will be alkylated and especially cysteine, which has an ionised thiol (SH) group very reactive to carbonium ions. Nucleotides can also be attacked at nitrogen atoms and hydroxyl groups of the bases where they are present and at ionised phosphate groups. These same centres will also be susceptible to atack when the molecules are polymerised to form enzymes, structural proteins and nucleic acids. There is thus little that is selective about the sites in the body that are alkylated, but it does appear that cytotoxicity is predominantly a result of reaction with DNA. The bases of DNA are alkylated under physiological conditions and cross-linking of complementary strands of DNA, which can only occur with difunctional agents, is perhaps the most cytotoxic reaction of all. A small amount of cross-linking can deactivate a large molecule of DNA, whereas because of their smaller molecular weight a much greater total reaction is required to deactivate completely all the molecules of a particular protein that may be present in the cell.

From their chemical properties, all the clinically used alkylating agents would be expected to react in a similar way, and very detailed studies of their toxicity and spectrum of antitumor action in animals and man[1-3] leave no doubt that, while there may be variations in their selectivity of antitumour action, all the alkylating agents have basically similar properties. The development of resistance to one alkylating agent is likely to mean that there will be a cross-resistance to all others; this has been seen in a number of experimental studies on resistance.[4]

There are also other agents in clinical use which, while not classed as alkylating agents, may break down *in vivo* or be converted enzymatically to metabolites with alkylating function. Sugar hexitols of the dibromomannitol type, which were first used clinically in 1961,[5] are now known to rearrange *in vivo*, at least in part, to diepoxides which can then react as difunctional alkylating agents (Fig. 2).[6,7] 5-(3, 3-dimethyl-1-triazeno) imidazole-4-carboxamide (DIC), and nitrosoureas such as 1,3-bis(2-chloroethyl)-1-nitrosourea (BCNU) and 1-(2-chloroethyl)-3-cyclohexyl-1-nitrosourea (CCNU) are known to break down or be converted to alkylating compounds, and while their spectrum of action, at least against animal tumours, is quite different from the spectrum of action of conventional alkylating agents, it is thought that their mechanism of action could involve alkylation.[8-10] Laboratory studies on the platinum compounds, one of which is at present on clinical trial, have shown that they attack the same cellular sites as the alkylating agents.[11,12] It is therefore a possibility that, if resistance to an alkylating agent arises on treatment, there will be a cross-resistance not only to other difunctional alkylating agents but also to the compounds just described. There is ample experimental and clinical evidence to show that this is not always the case, but resistance of animal tumours to melphalan is sometimes associated with cross-resistance to platinum compounds.[13] Table 1 shows the spectrum of action of a mouse lymphoma very sensitive to BCNU and triazenes of the DIC type. Methotrexate and cytosine arabinoside are also effective, and slight but significant extension of

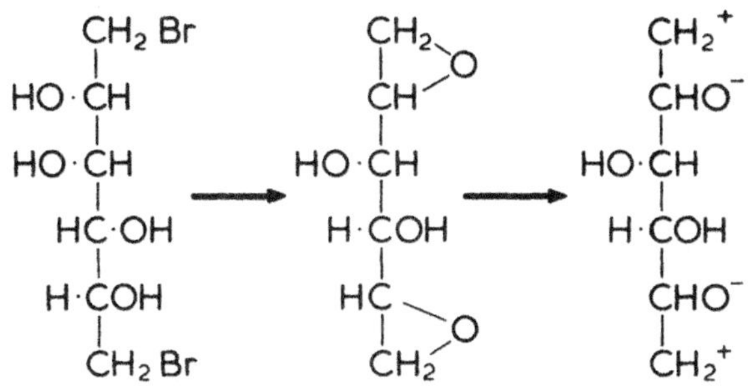

FIG. 2. Conversion of dibromomannitol to a bifunctional alkylating agent.

TABLE 1. SPECTRUM OF ACTION OF VARIOUS COMPOUNDS AGAINST TRANSPLANTED MOUSE LYMPHOMAS

	TLX5 (% ILS)	TLX5/R* (% ILS)
Triazene	67	0
BCNU	197	19
R_2 Pt Cl_2	15	0
Melphalan	19	23
Methotrexate	55	84
Ara-C	39	51

*Tumor with acquired resistance to a triazene 5-(3,3-dimethyl-1-triazeno)-4-carbethoxy-2-phenyl imidazole and cross-resistant to all triazenes. The triazene used in this experiment was 5-(3,3-dimethyl-1-triazeno)-4-carbethoxy-2-methyl imidazole and the platinum compound cis dichloro dicyclopentylamineplatinum (II). ILS = increase in median lifespan. See text for other abbreviations.

survival time is also obtained with melphalan and a platinum compound. A line with acquired resistance to the triazene shows almost complete cross-resistance to BCNU and to the platinum compound, but melphalan retains its slight antitumour effect. The resistant line of the tumour also shows an enhanced sensitivity to methotrexate and to cytosine arabinoside.

DEFINITION OF RESISTANCE

The clinical importance of fundamental studies on cells with acquired resistance to alkylating agents is that once the pathways leading to resistance are known, it may be possible to design ways of inhibiting them and so restore a cancer cell to its original sensitive condition.

A diminishing response of a tumour to successive doses of an alkylating agent may not necessarily be due to cells becoming resistant but to a host effect which reduces the amount of an alkylating agent reaching the tumour cell. It is a fairly simple matter, using animals with transplanted tumours, to demonstrate a true resistance, by obtaining dose–response curves for lethality and antitumour effect in both sensitive and resistant lines of the tumour. The sensitive tumour (Fig. 3) regresses completely at well tolerated dose levels, while there is no significant regression of the resistant tumour even at toxic doses. Host factors may be almost entirely ruled out by transplanting sensitive and resistant tumours bilaterally in the same animal. To confirm this resistance, the effect of the drug on the tumour lines is measured *in vitro*. A typical experiment is shown in Fig. 4. The growth of the sensitive tumour is inhibited at concentrations of the alkylating agent that have no effect on the growth of the resistant tumour.

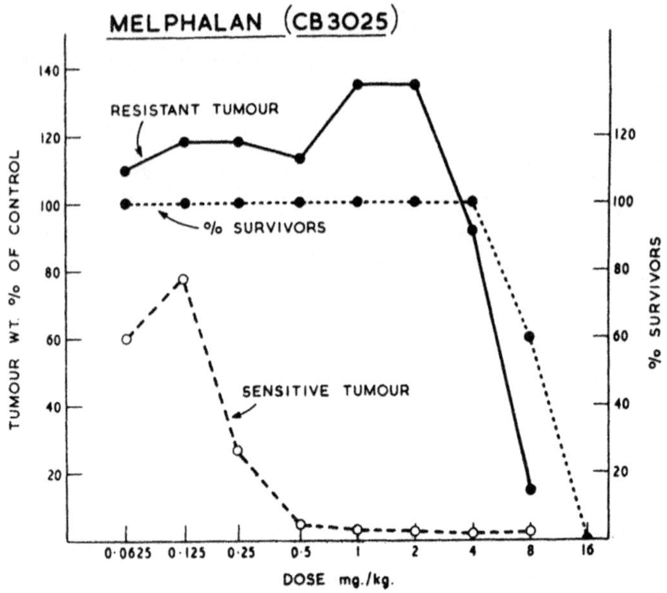

FIG. 3. Effect of melphalan on the growth of the sensitive and resistant Yoshida sarcomas and on host mortality. Groups of animals with established tumours (1 week old and about 1 g in weight) were treated intraperitoneally with a series of dose levels of melphalan. Sensitive and resistant tumours were transplanted bilaterally in one animal.

Clinically, however, it is not always easy to determine whether resistance arises because of some basic change in biochemical properties of the cancer cell or because of a less specific host effect. Some of the factors that may reduce the amount of drug reaching the vicinity of the tumour have already been described in earlier papers, but some specific examples relating to alkylating agents will be mentioned briefly.

Host effects giving rise to apparent resistance

Absorption from site of administration. It is well known that the same drug given by different routes of administration can vary greatly in its potency. HN2, for example when given intravenously, usually begins to produce signs of bone marrow damage in man at about 0.4 mg/kg. When it was given orally to patients, neither therapeutic effects nor bone marrow damage was observed at doses up to 1.3 mg/kg.[14] Obviously such wide differences in potency of the standard alkylating agents depending

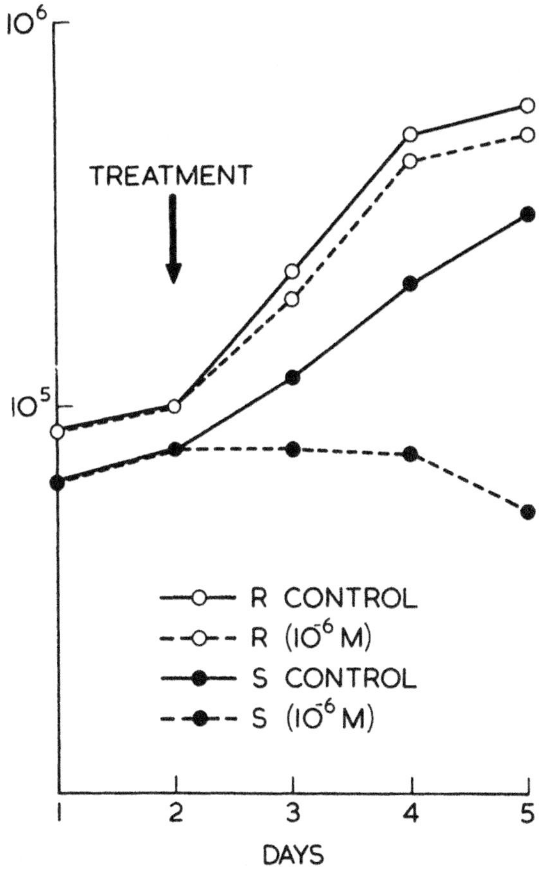

FIG. 4. Effect of melphalan on the growth of the sensitive and resistant Yoshida sarcomas *in vitro*. Both tumours grow at the same rate, but there is no effect on the growth of the resistant tumour at a dose level which kills all the sensitive cells. (K. R. Harrap, unpublished results).

on the route of administration will be well recognised by clinicians, but more subtle effects are known to occur which reduce absorption and give a false impression of the development of resistance. Orally, triethylenemelamine (TEM) may be ineffective unless given to fasting patients. The quantity of food in the stomach and the acidity are critical factors in determining the amount of active drug absorbed. This, no doubt, was one reason that caused the variability of this drug in man and led to its rejection as an anticancer agent, despite its very high selectivity in tumour-bearing animals. Prolonged administration of alkylating agents may also damage intestinal mucosa and alter the amount of drug absorbed.

Transport to the tumour. The concentration of serum proteins and chloride and the pH of blood can all influence the amount of active drug reaching the tumour site. Some alkylating agents, especially chlorambucil, bind strongly to serum albumin.[15] This binding reduces the hydrolysis of chlorambucil in the extracellular fluid and its excretion but does not apparently prevent access of the drug to the tumour, since complexes of albumin and alkylating agents have good antitumour effects.[16] Chlorambucil absorbed to a melanoma antiserum has, in fact, been used successfully to treat a case of melanoma.[17] The relatively high chloride content of serum would be expected to restrict considerably the rate of reaction of the nitrogen mustards,[18] and the reactivity of compounds like thio-TEPA, where ring opening and formation of carbonium ions are acid-catalysed, would be greatly influenced by the pH. Any extreme alteration in the properties of the serum may therefore alter the response of a tumour to an alkylating agent by influencing the amount of active drug reaching it.

Metabolism and excretion. Some alkylating agents are excreted mainly unchanged, and their antitumour action and toxicity may be greatly enhanced by compounds with an antidiuretic effect.[19] Most of the clinically used alkylating agents are metabolised to a large extent and may not be potentiated in anuric patients, although agents given in combination and causing diuresis could reduce the effectiveness of compounds with a long biological half-life.

Alkylating agents may be metabolised, principally in the liver, either to more active or to completely inactive derivatives. Some of these pathways are shown in Fig. 5. Specific enzymes may convert cyclophosphamide and azomustards to their active forms, and demethylate HN2 to a less potent compound, nor-HN2. An enzyme is also present in liver which dechloroethylates cyclophosphamide and aniline mustard, and which, if it acted generally on difunctional nitrogen mustards, would cause them to lose their antitumour effect by converting them to their monofunctional analogues. Any factor that interferes with liver function may be expected to influence the response of a tumour to agents that are metabolised by the liver. Phenobarbital, which enhances liver microsomal activity, has been shown in patients to increase 3-fold the rate of metabolism of cyclophosphamide.[20]

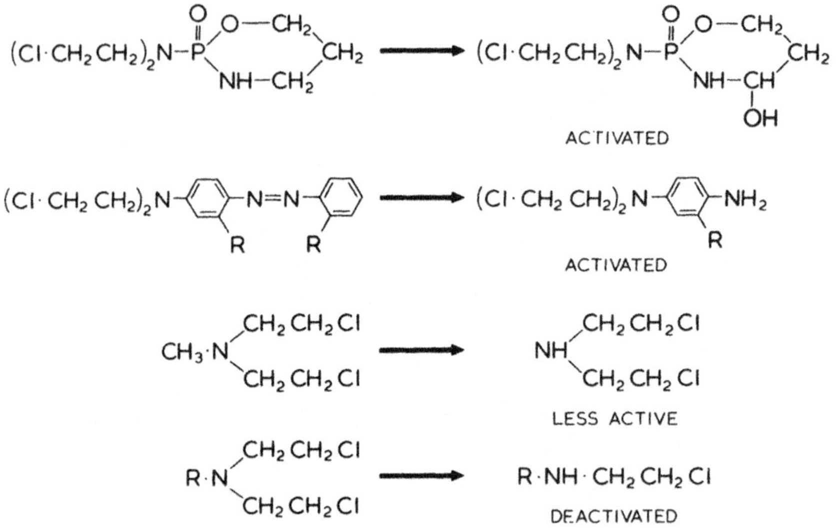

FIG. 5. Metabolism of alkylating agents by liver. Some metabolic pathways activate alkylating agents, but others can make them completely inactive.

Local distribution to the tumour. Host factors, e.g. poor absorption or enzymatic breakdown in the liver, that reduce the amount of drug reaching the tumour would be recognised if it were possible always to measure blood levels of administered agents or their active metabolites. There are situations, however, where the amount of agent reaching viable tumour cells may be reduced, even though the concentration of drug in the systemic blood remains high. Apart from the well known insensitivity of metastases involving the central nervous system because of the blood–brain barrier, there are other anatomical sites to which a tumour may metastasise during treatment and which are not accessible to the drug. A mouse tumour, for example, growing in the lung did not respond to alkylating agents, whereas the identical tumour growing subcutaneously was very sensitive.[21] When the lung tumour was transplanted to the flank, it responded to alkylating agents, showing that the failure to respond was a host effect.

Rapidly growing solid tumours may form necrotic areas distant from functional capillaries but containing viable cells. These cells may be hypoxic and nondividing,[22] and may be less sensitive to proliferation-dependent agents than cells in areas of good blood supply. Alkylating agents administered systemically may only reach them by a process of diffusion, and both factors will allow them to survive treatment and prevent complete tumour cell eradication, even though all the cells are inherently very sensitive to alkylating agents. It has been shown that the possibility of cure in animals bearing solid tumours is dependent on whether or not viable cells are present in necrotic areas.[23] Also, any treatment which allows the outgrowth of cells with altered kinetics may result in the development of resistance. Tumours becoming insensitive to treatment with alkylating agents, however, do not usually show a decreased growth rate, although it has been reported that L cells with acquired resistance to sulphur mustard had a 30 per cent increase in their doubling time.[24]

Clinical resistance

Although many host variables may give a false impression that resistance is developing, there is no doubt that in man resistance can also arise from an altered biochemical property of the tumour cell. Occasionally in animals, it is not possible to produce a resistant tumour line and in man there are also cases where patients with chronic myeloid leukaemia have been treated with Myleran for up to 10 years with no development of resistance. A more usual outcome, however, is the development of resistance and Fig. 6 shows a typical example of a patient with chronic lymphatic leukaemia. Initially, a good response to chlorambucil is obtained, but even though treatment is continued, the response diminishes. Once complete resistance has developed, a cross-resistance to cyclophosphamide is seen.

Mechanisms of resistance

Although the alkylating agents react with many molecules in the cell, the major target site is DNA. Any property of the cell which prevents alkylating agents from reaching this site or which leads to repair of alkylated DNA will lower the sensitivity of the cell to these compounds. Theoretically, there are a number of ways by which this may be achieved: (1) reduced uptake of the agent; (2) reduced activation of the agent; (3) increased breakdown of the agent; (4) increased production of target molecule of other nucleophile; (5) reduced sensitivity of target site; and (6) repair of

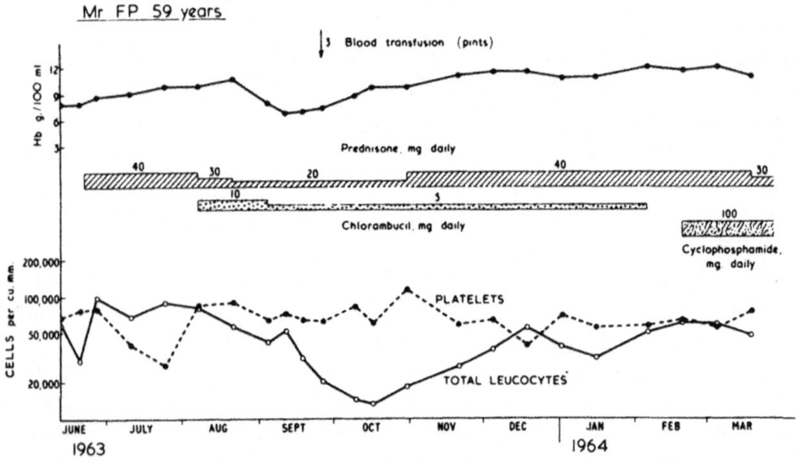

FIG. 6. Development of clinical resistance. (E. Wiltshaw, unpublished results.)

alkylated DNA. There is good evidence for some of these pathways in experimental models, but the importance of any particular one in determining resistance in man is yet to be established.

Reduced uptake of drug. An easy to understand mechanism of resistance and one which is readily demonstrable in bacteria with acquired resistance to antibiotics is a failure to take up the agent. In a large number of experiments it has been shown that alkylating agents distrubute fairly uniformly throughout the body and the concentration in tumours is usually less than that found in liver, spleen or kidney.[25–27] There is no evidence that any alkylating agent is taken up in man by active transport and only rarely have there been reports of their selective concentration in human tumours.[28] Reduction of the uptake of an alkylating agent where active transport mechanisms do not operate would presumably involve a nonspecific change in the permeability of the cell membrane. Nevertheless, it has often been reported that resistance of animal tumours to alkylating agents is associated with a reduced uptake of the drug.[29–36] In most cases the reduction in uptake is small compared with the degree of resistance, but it is such a frequent finding that it may well prove to be an important factor in the development of resistance.

Reduced activation of the agent. Resistance to purine and pyrimidine antagonists is commonly a result of loss of the enzyme necessary to convert the base analogues into their active nucleotides. Most alkylating agents are active in their own right, or are activated in the liver before reaching the tumour so that activating enzymes are not essential. However, in attempts to obtain greater selectivity, "latent" alkylating agents have been synthesised which are only poorly reactive and not cytotoxic, but which can be converted by known enzymatic pathways to highly reactive and cytotoxic metabolites.[37] A high level of the enzyme β-glucuronidase may be the reason why some tumours are sensitive to the glucuronide of aniline mustard.[38–40] Hepatocellular carcinoma cells have an azo reductase level as high as that of normal hepatocytes,* and

*G. P. Warwick, personal communication.

this has been the basis of attempts to treat this cancer by the design of nitrogen mustards activated by azo reductase.[41] In both these cases where selective antitumour effects are the result of enzyme activation, the loss of the enzyme could lead to resistance.

Increased catabolism of the agent. The breakdown of alkylating agents by liver into inactive or less active compounds has already been mentioned (Fig. 5). Tumours are generally poor in drug-metabolising enzymes, but induction of these enzymes could be a pathway for resistance. A line of the rat Yoshida sarcoma resistant to chlorambucil can metabolise it,[42] but the induction of such a specific enzyme cannot explain the cross-resistance of this tumour to other alkylating agents. Similarly, enzymes which demethylate HN2 or dechloroethylate nitrogen mustards will only account for the development of resistance to HN2 or to the nitrogen mustards generally; they cannot account for the cross-resistance to aziridines and other alkylating agents, which is a common feature of tumours developing resistance to one of these agents.[43]

Cyclophosphamide is one of the most selective alkylating agents, but its mechanism of action is not fully understood. Recent work* has given some idea as to how this selectivity may be achieved. Cyclophosphamide (I, Fig. 7) is an unreactive alkylating agent and is excreted mainly as the acid (III, Fig. 7) with small quantities of the 4-keto derivative (IV, Fig. 7)[44] and the monochloroethyl derivative.[45] All these compounds are chemically unreactive and inactive as antitumour agents. A derivative of the predicted primary metabolite (II, Fig. 7) has just been isolated and has been shown to

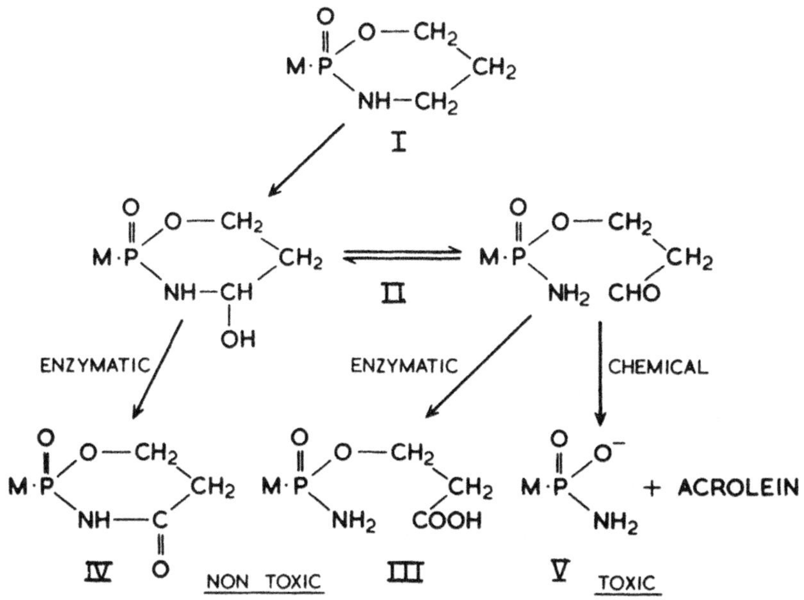

FIG. 7. Activation of Endoxan by liver. The primarily liver metabolite can be converted enzymatically to stable and nontoxic products. It is an unstable compound and, in the absence of enzymes, can break down to the tumour-inhibitory phosphamide mustard and to cytotoxic acrolein. Chemical breakdown in tumours lacking the detoxifying enzymes would give selectivity.

*T. A. Connors, P. J. Cox, P. B. Farmer, A. B. Foster and M. Jarman, *Biochem. Pharmac.* **23**, 115 (1974).

be highly toxic *in vitro*, probably by breakdown to the known toxic phosphoramide mustard (V, Fig. 7) and acrolein, which has been detected following cyclophosphamide activation *in vitro*.[46] It is thought that selectivity occurs because normal tissues convert the primary metabolite by dehydrogenases and aldehyde oxidases into the inactive and nontoxic acid and 4-keto derivatives. Tumours lacking in these enzymes take up the primary metabolite, which may decompose chemically inside the cells to form the active nitrogen mustard and the toxic acrolein. The nitrogen mustard may act synergistically with acrolein to cause a very selective killing of tumour cells. Resistance in this case could occur by induction of the appropriate detoxifying enzymes in the tumour, but again such an induction would not explain a cross-resistance to other alkylating agents.

Increased production of target molecule or other nucleophiles. Resistance to the antifolate methotrexate is in many cases a result of the production of an excess of the target enzyme so that the level of enzyme–antagonist binding remains the same, but sufficient unbound enzyme is left to metabolise the normal substrate. An analogous situation for the alkylating agents would be to increase the DNA content per cell. Interestingly enough, a correlation has been observed in some cases between the degree of ploidy and the development of resistance,[47] although this is by no means a general finding. The degree of resistance obtainable would be very small because of the large molecular size of DNA and its high sensitivity to alkylation.

Resistance could result much more efficiently from an increase in small molecular weight materials, which have a high affinity for alkylating agents and would thus compete with the target DNA for alkylation. Cysteine is one such compound and it can considerably reduce the antitumour properties of an alkylating agent if administered beforehand.[48] There are also several examples where animal tumours with acquired resistance to alkyating agents had a greater free thiol content than the sensitive line from which they were derived, although the total increase in thiol content was too small to account for the degree of resistance observed.[47, 49, 50]

Reduced sensitivity of target site. The structural specificity of functional DNA makes it unlikely that resistance could develop from any radical change in structure which would prevent access of alkylating agents to the most sensitive sites. It is of interest, however, that using polynucleotides as models for DNA, evidence has been obtained that DNA is much more readily alkylated in the unpaired state than in the helical form.[51] More subtle changes in relationship between DNA and nuclear protein could also reduce the amount of DNA alkylation and cause resistance. For instance, an ionised thiol of a nuclear protein, if close to a guanine base, might prevent alkylation of the latter by competing for the agent. Cross-linking between purine bases may, in this way, be replaced by protein–DNA linking. This type of cross-linking is known to occur, but whether it contributes to any large extent to cytotoxicity has not been established.

Repair of alkylated DNA. Studies on the light-sensitive skin disease, xeroderma pigmentosa, first showed that repair of damaged DNA was a normal physiological process.[52] Further studies have now shown that DNA damaged in a number of different ways may be repaired before irreversible toxicity occurs.[53,54] DNA damaged by alkylating agents is repaired probably by one of two mechanisms involving either enzymatic excision of alkylated bases followed by repair synthesis or by a process analogous to recombination in bacteria. Most experiments demonstrating repair of alkylated DNA in animal or human cells have used systems *in vitro*. Using sensitive and resistant tumour lines *in vivo*, it has not yet been quantitatively demonstrated that differences in sensitivity are due to a difference in ability to repair alkylated DNA. However, resistant tumours in animals will respond to alkylating agents if caffeine, a known inhibitor of DNA repair, is administered at the same time.[55]

CONCLUSIONS

Resistance to anticancer agents is often the result of a single biochemical difference between sensitive and resistant cells: increase in folate reductase enzymes for resistance to methotrexate, loss of a transferase enzyme for purine and pyrimidine antagonists, and induction of asparagine synthetase for resistance to asparaginase are examples. In such cases, the development of resistance is often rapid and due possibly to a single-step mutation or more likely to enzyme induction or repression, or to a selection of cells with the appropriate biochemical pathway.

Using animal tumours, the development of resistance to alkylating agents is often a much slower process and can never be shown to be due to a single biochemical difference. These findings imply that acquisition of resistance may require a number of biocnemical changes which, in combination, give a high degree of resistance. Small changes in thiol content and in permeability have been consistent findings associated with the development of resistance to alkylating agents. These pathways, combined with the induction of DNA repair enzymes, might operate together to give a highly resistant tumour which would not discriminate between individual alkylating agents and show cross-resistance to all, which is general feature of tumours resistant to these agents.

REFERENCES

1. L. M. SCHMIDT, R. FRADKIN, R. SULLIVAN and A. FLOWERS, *Cancer Chemother. Rep.* Suppl. 2, parts I, II and III (1965).
2. D. A. KARNOFSKY, *Fedn Proc.* **26**, 925 (1967).
3. R. B. LIVINGSTON and S. K. CARTER, *Single Agents in Cancer Chemotherapy*, Plenum, New York (1970).
4. G. P. WHEELER, *Cancer Res.* **22**, 651 (1962).
5. C. SELLEI, S. ECKHARDT and L. NEMETH, *Chemotherapy of Neoplastic Diseases*, Akad. Kiado (1970).
6. M. JARMAN and W. C. J. ROSS, *Chem. Ind.* 1789 (1967).
7. I. P. HORVATH, C. SELLEI, S. ECKHARDT and J. KRALOVANSZKY, *Abstracts Tenth Int. Cancer Congr.* abstr. no. 672 (1970).
8. Y. F. SHEALY, *J. pharm. Sci.* **59**, 1533 (1970).
9. S. K. CARTER and M. A. FRIEDMAN, *Eur. J. Cancer* **8**, 85 (1972).
10. S. K. CARTER, F. M. SCHABEL, L. E. BRODER and T. P. JOHNSTON, *Adv. Cancer Res.* **16**, 273 (1972).
11. J. J. ROBERTS and J. M. PASCOE, *Nature, Lond.* **235**, 282 (1972).
12. J. A. HOWLE and G. R. GALE, *Biochem. Pharmac.* **19**, 2757 (1970).
13. T. A. CONNORS, *Int. Congr. Chemother. Adv. Antimicrobial and Antineoblastic Chemotherapy* **2**, 237 (1972).
14. V. T. OLIVERIO and C. G. ZUBROD, *A. Rev. Pharmac.* **5**, 335 (1965).
15. J. H. LINFORD, *Can. J. Biochem. Physiol.* **41**, 931 (1963).
16. K. SHINKAI and M. MARUYAMA, *A. Rep. Sankyo Res. Lab.* **22**, 103 (1970).
17. T. GHOSE, S. T. NORVELL, A. GUCLU, D. CAMERON, A. BODURTHA and A. S. MACDONALD, *Br. med. J.* **3**, 495 (1972).
18. C. R. BALL and T. A. CONNORS, *Biochem. Pharmac.* **16**, 509 (1967).
19. T. A. CONNORS, L. A. ELSON and C. L. LEESE, *Biochem. Pharmac.* **13**, 963 (1964).
20. J. Y. JAO, W. J. JUSKO and J. L. COHEN, *Cancer Res.* **32**, 2761 (1972).

21. G. M. CONZELMAN and K. SPRINGER, *Cancer Chemother. Rep.* **53**, 105 (1969).
22. I. F. TANNOCK, *Cancer Res.* **30**, 2470 (1970).
23. R. J. GOLDACRE and B. SYLVEN, *Br. J. Cancer* **16**, 306 (1962).
24. B. D. REID and I. G. WALKER, *Cancer Res.* **26**, 1801 (1966).
25. G. P. WHEELER, B. J. BOWDEN and T. C. HERREN, *Cancer Chemother. Rep.* **42**, 9 (1964).
26. M. OCHOA and E. H. HIRSCHBERG, *Alkylating Agents in Experimental Chemotherapy* (Eds. R. J. SCHNITZER and F. HAWKING), Vol V, pp. 1–32. Academic Press, New York (1967).
27. R. K. MALLER, F. A. MCIVER and C. HEIDELBERGER, *Cancer Res.* **17**, 291 (1957).
28. W. BOLT, F. RITZL, R. TOUSSAINT and H. NAHRMANN, *Arzneimittel-Forsch.* **11**, 170 (1961).
29. I. HIRONO, H. KACHI and A. OHASHI, *Gann* **53**, 73 (1962).
30. T. YAMADA, Y. IWANAMI and T. BABA, *Gann* **54**, 171 (1963).
31. E. H. L. CHUN, L. GONZALES, F. S. LEWIS, J. JONES and R. J. RUTMAN, *Cancer Res.* **29**, 1184 (1969).
32. M. K. WOLPERT and R. W. RUDDON, *Cancer Res.* **29**, 873 (1969).
33. O. KLATT, J. S. STEHLIN, C. MCBRIDE and A. C. GRIFFIN, *Cancer Res.* **29**, 286 (1969).
34. M. INABA and Y. SAKURAI, *Int. J. Cancer* **7**, 430 (1971).
35. B. T. HILL, M. JARMAN and K. R. HARRAP, *J. med. Chem.* **14**, 614 (1971).
36. B. W. FOX, *Chem. Biol. Interact.* **3**, 149 (1971).
37. W. C. J. ROSS, *Biological Alkylating Agents.* Butterworths, London (1962).
38. M. E. WHISSON and T. A. CONNORS, *Nature, Lond.* **206**, 689 (1965).
39. T. A. CONNORS and M. E. WHISSON, *Nature, Lond.* **210**, 866 (1966).
40. C. YOUNG, A. YAGODA and E. BITTAR, *Abstr. Seventh American Meeting of Clinical Oncologists* Abstr. No. 58 (1971).
41. A. BUKHARI, T. A. CONNORS, A. M. GILSENAN, W. C. J. ROSS, M. J. TISDALE, G. P. WARWICK and D. E. V. WILMAN, *J. natn. Cancer Inst.* **50**, 243 (1973).
42. K. R. HARRAP and B. T. HILL, *Biochem. Pharmac.* **19**, 209 (1970).
43. G. P. WHEELER, *Cancer Res.* **23**, 1334 (1963).
44. R. F. STRUCK, N. C. KIRK, L. B. MELLETT, S. E. DAREER and D. L. HILL, *Molec. Pharmac.* **7**, 519 (1971).
45. J. E. BAKKE, V. J. FEIL, C. E. FJELSTUL and E. J. THACKER, *J. agric. Fd Chem.* **20**, 384 (1972).
46. R. A. ALARCON and J. MEIENHOFER, *Nature New Biol.* **233**, 250 (1971).
47. G. J. GOLDENBERG, *Ann. N. Y. Acad. Sci.* **163**, 936 (1969).
48. T. A. CONNORS, *Eur. J. Cancer* **2**, 293 (1966).
49. C. R. BALL, T. A. CONNORS, J. A. DOUBLE, V. UJHAZY and M. E. WHISSON, *Int. J. Cancer* **1**, 319 (1966).
50. I. HIRONO, *Gann* **52**, 39 (1961).
51. D. B. LUDLUM, *Biochim. biophys. Acta* **95**, 674 (1965).
52. R. B. SETLOW, J. D. REGAN, J. GERMAN and W. C. CARRIER, *Proc. natn Acad. Sci. U.S.A.* **64**, 1035 (1969).
53. R. F. BEERS, R. M. HERRIOT and R. C. TILGHMAN (Eds.), *Fifth Int. Symp. Molec. Biol.* Johns Hopkins University Press, Baltimore (1972).
54. F. K. SCHATTAUER, *DNA-Repair, Mechanisms. Symp. Schoss Remhargshausen/Rhein.* (Ed. H. ALTMANN). F. K. Schattauer Verglag, Stuttgart (1972).
55. D. GAUDIN and K. L. YIELDING, *Proc. Soc. exp. Biol. Med.* **131**, 1413 (1969).

Pp. 101—106, Supplement Number 2, 1974.
Biochemical Pharmacology. Printed in the U.S.A.

RESISTANCE TO FOLIC ACID ANTAGONISTS - CLINICAL ASPECTS*

JOSEPH R. BERTINO† and ROLAND T. SKEEL

Departments of Medicine and Pharmacology, Yale University School of Medicine
New Haven, Conn. 06510, U.S.A.

RESISTANCE of human neoplasms to folic acid antagonists, like resistance to other antineoplastic agents, may be natural or acquired. The paucity of data available to document mechanisms of resistance in man probably refelcts the difficulties in obtaining sufficient repetitive sampling of tumors and in correlating biochemical, pharmacological or kinetic observations with unequivocal clinical resistance. Information that is available has been derived mainly from patients with leukemia, since response or lack of response may be quantitated readily, and sampling of blood or bone marrow for tumor cell assays is easily accomplished.[1]

General considerations

Drug resistance may or may not relate to the mechanism of action of the agent. If a drug is not absorbed, excluded from the site of the tumor, not activated, or rapidly destroyed, then a tumor may appear clinically resistant despite biochemical sensitivity. Apart from the relative exclusion of methotrexate (MTX) from the central nervous system, these mechanisms do not play an important role in clinical resistance to folic acid antagonists. A more frequent mechanism of resistance to the folate antagonists relates to tumor cell population kinetics. Inasmuch as folate antagonists inhibit growth by preventing DNA synthesis, slow-growing tumors with a large proportion of cells in a G_0 or prolonged G_1 state might be expected to be naturally resistant to MTX, as well as to other inhibitors of DNA synthesis. Since treatment with an antimetabolite would not affect the majority of cells in G_0 or G_1, therapy would have to be continued for an inordinately long period of time to kill a significant fraction of the cell population which has such a slow rate of entry into the S or DNA synthesis phase. Examples of this type of neoplasm in man are chronic lymphatic leukemia and multiple myeloma.[2]

In order to consider other mechanisms of natural resistance to folic acid antagonists, the mechanism of action of this class of drugs must first be considered. Most of the clinically useful folate antagonists act by inhibiting the enzyme dihydrofolate reductase (DHFR).[3] Since this enzyme is located in the cytoplasm, the drug must first cross the cell membrane in order to interact with the target enzyme (Fig. 1). It is clear from studies of the L1210 and L5178Y mouse leukemias that MTX utilizes a transport system that normally appears to be responsible for the transport of reduced folates, in particular, 5-methyltetrahydrofolate and 5-formyltetrahydrofolate.[4–6]

*Supported by Grants CA08010 and CA08341 and from the U. S. Public Health Service.
†Carreer Development Awardee of the U. S. Public Health Service.

RESISTANCE TO METHOTREXATE

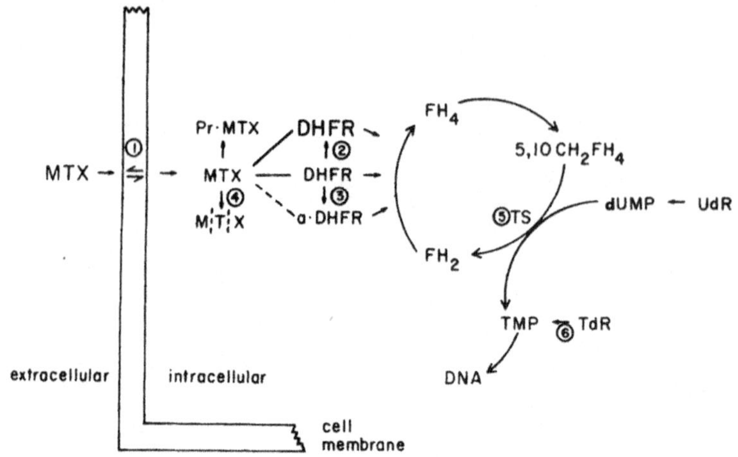

FIG. 1. Possible mechanisms of resistance to methotrexate. (1) Decreased transport; (2) increased DHFR; (3) altered DHFR; (4) metabolism of MTX to inactive compound; (5) increase or alteration of thymidylate synthetase; and (6) increase in thymidine (and purine and serine) from salvage pathways. Abbreviations used: methotrexate, MTX; dihydrofolate reductase, DHFR; N^5, N^{10}-methylene tetrahydrofolate, 5,10 CH_2FH_4; thymidylate synthetase, TS; deoxyuridine, UdR; deoxyuridine monophosphate, dUMP; thymidine, TdR; thymidine monophosphate, TMP; dihydrofolate, FH_2; tetrahydrofolate, FH_4.

The interaction with DHFR is concentration dependent, i.e. the amount of inhibitor relative to the amount of enzyme determines the degree of inhibition, and is also dependent upon the intracellular conditions, i.e. the pH and level of normal substrate present.[3] Thus, a cell with a high level of DHFR will be able to withstand a higher intracellular concentration of MTX than would a cell with a low level of this enzyme; in addition, inhibition of the enzyme is partly relieved as the pH becomes greater than 6.0.[7] If the enzyme is altered, by virtue of the induction of the neoplastic state or via a mutational event, resistance to folic acid antagonists may result if the inhibitor is bound less well by the mutant or neoplastic enzyme than by the normal tissue reductase. Other possible ways in which a cell may escape the effects of MTX and thus be "resistant" are also shown in Fig. 1. A cell that is able to obtain sufficient amounts of the products that are depleted because of the antifolate-induced block (i.e. thymidine, a purine and serine) from salvage pathways, may be able to continue DNA synthesis in the presence of MTX. Conceivably, an increase in activity of the enzyme thymidylate synthetase or a higher affinity of this enzyme for the folate cofactor N^5, N^{10}-methylenetetrahydrofolate could also lead to antifolate resistance, since thymidylate synthesis would continue in the face of decreased levels of folate coenzymes. MTX is a weak inhibitor of thymidylate synthetase and any direct inhibition of this enzyme[8] would also be lessened in this circumstance.

Resistance to MTX in experimental tumors

In experimental tumors, natural resistance to folate antagonists may be due to cell population kinetics or impaired drug uptake. The L1210 and the L5178Y murine tumors are sensitive to the effects of MTX when the cells are growing exponentially; when the cells are in plateau growth and have slower progression into the DNA synthetic phase, they are decimated to a far lesser degree.[9] This situation may be due not only to kinetic considerations, but also to biochemical differences between cell populations growing exponentially and in stationary phase. For example, cells in stationary phase may transport MTX less efficiently, and may have a larger pool size of folate coenzymes.* An example of decreased cellular uptake as an explanation for natural resistance to MTX is provided by the Walker 256 rat carcinoma.[10] However, this cell type transports pyrimidine folate antagonists (i.e. pyrimethamine) and a triazine folate antagonist (i.e. triazinate) very well,[11] and the tumor is sensitive to these drugs. It is of interest that the Walker tumor apparently also transports naturally occurring folates poorly, and is extremely sensitive to dietary folate deficiency[12] and enzymically induced folate deficiency with carboxypeptidase G_1.[13]

Acquired resistance to MTX in most of the mouse tumors studied has usually been attributed to an increase in the enzyme DHFR or to impaired uptake of the drug.[14,15] There are a few reports of a third mechanism of resistance to MTX, namely an altered dihydrofolate reductase with less affinity for MTX.[16,17] It should be pointed out, however, that these mechanisms have been detected after several passages of these mouse lines, *in vitro* or *in vivo*, in the presence of high levels of MTX. More studies of the type described by Schrecker *et al.*[18] are needed, in which resistance is studied *in vivo* after treatment of individual animals, a situation more analagous to the human problem.

Resistance to MTX in man

In man, except for studies in acute leukemia, relatively few studies have been done on resistance of neoplastic cells to folate antagonists. The relative natural resistance of patients with acute myelocytic leukemia (AML) to MTX may be due to several factors: a long generation time, a rapid "turnover" of DHFR, and a rise in this enzyme activity caused by stabilization of the enzyme by MTX.[19] Poor transport of MTX has also been implicated as a cause of natural drug resistance,[20] but testing *in vitro* showed no differences in inhibition of DNA synthesis by MTX between AML and the more MTX-sensitive acute lymphocytic leukemia (ALL) cells.[19] ALL cells appear to be naturally "sensitive" to MTX therapy, presumably because they accumulate levels of the drug sufficient to inhibit DHFR completely. In addition, the stem cells from patients with ALL may have a shorter generation time with less rapid turnover of DHFR.

Acquired resistance to MTX, one of the key agents in the therapy of ALL, still remains an important clinical problem, despite improved combination chemotherapy programs. A valuable screening test *in vitro* that may detect biochemical resistance in these patients is the measurement of DNA synthesis, using ^{3}H-deoxyuridine as the DNA label, in the presence and absence of MTX.[19] During the past several years, patients with ALL have been studied before and after development of resistance to MTX. Six of these patients have shown a decreased sensitivity to this drug after

*A. Nahas, R. Capizzi and J. R. Bertino, in preparation.

development of clinical MTX resistance. These patients were then studied for possible mechanisms of drug resistance: MTX transport, level of DHFR and sensitivity of this enzyme to MTX. None of these patients had a significantly increased level of DHFR associated with MTX resistance. We have recently described the results of studies on one adult who developed MTX resistance after a year of therapy with high level infusions and intrathecal MTX.[21] Uptake of deoxyuridine into DNA of leukemia cells taken from this patient was inhibited only 50 per cent by levels (10^{-5} M) ordinarily resulting in greater than 95 per cent inhibition (Fig. 2). Transport of ^{3}H-MTX by these cells was within the range observed for untreated ALL patients, and the level of DHFR was not elevated. However, DHFR activity was much less inhibited by MTX than was expected from previous studies of other patients with untreated ALL. Limited amounts of material available from this patient precluded further characterization of this apparently altered enzyme, but this explanation for drug resistance deserves further study.

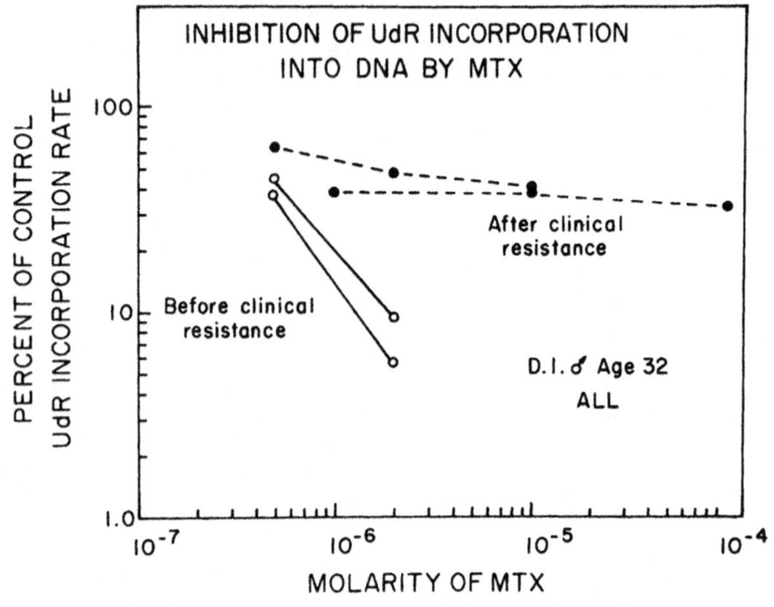

FIG. 2. Inhibition of ^{3}H-UdR incorporation into DNA by MTX before and after clinical resistance. Peripheral blood blasts were incubated in Eagle's MEM with 10% horse serum with 9×10^{-7} M ^{3}H-UdR with and without MTX. The incorporation of radiolabel into DNA is determined at intervals[19] and the rate of incorporation in the presence of MTX, expressed as a per cent of the control incorporation is used as a measure of the inhibition by MTX.

Prevention and exploitation of folate antagonist resistance

Emergence of a resistant population from a previously sensitive one depends upon several factors that include: (1) the number of cells initially present, (2) the sensitivity of these cells to the drug, (3) the concentration or dose of the drug employed and the frequency of its administration, (4) the mutant frequency conferring resistance to the drug, and (5) the mutagenicity of the drug itself. Studies by Fischer[22] using L5178Y cells indicate that L5178Y cells in culture have a mutant frequency of about 2 per 10^6 cells when cells are exposed to 10^{-7} M MTX. Lower levels of MTX produced a higher number of MTX-resistant clones.

Only two ways to delay or prevent drug resistance are suggested by the above considerations: (1) the use of intensive, high dose treatment, if the tumor is growing rapidly, and (2) the use of drugs with different mechanisms of action in combination so that common resistant mutants are not likely to be selected out. Recently, evidence has been obtained by Schabel and Skipper,* in the L1210 system, to show that the use of two drugs in combination may prevent drug resistance. However, in this system, if the cell number is very large, even a two-drug combination does not prevent mutant clones from developing. Since human tumor cell populations initially considered for chemotherapy may have cell numbers on the order of $10^{11}-10^{12}$ cells, more than two drugs in combination may be necessary to prevent the emergence of drug-resistant mutants.

An attractive yet little exploited potential for dealing with biochemical drug resistance is the design of chemotherapy specific for resistant cells. Drug-resistant cells may be more immunogenic, and recent evidence indicates that in some circumstances this may be the explanation for the phenomenon of collateral sensitivity, i.e. increased sensitivity of a drug-resistant tumor to another drug.[23,24] Since drug resistance may be associated with a biochemical change in the tumor cell unique to that cell, the opportunity for rationally designed chemotherapy exists. For example, if resistance occurs to MTX by virtue of an altered DHFR with a decreased affinity for MTX, then new inhibitors might be synthesized with greater affinity for the altered tumor enzyme than for the host cell enzyme. Similarly, if membrane changes occur that results in impaired MTX transport, folate analogs of different structure might be transported better by these cells than normal replicating cells. Friedkin[25] has suggested that resistance to MTX caused by an increased level of DHFR might be exploited by the use of analogs that are substrates for DHFR and are inhibitors of thymidylate synthetase.

These considerations serve to emphasize that more investigations of ways to detect drug resistance in man are clearly warranted.

*F. M. Schabel and H. Skipper, personal communication.

REFERENCES

1. J. R. BERTINO and R. T. SKEEL, *Proc. Fifth Int. Congress on Pharmacology,* Vol. III, in press.
2. J. R. BERTINO and W. M. HRYNIUK, in *Clinical Pharmacology. Basic Principles in Therapeutics* (Eds. K. L. MELMON and H. F. MORRELLI), pp. 511–533. Macmillan, New York (1972).
3. J. R. BERTINO and D. G. JOHNS, in *Twenty-Second Hahnemann Symposium* (Eds. I. BRODSKY, S. B. KAHN and J. H. MOYER), pp. 9–22. Grune & Stratton, New York (1972).
4. A. NAHAS, P. F. NIXON and J. R. BERTINO, *Cancer Res.* **32**, 1416 (1972).
5. A. NAHAS, P. F. NIXON and J. R. BERTINO, *Fedn Proc.* **28**, 389 (1969).
6. I. D. GOLDMAN, N. S. LICHTENSTEIN and V. T. OLIVERIO, *J. biol. Chem.* **243**, 5007 (1968).
7. J. R. BERTINO, B. A. BOOTH, A. CASHMORE, A. L. BIEBER and A. C. SARTORELLI, *J. biol. Chem.* **239**, 479 (1964).
8. J. BORSA and G. F. WHITMORE, *Molec. Pharmac.* **5**, 318 (1969).
9. W. A. HRYNIUK, G. A. FISCHER and J. R. BERTINO, *Molec. Pharmac.* **5**, 557 (1969).
10. F. ROSEN, H. SOTOBAYASHI and C. A. NICHOL, *Proc. Am. Ass. Cancer Res.* **5**, 54 (1964).

11. R. T. SKEEL, A. CASHMORE and J. R. BERTINO, *Proc. Am. Ass. Cancer Res.* **14**, 52 (1973).
12. F. ROSEN and C. A. NICHOL, *Cancer Res.* **22**, 495 (1962).
13. B. CHABNER, P. L. CHELLO and J. R. BERTINO, *Cancer Res.* **32**, 2114 (1972).
14. G. A. FISCHER, *Biochem. Pharmac.* **7**, 75 (1961).
15. G. A. FISCHER, *Biochem. Pharmac.* **11**, 1233 (1962).
16. J. L. BIEDLER, A. M. ALBRECHT, J. D. HUTCHISON and B. A. SPENGLER, *Cancer Res.* **32**, 153 (1972).
17. G. BLUMENTHAL and D. M. GREENBERG, *Oncology* **24**, 223 (1970).
18. A. W. SCHRECKER, J.. A. R. MEAD, N. H. GREENBERG and A. GOLDIN, *Biochem. Pharmac.* **20**, 716 (1971).
19. W. M. HRYNIUK and J. R. BERTINO, *J. clin. Invest.* **48**, 2140 (1969).
20. D. KESSEL, T. C. HALL and D. ROBERTS, *Cancer Res.* **28**, 564 (1968).
21. R. T. SKEEL and J. R. BERTINO, *Blood* **40**, 934 (1972).
22. G. A. FISCHER, *Natn Cancer Inst. Monogr.* **34**, 131 (1971).
23. P. A. SCHMID and D. J. HUTCHISON, *Cancer Res.* **32**, 808 (1972).
24. E. BONMASSAR, A. BONMASSAR, S. VADLAMUDI and A. GOLDIN, *Proc. natn. Acad. Sci. U.S.A.* **66**, 1089 (1970).
25. M. FRIEDKIN, *J. biol. Chem.* **242**, 1466 (1967).

Pp. 107—117, Supplement Number 2, 1974.
Biochemical Pharmacology. Printed in the U.S.A.

RESISTANCE TO PURINE ANALOGS

ROBERT W. BROCKMAN

Southern Research Institute, Birmingham, Ala. U.S.A.

"THE PROBLEM of resistance in neoplastic cells, as in micro-organisms, will remain a most important perpetual threat to the successful use of therapeutic agents." Dr. Lloyd Law made this statement in 1956[1] and laboratory investigations repeatedly have confirmed its validity. Resistance to all of the major classes of anticancer agents has been recognized. As long as cancer cells are able to divide, the processes of mutation and selection evidently are possible, and drug resistance casts its shadow over cancer chemotherapy. This presentation will be mainly about resistance to purine analogs with particular emphasis on resistance in mammalian cells, including human tumor cells.

*Resistance to purine base analogs accompanied by marked decrease or loss of purine phosphoribosyltransferase activities.** Fundamental to studies of resistance to purine analogs was the identification of 5-phosphoribosyl-1-pyrophosphate and the enzyme-catalyzed reaction of this compound with purine bases (Fig. 1). This discovery was made in the laboratories of Lieberman, Kornberg and Simms[2-4] and Remy *et al.*[5] It was recognized by Lukens and Herrington[6] and by Way and Parks[7] that purine analogs also could serve as substrates for purine phosphoribosyltransferases. It was soon demonstrated that bacterial cells[8-10] and neoplastic cells[8,11-14] resistant to 6-mercaptopurine and to 8-azaguanine lacked the capacity to form nucleotides of these analogs and that this failure was a consequence of a marked decrease or loss of H-GPRT activity in some of these resistant cell lines.[15] A corollary of this finding was that nucleotide derivatives of purine analogs were the active metabolic inhibitors.

Does this mechanism of resistance play a role in the failure of 6-mercaptopurine to maintain remissions in human leukemia? This question was discussed a decade ago when the results of a careful study by Davidson and Winter[16] were considered. These

*It should be noted that the purine phosphoribosyltransferases of mammalian cells, namely those enzymes which catalyze the formation of nucleotides from adenine, hypoxanthine and guanine, originally were named purine nucleotide pyrophosphorylases, and this designation was used until recently. This nomenclature implies a degradative function when, in fact, the enzymes catalyze the synthesis of nucleotides of purines and analogs. The specificities generally recognized for mammalian cell enzymes are as follows:

Enzyme	Abbreviation	Product
Adenine phosphoribosyltransferase	APRT	AMP
Hypoxanthine–guanine phosphoribosyltransferase	H-GPRT	IMP GMP
Xanthine phosphoribosyltransferase	XPRT	XMP

Adenine analogs, such as 2-fluoroadenine, 4-aminopyrazolo(3,4-d)pyrimidine, and 2,6-diaminopurine are substrates for APRT. Hypoxanthine and guanine analogs, such as 6-mercaptopurine, 6-thioguanine and 8-azaguanine, serve as substrates for H-GPRT. XPRT activity appears to be weak in most mammalian cells examined.

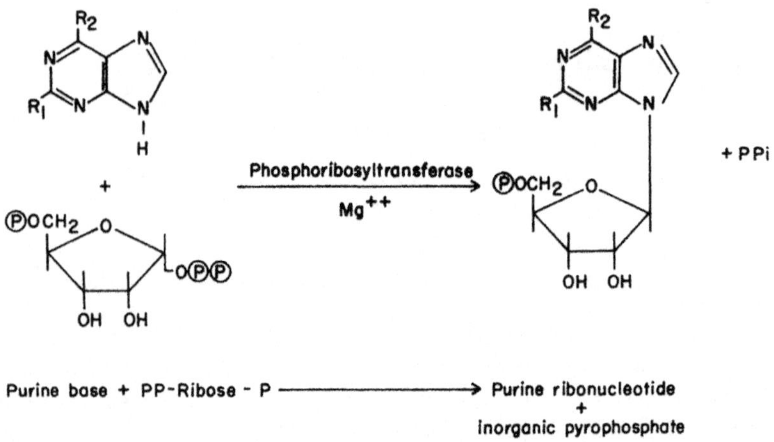

FIG. 1. Enzymatic conversion of purine bases and analogs to ribonucleotides by reaction of bases with 5-phosphoribosyl-1-pyrophosphate. R_1 = H, R_2 = NH_2; adenine. R_1 = H, R_2 = OH; hypoxanthine. R_1 = NH_2, R_2 = OH; guanine. R_1 = H, R_2 = SH; 6-mercaptopurine. R_1 = NH_2, R_2 = SH; 6-thioguanine.

investigators were able to demonstrate a marked decrease in the H-GPRT activity in human leukemia cells clinically resistant to 6-mercaptopurine in only one of fifteen cases, of which six were classified as highly resistant.* Resistance to 6-mercaptopurine in human leukemia cells as a consequence of loss of H-GPRT activity was considered to be a relatively rare occurrence;[22] a recent study supports this view.[23] Results of the Davidson and Winter study demonstrated that loss of H-GPRT activity does occur in human leukemia cells; therefore, this should be recognized as a clinical resistance mechanism.[24] The results of a study by Kessel and Hall[25] may be taken to support this view. These investigators observed greater retention *in vitro* of 6-mercaptopurine (presumably as the nucleotide) in human leukemia cells sensitive to 6-mercaptopurine than in thiopurine-resistant cells.

Resistance to adenine analogs, such as 2,6-diaminopurine, 8-aza-adenine and 2-fluoroadenine, is known to be accompanied by decrease or loss of APRT activity in micro-organisms[26–28] and in tumor cells.[29,30] Bennett *et al.*[31] have made use of neoplasms in cell culture that are deficient in purine phosphoribosyltransferases and also in adenosine kinase activity (see below) as a means of examining pathways of anabolism of analogs of purines and nucleosides.

Resistance to adenosine analogs accompanied by decrease or loss of adenosine kinase. 6-Methylmercaptopurine ribonucleoside was recognized as an active inhibitor of purine nucleotide biosynthesis.[32–34] This nucleoside acted as a feedback inhibitor and was inhibitory to growth of 6-thiopurine-resistant cells that lacked H-GPRT, suggesting that it might be phosphorylated by the action of a kinase.[34] This postulate was found to be correct;[35,36] adenosine kinase purified from mammalian cells utilized as substrates, adenosine, 6-methylmercaptopurine ribonucleoside and other adenosine analogs,[37,38] and tumor cells selected for resistance to 6-methylmercaptopurine ribo-

*APRT activity was observed to increase in cell lines that were deficient in H-GPRT activity. This was found to occur in thiopurine-resistant human leukemia[16,17] and in certain patients with abnormalities of purine metabolism.[18–21] nucleoside were deficient in adenosine kinase.[35,39] A subline of human epidermoid carcinoma cells (H.Ep-2) in culture was selected for resistance to both 2-fluoroadenine and 2-fluoroadenosine, and this doubly resistant mutant was found to be deficient in both adenine phosphoribosyltransferase and in adenosine kinase.[30]

6-Methylmercaptopurine ribonucleotide is a potent inhibitor of phosphoribosylpyrophosphate amidotransferase,[40] the site of feedback inhibition by natural purine nucleotides (Fig. 2). It is, therefore, significant that 6-mercaptopurine can be metabolized to 6-methylmercaptopurine ribonucleotide in cells that possess H-GPRT activity, and it has been suggested that the methylated derivative may be responsible for the feedback inhibition produced by 6-mercaptopurine.[41]

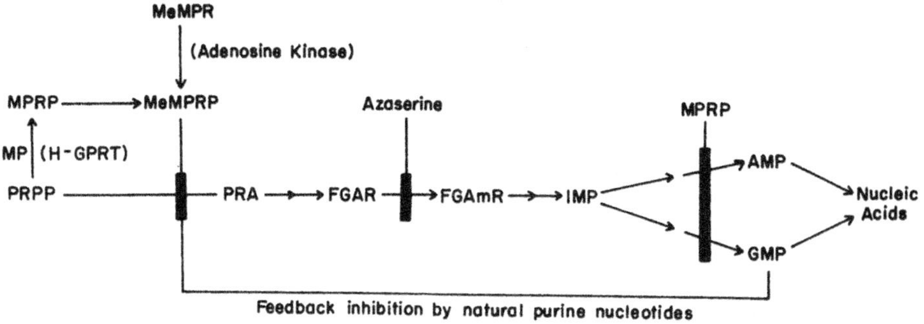

FIG. 2. Inhibition of purine nucleotide synthesis *de novo* by purines and 6-thiopurines. The conversion of 6-mercaptopurine (MP) to 6-mercaptopurine ribonucleotide (MPRP) and the methylation of MPRP to yield 6-methylmercaptopurine ribonucleotide (MeMPRP) are depicted. MeMPRP also can be formed by phopsphorylation of 6-methylmercaptopurine ribonucleoside (MeMPR). The synthesis of phosphoribosylamine (PRA) by reaction of 5-phosphoribosyl-1-pyrophosphate (PRPP) and glutamine is inhibited by natural purine nucleotides and also by MPRP, MeMPRP and 6-thioguanylic acid (not shown). The conversion of formylglycinamide ribonucleotide (FGAR) to formylglycinamidine ribonucleotide (FGAmR) is inhibited by azaserine, providing a tool for evaluating feedback inhibition. The conversion of IMP to AMP and GMP also is inhibited by MPRP.

It is of interest that loss of a kinase activity accompanying resistance in human leukemia recently has been described. Gailani and Nussbaum[42] observed loss of capacity to phosphorylate arabinosylcytosine in leukemia cells from a patient initially responsive but later refractory to therapy with this agent.*

Altered purine phosphoribosyltransferase and resistance to purine analogs in mammalian cells. Considerable interest in H-GPRT was engendered by the discovery that a genetic deficiency of this enzyme[18,43] was associated with the Lesch–Nyhan syndrome.[44] Studies of abnormalities of purine metabolism have led to observations of partial deficiencies of H-GPRT[19,20,45] and of kinetically altered enzyme.[46,47]

Benke *et al.*,[47] in their studies of erythrocytes derived from a hyperuricemic patient exhibiting accelerated purine nucleotide biosynthesis, observed unusual sensitivity of H-GPRT to sodium fluoride and to sodium pyrophosphate in comparison with the enzyme from normal cells. These findings are reminiscent of those of Adye and Gots[48] who observed altered enzyme kinetics and increased sensitivity to *p*-chloromercuribenzoate of H-GPRT from resistant mutants of *Salmonella typhimurium*. Of particular

*S. Gailani, personal communication.

interest for the present discussion is the observation of DeMars and Held[49] that spontaneous 8-azaguanine-resistant mutants derived from diploid human fibroblasts exhibited H-GPRT activity ranging from loss of activity to normal levels of enzyme activity.* Many of these mutant strains were partially sensitive to 8-azaguanine and could utilize hypoxanthine for growth. These investigators were aware of Benke's observation, and they also found that H-GPRT activity from certain of their resistant mutants was unusually sensitive to sodium fluoride.

McDonald and Kelley[46] found that the apparent K_m of H-GPRT for PRPP and for hypoxanthine and guanine was an order of magnitude greater for enzyme from a patient with Lesch–Nyhan syndrome than for a normal subject (Table 1). Benke *et al.*[47] found a similar increase in the apparent K_m for PRPP in cells from a patient with abnormal purine metabolism but, in contrast to the observation of McDonald and Kelley, found no significant change in the K_m for hypoxanthine.

TABLE 1. COMPARISON OF KINETIC PROPERTIES OF NORMAL AND MUTANT HYPOXANTHINE–GUANINE PHOSPHORIBOSYLTRANSFERASE IN HUMAN ERYTHROCYTES AND FIBROBLASTS

			Apparent K_m for PRPP (M)			
Enzyme source	Cell type	H-GPRT activity	Guanine	Hypoxanthine	Sensitivity to NaF	Reference
Fibroblast*	Normal	Normal	1×10^{-4}			McDonald
	Mutant	Deficient	$>2 \times 10^{-3}$			and Kelley[46]
Erythrocyte*	Normal	Normal	2.5×10^{-4}			46
	Mutant	Deficient	3.2×10^{-3}	2.8×10^{-3}		
Erythrocyte†	Normal	Normal		$1.1–1.4 \times 10^{-4}$	–	Benke *et al.*[47]
	Mutant	Normal		$1.0–1.4 \times 10^{-3}$	+	
Fibroblast‡	Normal	Normal			–	DeMars and
	AG-resistant	Normal			+	Held[49]

*These cells were from a patient with Lesch-Nyhan syndrome. H-GPRT activity ranged from 8–34 per cent of normal levels at high PRPP concentrations in the enzyme reaction medium.
†These cells were from a hyperuricemic patient with accelerated purine production. H-GPRT activity was apparently normal at high PRPP concentrations.
‡These cells were selected for resistance to 8-azaguanine from cultures of human fibroblasts.

Rosman and Williams[17] recently reported results of a study of resistance to 6-thiopurines in human leukemia, and their findings appear to be related to those just discussed. H-GPRT activity was examined in leukemic leukocytes from a patient who

*Most of the mutants isolated by DeMars and Held[49] retained H-GPRT activity; a minority exhibited loss of enzyme activity. Morrow *et al.*[50] and Shin *et al.*[51] also selected 8-azaguanine-resistant hamster and mouse cell lines in culture that were not deficient in H-GPRT activity by growing resistant cells in media containing hypoxanthine, amethopterin and thymidine, i.e. HAT medium. Cells deficient in H-GPRT activity thus were eliminated. Altered enzyme kinetics with respect to purine base, PRPP, or both, as described by McDonald and Kelley[46] and by Benke *et al.*[47] may offer a basis for understanding azaguanine resistance in these cell lines. Sato *et al.*[52] obtained H-GPRT-deficient mutants from human lymphoblasts exposed to ethylmethane sulfonate and then cultured in the presence of 6-thioguanine.

was no longer responsive to therapy with 6-thioguanine. The concentration of PRPP required to give one-half maximum velocity of conversion of 6-mercaptopurine to the nucleotide was significantly higher (approximately 6-fold) with enzyme from resistant leukemic leukocytes than it was from normal leukemic leukocytes. In the light of similar observations of McDonald and Kelley and of Benke, it appears that altered H-GPRT, in which the affinity of enzyme for PRPP is decreased, could be a significant factor in resistance to purine analogs in mammalian cells, including human neoplastic cells.

The concentration of PRPP in tumor cells, such as Ehrlich and Sarcoma 180, was found to range from 1×10^{-5} M to 6×10^{-4} M;[53–55] PRPP levels measured in erythrocytes were in the range of 10^{-6} to 10^{-5} M.[56,57] Treatment of such tumor cells with 6-methylmercaptopurine ribonucleoside, which inhibits the utilization of PRPP for purine nucleotide biosynthesis (see Fig. 2), can result in as much as a 10-fold increase in the intracellular level of PRPP.[54,55] These observations lead one to consider the merits of a combination of 6-methylmercaptopurine ribonucleoside and 6-thiopurines in cells, such as those described above, that have altered H-GPRT enzyme with a higher K_m for PRPP. Such combinations are known to increase the level of 6-thiopurine nucleotides in tumor cells.[54,55,58,59]

Resistance to purine analogs as a consequence of increased degradation. One of the biochemical mechanisms by which cells might become resistant to purine analogs is the development of increased capacity to degrade the base analog. Elion[60] has summarized catabolism of 6-thiopurines in mammalian cells. Sartorelli *et al.*[61] selected a subline of Ehrlich ascites carcinoma cells that was resistant to 6-thioguanine and cross-resistant to 6-mercaptopurine. Less analog nucleotide was present in the resistant line compared to the sensitive line after a standard dose of 6-thioguanine. Pretreatment of tumor-bearing animals with azaserine followed by 6-thioguanine eliminated this difference, indicating that the resistant line possessed adequate capacity to metabolize 6-thioguanine to nucleotide derivatives. Resistant cells appeared to be more active than the parent sensitive cells in the degradation of 6-thioguanine to 6-thioxanthine and 6-thiouric acid; this was considered to be a basis for resistance in this cell line.[61]

In the light of recent studies on altered H-GPRT in mutant cells, discussed above, one might speculate as to whether altered H-GPRT might be a factor in resistance to 6-thiopurines in this Ehrlich cell line. Azaserine pretreatment would result in an increased level of PRPP as a consequence of inhibition of purine nucleotide biosynthesis (see Fig. 2). An increased K_m for PRPP was one of the changes observed in some of the mutant cell lines characterized by altered H-GPRT. The increased levels of PRPP produced by azaserine pretreatment might then be sufficient to increase the rate of synthesis of thiopurine nucleotides from the corresponding bases.

Another possible degradative route for 6-thiopurines is their conversion to 6-hydroxypurines by desulfurization. This has been observed in micro-organisms,[62–64] in mammalian tissue,[65] including neoplasms,[61] and has been reported to occur in human leukemia cells by conversion of 6-mercaptopurine ribonucleotide to inosinic acid.[66] This latter reaction would provide an effective way for a cell to resist the inhibitory effects of 6-mercaptopurine, since the IMP formed would bypass the inhibition of purine nucleotide biosynthesis produced by 6-thiopurine nucleotides.

Another degradative mechanism by which cells may become resistant to purine analogs is by increased catabolism of the analog nucleotide. Bieber and Sartorelli[67] suggested that this was a factor in resistance to 6-thioguanine in Sarcoma 180 cells and Bennett *et al.*[68] concluded that resistance to 4-aminopyrazolo-(3,4-d)pyrimidine in neoplastic cells in culture was associated with a higher rate of degradation of the analog ribonucleotide in resistant cells. Recently Wolpert *et al.*[69] found that cell-free extracts of a 6-thioguanine-resistant Sarcoma 180 line possessed increased alkaline phosphatase activity relative to the parent-sensitive line (Fig. 3). Such phosphatase activity in sensitive and resistant cells was similar at lower pH values; under more alkaline conditions of enzyme assay (pH 9.2), phosphatase activity decreased in enzyme preparations from sensitive cells but increased in those from resistant cells. In considering this as a resistance mechanism, one must rationalize the significance of differences between enzyme activity from sensitive and resistant cells observed at a pH value so far removed from physiological conditions. Also, it is presumed that natural purine and pyrimidine nucleotides would be partially protected from degradation by alkaline phosphatase activity, since they are present predominantly as nucleoside triphosphates. 6-Mercaptopurine ribonucleoside 5′-monophosphate is not phosphorylated to the di- or triphosphate,[70] and the intracellular pool of 6-thioguanine nucleotides is known to consist predominantly of 6-thioguanosine 5′-monophosphate.[55,61] Nucleoside 5′-monophosphates are good substrates for alkaline phosphatase. Activity of this tumor cell alkaline phosphatase for nucleoside triphosphates should be evaluated, however, since alkaline phosphatases from bacterial cells[71] and mammalian cells[72] can degrade nucleoside di- and triphosphates although, in mammalian cells, the triphosphates serve less well as substrates than do the monophosphates.

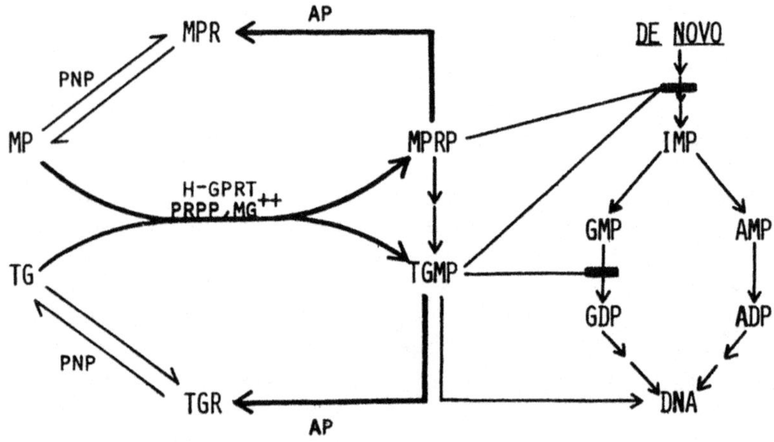

FIG. 3. Conversion of MP and 6-thioguanine (TG) to the corresponding nucleotides. MPRP can be metabolized to 6-thioguanylic acid (TGMP) which, after reduction to 6-thiodeoxyguanylic acid, can be incorporated into DNA. Resistance to purine analogs in a TG-resistant subline of Sarcoma 180 is accompanied by increased alkaline phosphatase (AP) activity.[69] The nucleosides of MP and TG, MPR and TGR, then can be hydrolyzed by purine nucleoside phosphorylase (PNP) to yield the bases.

Nelson and Parks[55] observed that the half-life of 6-thioguanine nucleotides was about 3 hr in the 6-thioguanine-resistant Sarcoma 180 cells compared to a half-life of about 7 hr in the sensitive tumor. It is interesting that pretreatment with 6-methylmercaptopurine ribonucleoside prolonged the half-life of acid-soluble metabolites of 6-thioguanine in the resistant tumor to 6.6 hr, almost the value observed in the sensitive tumor in the absence of such pretreatment. It is tempting to assume that the effect of 6-methylmercaptopurine ribonucleoside was to increase PRPP levels with consequent increased synthesis of 6-thioguanylic acid. However, azaserine pretreatment, which also should result in increased intracellular levels of PRPP, had no effect on the half-life of 6-thioguanine nucleotides. Thus, it was concluded that 6-methylmercaptopurine ribonucleotide inhibited the degradation of 6-thioguanine ribonucleotides by inhibiting phosphatase activity in the resistant tumor cells, probably as a consequence of competition for the enzyme.

Decreased feedback inhibition of purine nucleotide biosynthesis and decreased sensitivity to purine analogs. Henderson *et al.*[73] observed decreased inhibition of purine nucleotide biosynthesis in 6-methylmercaptopurine-resistant Ehrlich ascites tumor cells that were not deficient in adenosine kinase. Indirect evidence suggested that the early step in the purine nucleotide biosynthetic pathway, phosphoribosylpyrophosphate amidotransferase, was less subject to feedback regulation by 6-methylmercaptopurine ribonucleotide and by GMP in the resistant line than it was in the sensitive line (see Fig. 2). Feedback regulation by adenine nucleotides appeared to be identical in the two lines.

Dixon *et al.*[74] suggested decreased feedback inhibition as a basis for understanding observed differences in sensitivity of Sarcoma 180 and Adenocarcinoma 755 tumor cells growing in culture. These neoplasms possessed comparable H-GPRT activity. Adenocarcinoma 755 cells in culture were more sensitive to purine analogs than were the Sarcoma 180 cells;[74] this also was observed *in vivo.*[75] Purine nucleotide synthesis *de novo* was blocked by azaserine in tumor cells growing in culture, and ^{14}C-formylglycinamide ribonucleotide accumulated in cells grown in medium containing ^{14}C-formate; candidate feedback inhibitors were evaluated by their capacity to inhibit such accumulation[76] (Fig. 2). Adenine, hypoxanthine, 6-mercaptopurine and 6-thioguanine, after conversion to nucleotides, were more effective inhibitors in Adenocarcinoma 755 cells than in Sarcoma 180 cells. However, actual differences in kinetic behavior of phosphoribosylamidotransferase prepared from sensitive and resistant cells have not been demonstrated, nor has this mechanism of resistance been described in clinical resistance to purine analogs.

Resistance to 6-thiopurines accompanied by decreased incorporation of analog nucleotide into polynucleotides. LePage[77] found that 6-thioguanine is incorporated as the nucleotide into RNA and DNA of tumor cells. Incorporation of the analog into the DNA of sensitive tumors was found to be greater than that of resistant tumors, which suggested that this incorporation was involved in the antitumor effect of 6-thioguanine. LePage and Jones[78] described thioguanine-insensitive lines of tumor cells that were not deficient in the synthesis of 6-thioguanylic acid, but which incorporated less thioguanine into DNA than did sensitive neoplasms. Radioactivity from 2′-deoxy-6-thioguanosine-8-^{14}C was incorporated into acid-soluble nucleotides and into DNA[79] of such a thioguanine-insensitive neoplasm, the Mecca lymphosarcoma, and this neoplasm gave some response to treatment with 6-thiodeoxyguanosine. The interesting suggestion was made that this neoplasm might be deficient in the capacity to reduce 6-thioguanosine 5′-diphosphate to the corresponding deoxyribonucleotide; an altered specificity of DNA polymerase also could account for these results.

Failure of the analog to gain entry into resistant cells. Paterson[80] isolated a 6-mercaptopurine-resistant subline of Ehrlich carcinoma which failed to form nucleotides of 6-mercaptopurine in intact cells, but which clearly possessed H-GPRT activity and formed 6-mercaptopurine ribonucleotide enzymatically in the presence of base analog and PRPP.[81] The synthesis of nucleotides from adenine, guanine and hypoxanthine in intact cells of sensitive and resistant lines was similar.[82] The conclusion drawn from these studies was that 6-mercaptopurine failed to gain access to the site of nucleotide synthesis in intact resistant cells, presumably as a consequence of failure of 6-mercaptopurine to gain entry into the cells.

In *Escherichia coli,* the uptake of purines has been related to the activity of purine phosphoribosyltransferase activities associated with cell membranes.[83,84] Recently, Benke *et al.*[85] have reported decreased uptake of hypoxanthine in cells with mutant H-GPRT enzyme; there was almost no uptake in cells from patients with Lesch–Nyhan syndrome which lacked H-GPRT activity. It cannot be said that H-GPRT is a membrane-associated enzyme in mammalian cells, but Benke's results do show a relationship between intracellular H-GPRT activity and uptake of a substrate for this enzyme. This is due in part to the conversion of base to nucleotide, which would displace equilibrium between the external and the intracellular concentration of hypoxanthine with resultant increased uptake of the substrate into cells competent to utilize it. However, his explanation does not appear to hold in the case of resistance that Paterson describes, since his resistant line possessed H-GPRT activity comparable to that in the sensitive line.

Other mechanisms of resistance. One must leave a discussion of mechanisms of resistance to inhibitors of cell growth open-ended simply because of the versatility of cells to adapt to adverse conditions posed by the presence of an inhibitor. Undoubtedly other mechanisms of resistance to metabolic inhibitors, such as the purine analogs, are yet to be described. For example, Bieber *et al.*[86] described a 6-mercaptopurine-resistant subline of Adenocarcinoma 755 which incorporated radioactivity from 6-mercaptopurine-^{35}S into nucleic acids more extensively than did the parent sensitive line. It was later demonstrated that 6-mercaptopurine-8-^{14}C was metabolized and incorporated into the DNA of this resistant line as 6-thiodeoxyguanylic acid;[87] therefore, there was no impairment in the pathway of anabolism of 6-mercaptopurine (Fig. 3). An understanding of the manner in which this tumor cell line achieved resistance probably will provide yet another mechanism of resistance to thiopurine.

CONCLUSIONS

In considering resistance to purine analogs, as this problem bears on clinical cancer, emphasis necessarily is placed on the 6-thiopurines that have found use in the treatment of leukemia, namely 6-mercaptopurine, 6-thioguanine and 6-methylmercaptopurine ribonucleoside. Resistance to all three of these agents can be achieved both in experimental neoplasms and in clinical disease by the loss of activity of those enzymes that convert the analog bases and nucleosides to nucleotides. Decrease or loss of hypoxanthine–guanine phosphoribosyltransferase activity results in decrease or loss of capacity to form nucleotides of 6-mercaptopurine and 6-thioguanine. This mechanism of resistance has been observed in clinical cases of leukemia. Decrease or loss of adenosine kinase activity results in diminished capacity to phosphorylate 6-methylmercaptopurine ribonucleoside. Although loss of adenosine kinase associated with resistance to MeMPR has not been described in clinical cancer, an analogous loss of the capacity to phosphorylate arabinosylcytosine has been observed in clinical leukemia resistant to this agent.[42,*]

Interesting observations have been made on alterations in the kinetic behavior of H-GPRT in cells exhibiting abnormal purine nucleotide metabolism, particularly increased K_m value for 5-phosphoribosyl-1-pyrophosphate. It appears that a similar alteration may occur in examples of experimental and clinical resistance to purine analogs. In such cases, it may prove feasible to circumvent resistance by elevation of PRPP levels with an inhibitor of purine nucleotide synthesis, such as 6-methylmercaptopurine ribonucleoside.

The development of resistance to one agent can result in increased sensitivity to another agent which acts by a different mechanism. For example, tumor cells made resistant to purine analogs exhibited increased sensitivity to amethopterin.[88] Recently we observed an unusual increase in sensitivity to the uridine analog 3-deazauridine in L1210 cells selected for resistance to arabinosylcytosine.[89] In the present discussion, it was seen that cells deficient in H-GPRT activity frequently exhibit an elevated APRT activity; this effect also was noted in human leukemia cells resistant to 6-mercaptopurine.[16] Such cells should be more vulnerable to attack by adenine analogs that are converted to inhibitory nucleotides by APRT, as suggested by Rosman and Williams.[17] These few examples may serve to point out the long recognized possibility that, even though resistant to one drug, cells may become more susceptible to the inhibitory effects of other drugs than were the parent cells.[90,91]

In conclusion, I would like to comment briefly on combination chemotherapy of cancer. From both a theoretical and a pragmatic viewpoint, combination chemotherapy appears to be a logical way to minimize, if not circumvent, the ever present problem of the development of resistance to therapy with a single agent. It is to be hoped that conferences such as this one may stimulate exchange of views between experimental and clinical cancer chemotherapists with the outcome being better ways for selecting combinations of agents for clinical trials.

*S. Gailani, personal communication.

Acknowledgement – The author is indebted to Dr. Paul Benke, McArdle Laboratory and Department of Pediatrics and Pathology, University of Wisconsin, for valuable discussions of aspects of his work and to colleagues at Southern Research Institute for stimulating discussions of aspects of resistance to purine analogs.

REFERENCES

1. L. W. LAW, *Cancer Res.* **16**, 698 (1956).
2. I. LIEBERMAN, A. KORNBERG and E. S. SIMMS, *J. Am. chem. Soc.* **76**, 2844 (1954).
3. I. LIEBERMAN, A. KORNBERG and E. S. SIMMS, *J. biol. Chem.* **215**, 403 (1955).
4. A. KORNBERG, I. LIEBERMAN and E. S. SIMMS, *J. biol. Chem.* **215**, 417 (1955).
5. C. N. REMY, W. T. REMY and J. M. BUCHANAN, *J. biol. Chem.* **217**, 885 (1955).
6. L. N. LUKENS and K. A. HERRINGTON, *Biochim. biophys. Acta* **24**, 432 (1957).
7. J. L. WAY and R. E. PARKS, JR., *J. biol. Chem.* **231**, 467 (1958).

8. R. W. BROCKMAN, M. C. SPARKS and M. S. SIMPSON, *Biochim. biophys. Acta* **26**, 671 (1957).
9. M. E. BALIS, V. HYLIN, M. K. COULTAS and D. J. HUTCHISON, *Cancer Res.* **18**, 220 (1958).
10. R. W. BROCKMAN, C. SPARKS, D. J. HUTCHISON and H. E. SKIPPER, *Cancer Res.* **19**, 177 (1959).
11. R. W. BROCKMAN, L. L. BENNETT, JR., M. S. SIMPSON, A. R. WILSON, J. R. THOMSON and H. E. SKIPPER, *Cancer Res.* **19**, 856 (1959).
12. R. W. BROCKMAN, *Cancer Res.* **20**, 643 (1960).
13. R. W. BROCKMAN, G. G. KELLEY, P. STUTTS and V. COPELAND, *Nature, Lond.* **191**, 469 (1961).
14. R. W. BROCKMAN, R. A. ROOSA, L. W. LAW and P. L. STUTTS, *J. Cell Biol.* **60**, 65 (1962).
15. R. W. BROCKMAN, *Adv. Cancer Res.* **7**, 129 (1963).
16. J. D. DAVIDSON and T. S. WINTER, *Cancer Res.* **24**, 261 (1964).
17. M. ROSMAN and H. E. WILLIAMS, *Cancer Res.* **33**, 1202 (1973).
18. J. E. SEEGMILLER, F. M. ROSENBLOOM and W. N. KELLEY, *Science, N.Y.* **155**, 1682 (1967).
19. W. N. KELLEY, M. L. GREENE, F. M. ROSENBLUM, J. F. HENDERSON and J. E. SEEGMILLER, *Ann. intern. Med.* **70**, 155 (1969).
20. M. D. KOGUT, G. N. DONNELL, W. L. NYHAN and L. SWEETMAN, *Am. J. Med.* **48**, 148 (1970).
21. P. J. BENKE and N. HERRICK, *Am. J. Med.* **52**, 547 (1972).
22. J. D. DAVIDSON, *Cancer Res.* **25**, 1606 (1965).
23. J. L. SMITH, G. A. OMURA, I. H. KRAKOFF and M. E. BALIS, *Proc. Soc. exp. Biol. Med.* **136**, 1299 (1971).
24. R. W. BROCKMAN, *Cancer Res.* **25**, 1596 (1965).
25. D. KESSEL and T. C. HALL, *Cancer Res.* **29**, 2116 (1969).
26. G. P. KALLÉ and J. S. GOTS, *Biochim. biophys. Acta* **51**, 130 (1961).
27. R. W. BROCKMAN, C. S. DEBAVADI, P. STUTTS and D. J. HUTCHISON, *J. biol. Chem.* **236**, 1471 (1961).
28. R. F. PITTILLO, C. MONCRIEF, R. W. BROCKMAN and P. CHAMBERS, *Antimicrobial Agents and Chemotherapy – 1964*, 474 (1965).
29. I. LIEBERMAN and P. OVE, *J. biol. Chem.* **235**, 1765 (1960).
30. L. L. BENNETT, JR., M. H. VAIL, S. CHUMLEY and J. A. MONTGOMERY, *Biochem. Pharmac.* **15**, 1719 (1966).
31. L. L. BENNETT, JR., M. H. VAIL, P. W. ALLAN and S. C. SHADDIX, *Biochem. Pharmac.* **22**, 1221 (1973).
32. J. F. HENDERSON, *Biochem. Pharmac.* **12**, 551 (1963).
33. J. F. HENDERSON and M. K. Y. KHOO, *J. biol. Chem.* **240**, 3104 (1965).
34. L. L. BENNETT, JR., R. W. BROCKMAN, H. P. SCHNEBLI, S. CHUMLEY, G. DIXON, F. M. SCHABEL, JR., E. A. DULMADGE, H. E. SKIPPER, J. A. MONTGOMERY and H. J. THOMAS, *Nature, Lond.* **205**, 1275 (1965).
35. L. L. BENNETT, JR., H. P. SCHNEBLI, M. H. VAIL, P. W. ALLAN and J. A. MONTGOMERY, *Molec. Pharmac.* **2**, 432 (1966).
36. I. C. CALDWELL, J. F. HENDERSON and A. R. P. PATERSON, *Can. J. Biochem. Physiol.* **44**, 229 (1966).
37. H. P. SCHNEBLI, D. L. HILL and L. L. BENNETT, JR., *J. biol. Chem.* **242**, 1997 (1967).
38. B. LINDBERG, H. KLENOW and K. HANSEN, *J. biol. Chem.* **242**, 350 (1967).
39. I. C. CALDWELL, J. F. HENDERSON and A. R. P. PATERSON, *Can. J. Biochem. Physiol.* **45**, 735 (1967).
40. D. L. HILL and L. L. BENNETT, JR., *Biochemistry, N.Y.* **8**, 122 (1969).
41. L. L. BENNETT, JR. and P. W. ALLAN, *Cancer Res.* **31**, 152 (1971).
42. S. GAILANI and A. NUSSBAUM, *Proc. Am. Ass. Cancer Res.* **14**, 100 (1973).
43. W. N. KELLEY, *Fedn Proc.* **27**, 1047 (1968).
44. M. LESCH and W. L. NYHAN, *Am. J. Med.* **36**, 561 (1964).
45. O. SPERLING, M. FRANK, R. OPHIR, U. A. LIBERMAN, A. ADAM and A. DE VRIES, *Eur. J. clin. biol. Res.* **15**, 942 (1970).
46. J. A. MCDONALD and W. N. KELLEY, *Science, N.Y.* **171**, 689 (1971).
47. P. J. BENKE, N. HERRICK and A. HERBERT, *J. clin. Invest.*, **52**, 2234 (1973).
48. J. C. ADYE and J. S. GOTS, *Biochim. biophys. Acta* **118**, 344 (1966).
49. R. DEMARS and K. R. HELD, *Humangenetik* **16**, 87 (1972).
50. J. MORROW, J. COLOFIORE and D. RINTOUL, *J. Cell Biol.* **81**, 97 (1972).

51. S. SHIN, R. CANEVA, C. L. SCHILDKRAUT, H. P. KLINGER and M. SINISCALCO, *Nature New Biol.* **241**, 194 (1973).
52. K. SATO, R. S. SLESINSKI and J. W. LITTLEFIELD, *Proc. natn Acad. Sci.* U.S.A. **69**, 1244 (1972).
53. J. F. HENDERSON and M. K. Y. KHOO, *J. biol. Chem.* **240**, 2363 (1965).
54. A. R. P. PATERSON and M. C. WANG, *Cancer Res.* **30**, 2379 (1970).
55. J. A. NELSON and R. E. PARKS, JR., *Cancer Res.* **32**, 2034 (1972).
56. I. H. FOX and W. N. KELLEY, *Ann. intern. Med.* **74**, 424 (1971).
57. O. SPERLING, G. EILAM, S. PERSKY-BROSH and A. DE VRIES, *J. Lab. clin. Med.* **79**, 1021 (1972).
58. E. M. SCHOLAR, P. R. BROWN and R. E. PARKS, JR., *Cancer Res.* **32**, 259 (1972).
59. C. T. WARNICK and A. R. P. PATERSON, *Cancer Res.* **33**, 1711 (1973).
60. G. B. ELION, *Fedn Proc.* **26**, 898 (1967).
61. A. C. SARTORELLI, G. A. LE PAGE and E. C. MOORE, *Cancer Res.* **18**, 1232 (1958).
62. M. E. BALIS, V. HYLIN, M. K. COULTAS and D. J. HUTCHISON, *Cancer Res.* **18**, 440 (1958).
63. N. H. CAREY and H. G. MANDEL, *Biochem. Pharmac.* **5**, 64 (1960).
64. J. H. COGGIN, M. LOOSEMORE and W. R. MARTIN, *J. Bact.* **92**, 446 (1966).
65. G. B. ELION, S. BIEBER and G. H. HITCHINGS, *Ann. N.Y. Acad. Sci.* **60**, 297 (1954).
66. W. R. MARTIN, I. K. CRICHTON, R. C. YANG and A. E. EVANS, *Proc. Soc. exp. Biol. Med.* **140**, 423 (1972).
67. A. L. BIEBER and A. C. SARTORELLI, *Cancer Res.* **24**, 1210 (1964).
68. L. L. BENNETT, JR., P. W. ALLAN, D. SMITHERS and M. H. VAIL, *Biochem. Pharmac.* **18**, 725 (1969).
69. M. K. WOLPERT, S. P. DAMLE, J. E. BROWN, E. SZNYCER, K. C. AGRAWAL and A. C. SARTORELLI, *Cancer Res.* **31**, 1620 (1971).
70. A. R. P. PATERSON, *Can. J. Biochem. Physiol.* **37**, 1011 (1959).
71. L. A. HEPPEL, D. HARKNESS and R. HILMOE, *J. biol. Chem.* **237**, 841 (1962).
72. D. R. HARKNESS, *Archs Biochem. Biophys.* **126**, 513 (1968).
73. J. F. HENDERSON, I. C. CALDWELL and A. R. P. PATERSON, *Cancer Res.* **27**, 1773 (1967).
74. G. J. DIXON, E. A. DULMADGE, R. W. BROCKMAN and S. C. SHADDIX, *J. natn Cancer Inst.* **45**, 681 (1970).
75. H. E. SKIPPER, J. A. MONTGOMERY, J. R. THOMSON and F. M. SCHABEL, JR., *Cancer Res.* **19**, 425 (1959).
76. A. C. SARTORELLI and G. A. LE PAGE, *Cancer Res.* **18**, 1329 (1958).
77. G. A. LE PAGE, *Cancer Res.* **20**, 403 (1960).
78. G. A. LE PAGE and M. JONES, *Cancer Res.* **21**, 1590 (1961).
79. G. A. LE PAGE, I. G. JUNGA and B. BOWMAN, *Cancer Res.* **24**, 835 (1964).
80. A. R. P. PATERSON, *Can. J. Biochem. Physiol.* **38**, 1117 (1960).
81. A. R. P. PATERSON, *Can. J. Biochem. Physiol.* **40**, 195 (1962).
82. A. R. P. PATERSON and A. HORI, *Can. J. Biochem. Physiol.* **40**, 181 (1962).
83. J. HOCHSTADT-OZER and E. R. STADTMAN, *J. biol. Chem.* **246**, 5304 (1971).
84. J. HOCHSTADT-OZER and E. R. STADTMAN, *J. biol. Chem.* **246**, 5312 (1971).
85. P. J. BENKE, N. HERRICK and A. HERBERT, *Biochem. Med.*, **8**, 309 (1973).
86. S. BIEBER, L. S. DIETRICH, G. B. ELION, G. H. HITCHINGS and D. S. MARTIN, *Cancer Res.* **21**, 228 (1961).
87. J. P. SCANNELL and G. H. HITCHINGS, *Proc. Soc. exp. Biol. Med.* **122**, 627 (1966).
88. L. W. LAW, *Ann. N.Y. Acad. Sci.* **60**, 244 (1954).
89. R. W. BROCKMAN, S. C. SHADDIX, M. WILLIAMS, W. R. LASTER, JR. and F. M. SCHABEL, JR., *Proc. Am. Ass. Cancer Res.* **14**, 16 (1973).
90. D. J. HUTCHISON, *Adv. Cancer Res.* **7**, 235 (1963).
91. D. J. HUTCHISON, *Cancer Res.* **25**, 1581 (1965).

Pp. 119—127, Supplement Number 2, 1974.
Biochemical Pharmacology. Printed in the U.S.A.

CLINICAL RESISTANCE TO ANTIPYRIMIDINE ANTICANCER DRUGS*

THOMAS C. HALL†

Cancer Center and Departments of Medicine and Biochemistry
Los Angeles County – University of Southern California Medical Center
Los Angeles, Calif. 90033, U. S. A.

RESISTANCE to anticancer drugs can be classified as either absolute or relative. Absolute resistance is demonstrated by inactivity of the drug against both normal host tissues and target cancer tissues. The lack of toxicity of methotrexate in the rabbit or of the spindle-fiber poisons in the hamster are examples of species-determined absolute lack of sensitivity to these drugs. In clinical practice, resistance is almost always relative, i.e. it depends upon the degree of increased selective toxicity observed in the target tumor tissues over that induced in normal host tissues. If the degree of toxicity is about equal, then a drug is relatively ineffective, i.e. the tumor cells, having insufficient greater sensitivity to permit a differential drug effect upon them, are called "drug resistant." It is well to keep this clinical relativity in mind, since it might still be possible to deliver such a drug to a localized tumor-bearing area of the body in high concentrations and avoid systemic host toxicity, or to engage in other pharmacologic manipulations designed to maximize drug effect upon tumor.

Clinical resistance can be classified into three subtypes: innate, acquired and collateral. Tumors which have never been exposed to a drug are found not to respond at the first exposure can be considered innately resistant (Table 1). This is by far the

TABLE 1. INNATE CLINICAL RESISTANCE TO ANTIPURINES

Tumor type*	5-FU (%)	Cytarbine (%)
ALL	95	20
AML	95	50
CLL	100	?
Breast	75	90
Colon	75	90
Lung	90	90
Hodgkin's	95	65
Renal cell	95	?

*Abbreviations used: 5-FU, 5-fluorouracil; ALL, acute lymphocytic leukemia; AML, acute myelocytic leukemia; CLL, chronic lymphocytic leukemia.

*Supported in part by NCI Grant CA 11198.
†American Cancer Society Professor of Medicine and Biochemistry.

biggest problem in cancer chemotherapy. Probably the only solution for innate clinical resistance is better drugs. Acquired resistance is observed when a tumor which has been observed initially to respond to a drug, later grows again in the face of continued or intensified drug treatment. Possible implications here are: (1) the tumor may have been heterogeneous with respect to drug sensitivity, with a small residual population of initially resistant cells growing continuously (emergent clone); (2) most or all of the cells were initially sensitive, but their unstable genomes mutated to a resistant phenotype under the pressure of the drug (stepwise resistance); (3) the normal host cells may have become more drug sensitive, thus reducing the relative greater susceptibility of the tumor cell (this has not to my knowledge been described); or (4) the host tissues have developed mechanisms for inactivating the drug and prevented it from reaching and affecting the tumor. However, in almost no instances does one observe the development of resistance by normal host tissues to anitcancer drugs, although the regrowth of hair during continued administration of cyclophosphamide may be an unusual example of this.

Whether innate or acquired, absolute or relative, there are a limited number of general biochemical mechanisms of drug resistance (Table 2). The two clinically most important antipyrimidines today are fluorouracil (FU) and cytarabine (cytosine arabinoside, Ara-C). I will address my remarks to these agents although considerable data are also on hand as to the mechanism of resistance, mostly in animal systems to 6-azauracil and 5-azacytidine.

TABLE 2. MECHANISMS OF DRUG RESISTANCE*

1. Inaccessibility of target site to drug:
   (a) High plasma protein binding – DCM in man
   (b) Rapid excretion – TMT in man
   (c) Host catabolism – hepatic deamination of cytarabine
   (d) Poor plasma membrane transport – methotrexate
2. Lack of anabolism to active nucleotide:
   (a) FU and FUdR; other halopyrimidines
   (b) Ara-C
   (c) 6-AZUR and 5-AZCR
   (d) Antipurines
3. Rapid catabolism:
   (a) Phosphatase – 6-MP
   (b) Deaminase – Ara-C, 8-AG
4. Target of drug is noncritical pathway:
   (a) Target enzyme altered – Thymidylate synthetase
   (b) Alternate pathway used – Thymidine salvage
   (c) Repair processes efficient
   (d) Precursors pile up and break through

*Abbreviations used: DCM, 3′, 5′-dichloromethotrexate; TMT, triamterene; FU, 5-fluorouracil; Ara-C, cytosine arabinoside; 6-AZUR, 6-azauridine; 5-AZCR, 5-azacytidine; 6-MP, 6-mercaptopurine; 8-AG, 8-azaguanine.

Fluorouracil

In animal systems, innately resistant tumors appear to differ from initially sensitive tumors usually in only one or a very few aspects. Thus, it appears that mouse ascites tumors of different FU sensitivities vary largely in the degree of activity of a phosphoribosyltransferase, described by Kasbekar and Greenberg,[1] and later found by Reyes and Hall[2] to catalyze the one-step conversion of FU to FUMP. Figure 1 shows some of the possible mechanisms of resistance to FU. Recent studies in our lab (Fig. 2)

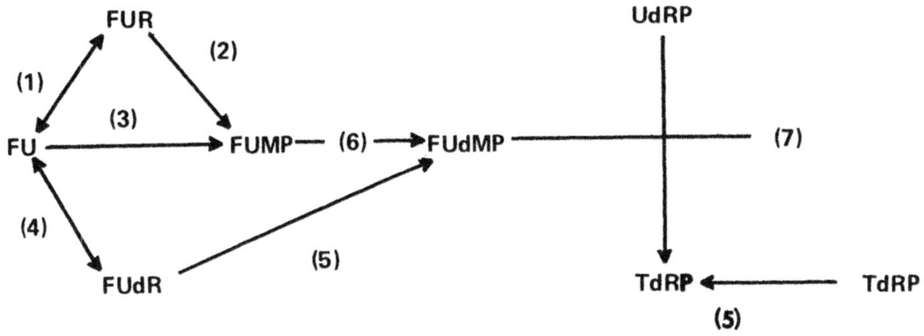

(1)	Uridine phosphorylase	↓Heidelberger, Hall
(2)	Uridine kinase	↓Reichard
(3)	Phosphoribosyltransferase	↓Brockman, Reyes
(4)	Deoxyuridine phosphorylase	↑Burchenal
(5)	Thymidine kinase	↑Kessel
		↓Heidelberger
(6)	Ribonucleotide reductase	→Reichard
(7)	Thymidylate synthetase	△Heidelberger

FIG. 1. Possible mechanisms for fluorouracil resistance.

show that the percentage of human colon tumors with high levels of the enzyme, as compared with adjacent normal tissue, is about the same as the percentage of patients whose tumors respond clinically to FU (25 per cent). Further follow-up studies now in progress should enable us to see whether this is the same 25 per cent. There is evidence that mouse ascites tumors vary in their ability to phosphorylate and utilize preformed thymidine, and that the greater this capacity, as measured by thymidine kinase activity, the less their sensitivity to FU[3] and FUDR.[4] This was not predictable, since this is the same enzyme that phosphorylates FUDR, and high levels of enzyme activity were, therefore, expected by Heidelberger[5] to have the opposite effect. This possibility has been examined in Fig. 3 for human colon and there are differences in enzyme activity of tumor obtained at surgery in the resonse rate to FU. Relative resistance of normal marrow to FUDR, given in doses that sometimes cause the breast cancer of the same host to respond, and the relative resistance of all leukemias to FU and FUDR

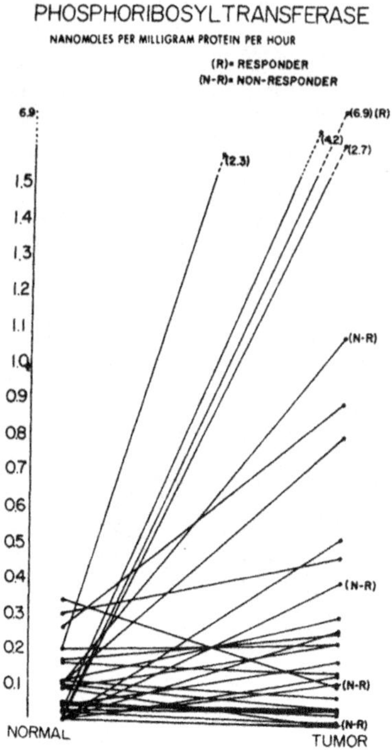

FIG. 2. Phosphoribosyltransferase activity of human colon tumors and adjacent normal tissues.

suggest that bone marrow may differ in some fundamental respect from solid tumors. Such a possibility is outlined on Fig. 4.

It appears that human leukemic and normal white cells may be quite different from human solid tumors and rodent ascites tumors. In hemopoietic malignancy, deletion of both uridine phosphorylase and pyrimidine phosphoribosyltransferase is involved, whereas in the "solid" tumors and rodent ascites the varying activity of the phosphoribosyltransferase is of greatest importance.[6–8]

Patterns of acquired resistance have been more commonly studied in animals and less commonly studied in man. This seems to be due to a number of unfortunate biases of our experimental approaches. The first is the biochemist's habit of comparing drug metabolism in a sensitive tumor and in its derived resistant clone, instead of in a number of differentially sensitive and resistant tumors. The second is the clinician's difficulty in working with human tissue after clinical drug resistance has occurred. It is difficult, but not impossible, to obtain fresh tissue at initial surgery for analysis of differences between patients' tumors relating to initial drug sensitivity. However, in the patients who relapse later, especially in the case of patients with solid tumor, it is difficult to get intravitum or usable post-mortem tissue samples to determine what biochemical changes have accompanied the development of resistance. A final difficulty is the well known impatience, on the part of those concerned with drug development, with mode-of-action studies. Particularly, this is so in the case of ineffective drugs. The

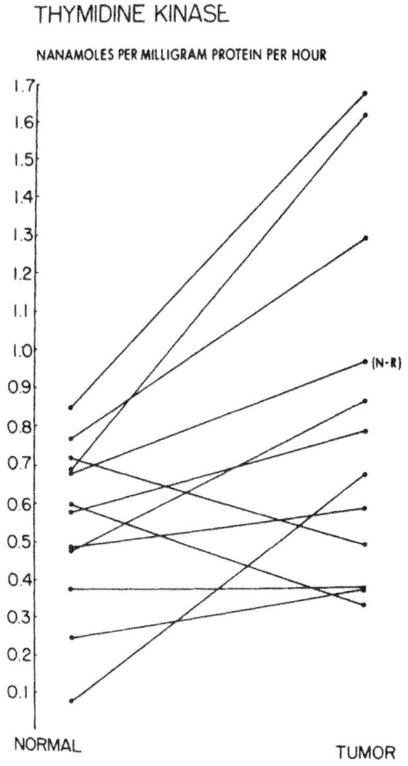

FIG. 3. Thymidine kinase activity of human colon tumors and adjacent normal tissue.

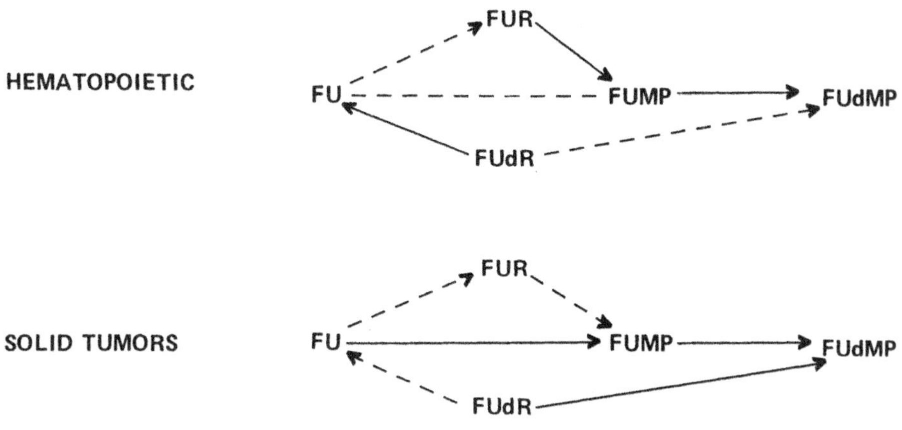

FIG. 4. Differences between hematopoietic and parenchymatous tissue sensitivity to fluorouracil. Therapeutically important, ⟶; therapeutically inoperative, --→.

attitude of, "Let's not spend money on knowing why a drug is no good, let's look for a better drug," is all too prevalent.

We can, however, get some leads regarding acquired FU resistance from the rodent work which may be of help. Reichard *et al.*[9] reported that deletion of uridine kinase occurred as they induced specific resistance to FU. Data from our own laboratories also suggest that increased use of the salvage pathways and loss of the capacity to phosphorylate FU are involved. Such assays have rarely been done in man, but should be done more often.

The problem of defining acquired resistance also seems more difficult than for innate resistance, because acquired resistant tumors seem commonly to express multiple simultaneous biochemical mechanisms. In addition to these, the host may also develop important drug-related changes. Thus, in the case of methotrexate, while innate resistance seems to be based primarily upon differences in cell membrane transport, acquired resistance seems to involve loss of transport into cells, selection of high dihydrofolate reductase (dHFR) clones, use of more thymidine as a DNA precursor, and "induction" of dHFR in normal host tissues. To cover such possibilities adequately, the examination of acquired drug resistance to FU in human colon or breast tissue should involve assay of multiple enzymatic activities, i.e. thymidine kinase, uridine kinase, uridine phosphorylase, phosphoribosyltransferase and thymidylate synthetase.

Cytarabine

Figure 5 shows some of the possible mechanisms for resistance to cytarabine. Innate resistance to cytarabine is also not accompanied by any limitation of transport into the

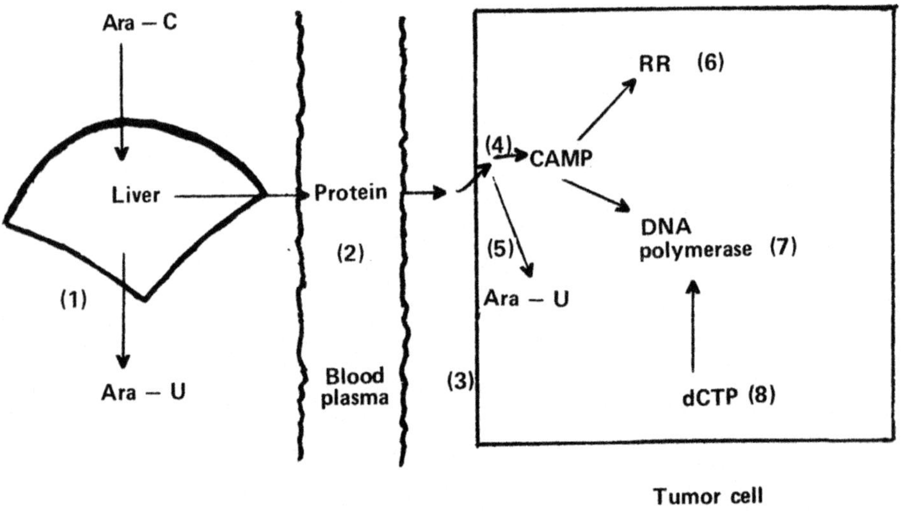

FIG. 5. Possible pathways of resistance to cytarabine. Abbreviations: Ara-C, arabinosylcytosine; Ara-U, arabinosyluridine; CAMP, arabinosylcytosine, 5′-phosphate; dCTP, deoxycytidine triphosphate; RR, ribonucleotide reductase.

cell[10] or plasma protein binding. In a few instances, very short plasma drug half-lives have been described. This suggests that hepatic deamination by the host is important in some cases. If so, pharmacokinetic studies might be of help in determining possible drug sensitivity for some patients. This is noteworthy because repeated studies suggest that it is not worthwhile to study the drug uptake, distribution and blood levels of those antimetabolites which need to be activated by intracellular enzymes. As Dr. Zaharko pointed out, one can extrapolate from mouse to man, but except in the case of a nonmetabolized drug such as methotrexate, the effort is usually not worthwhile.

Phosphorylation and retention of the nucleotide is the primary determinant of innate cytarabine sensitivity.[11] Figure 6 shows that, although the drug can be deaminated by enzymatic action within the cell,[12] the cellular concentration of this

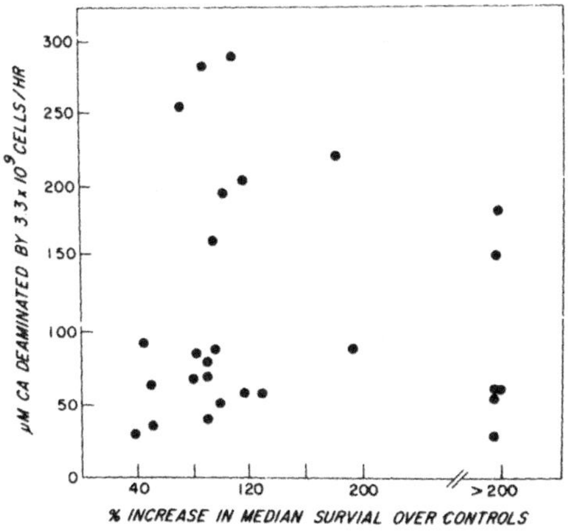

FIG. 6. Drug sensitivity and cytosine arabinoside deamination by mouse ascites tumors.

enzyme in the tumor does not determine resistance in rodent ascites tumors, nor in human cells, as shown in Fig. 7. Several authors have published ratios of cytarabine phosphorylation and deamination without discerning that the differences in ratio they described were largely due to changes in phosphorylation.[13,14] In our studies and in our interpretation of those of Stewart and Burke[14] and of Ho,[13] lack of phosphorylation alone determines innate resistance in leukemia. Insufficient data have been reported on the deoxycytidine kinase levels of solid tumors to determine whether levels of activity of this enzyme are responsible for the marked insensitivity shown by most solid tumors.[15]

Acquired resistance to cytarabine has not been adequately studied. Human leukocyte lines grown *in vitro* in the presence of cytarabine over many generations (courtesy of Dr. George E. Moore) showed no evidence of "induced" deamination. Rodent tumors made resistant to the drug by continuous exposure showed less activity of deoxycytidine kinase. The same was true for initially sensitive patients whose leukemia became resistant to the drug after continued administration. Other possibilities described for non-human systems, which need to be examined in the clinical situation, include resistance based upon an altered deoxycytidine kinase, suggested by Schrecker and Urshell,[16] altered DNA polymerase, hypothesized by Bach,[17] or a

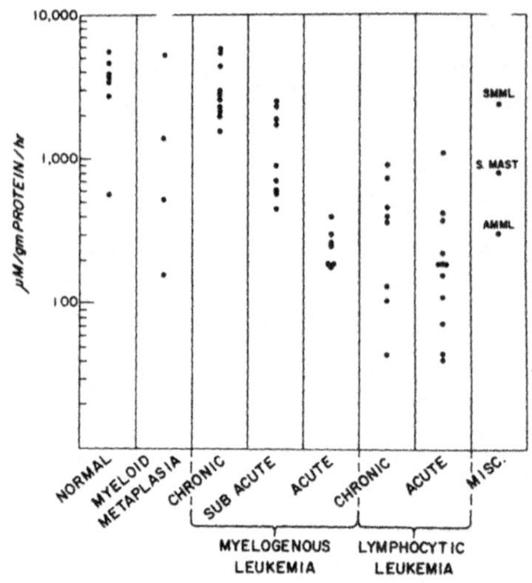

FIG. 7. Cytidine deaminase in human leukocytes.

change in ribonucleoside diphosphate reductase, recently proposed by Momparler *et al.*[18] and by Smith and Chu[19] in a strain of hamster cells *in vitro*.

Clinical pharmacologic attacks on pyrimidine-resistant tumors

If one could examine the untreated tumor and describe the enzymatic drug-handling pattern of each malignancy, it should be possible to select drugs or combinations which would circumvent the innate drug resistance. For example, if there were little uridine phosphorylase, FUR might be an effective drug. Figure 8 shows that it is often

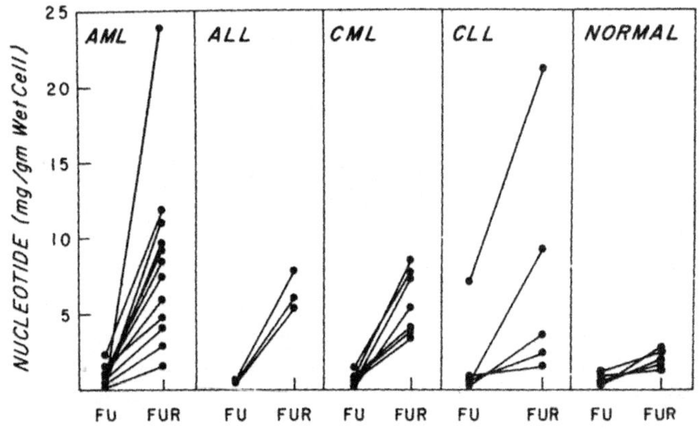

FIG. 8. Nucleotide formation from 5-fluorouracil (FU) and 5-fluorouridine (FUR) by human leukocytes.

phosphorylated better *in vitro* than is FU by human white cells. If there were very low deoxycytidine kinase, a cyclic internal nucleoside of cytarabine might be tried.[20] If radioautography showed only a fraction of the tumor cells to phosphorylate an antimetabolite, then a second drug might affect the other population.

In the case of acquired host deamination of cytarabine, 5-fluorocytarabine might work, since the product would be the highly active 5-fluorouracil arabinoside.* Or, in the few patients in whom a shortened plasma half-life plus persistant cellular phosphorylation of drug could be shown, a trial of tetrahydrouridine[21] could permit cytarabine to travel intact through the plasma to the target cell.

Since the development of acquired resistance depends upon the production of new proteins which act as inducer or repressor molecules, or "induced" enzymes, treatment with drugs which interfere with the translation of such genomal information might be considered for all patients who enter remission. Such drugs might include actinomycin D, puromycin and choloroquin.

In summary, the bases for almost all instances of pyrimidine drug resistance in man are alterations in intracellular drug metabolism, and have little to do with cytokinetics or pharmacokinetics. In most instances, the human phenomena resemble those seen in rodents. Innate drug resistance is commonly based upon a single difference from the sensitive cell, while drug-induced resistance results from multiple biochemical alterations. Knowledge of the biochemical bases for human drug resistance is critical if we are to design more effective drugs and regimens for induction and maintenance of remissions.

*D. Kessel and T. C. Hall, unpublished results.

Acknowledgement – The original data presented here represent fruitful collaboration over the years with Drs. David Kessel, Philip Reyes, Edwin Savlov and DeWayne Roberts.

REFERENCES

1. D. K. KASBEKAR and D. M. GREENBERG, *Cancer Res.* **23**, 818 (1963).
2. P. REYES and T. C. HALL, *Biochem. Pharmac.* **18**, 2589 (1969).
3. D. KESSEL and I. WODINSKY, *Biochim. biophys. Acta* **211**, 88 (1970).
4. D. KESSEL, P. REYES and T. C. HALL, *Med. Pharmac.* **6**, 251 (1970).
5. C. HEIDELBERGER, *A. Rev. Pharmac.* **7**, 101 (1967).
6. T. C. HALL (for the Eastern Cooperative Oncology Group), *J. Am. med. Ass.* **200**, 770 (1967).
7. C. G. MOERTEL, R. J. REITEMEYER and R. G. HAHN, in *Advanced Gastrointestinal Cancer*, pp. 108–18. Harper & Row, New York (1969).
8. D. KESSEL and T. C. HALL, *Biochem. Pharmac.* **16**, 2395 (1967).
9. P. REICHARD, O. SKÖLD, G. KLEIN, L. RÉVÉSZ and P-H. MAGNUSSON, *Cancer Res.* **21**, 110 (1961).
10. D. KESSEL, T. C. HALL and I. WODINSKY, *Science, N.Y.* **156**, 1240 (1967).
11. D. KESSEL, T. C. HALL and D. ROSENTHAL, *Cancer Res.* **29**, 459 (1969).
12. G. W. CAMIENER and C. G. SMITH, *Biochem. Pharmac.* **14**, 1405 (1965).
13. D. H. W. HO, *Proc. Am. Ass. Cancer Res.* 37 (1970).
14. P. J. STEWART and P. J. BURKE, *Nature New Biol.* **242**, 139 (1971).
15. P. J. BURKE (for Eastern Cooperative Oncology Group), *Cancer Res.* **30**, 1512 (1970).
16. A. W. SCHRECKER and M. J. URSCHELL, *Cancer Res.* **28**, 793 (1968).
17. M. K. BACH, *Cancer Res.* **29**, 1036 (1969).
18. R. L. MOMPARLER, M. Y. CHU and G. A. FISCHER, *Biochim. biophys. Acta* **161**, 481 (1968).
19. D. B. SMITH and E. H. Y. CHU, *Cancer Res.* **32**, 1651 (1972).
20. A. HOSHI, F. KANZAWA, K. KURETANI, M. SANEOYOSHI and Y. ARAI, *Gann* **62**, 145 (1971).
21. G. W. CAMIENER, *Biochem. Pharmac.* **17**, 1981 (1968).

Pp. 129—139, Supplement Number 2, 1974.
Biochemical Pharmacology. Printed in the U.S.A.

BIOCHEMICAL AND PHARMACOLOGICAL PRINCIPLES OF COMBINATION CHEMOTHERAPY

ALAN C. SARTORELLI

Department of Pharmacology, Yale University School of Medicine, New Haven, Conn. 06510, U.S.A.

THE USE of combination chemotherapy has added significant dimension to the treatment of neoplasia of man. The selection of mixtures of drugs to employ in combination can be devised and used on the basis of toxicological, kinetic, biochemical and pharmacological considerations. Drugs with different degrees of toxicity to various host tissues can be employed in admixture without reducing the optimal dosage of each so as to intensify toxicity to the neoplastic cell population without significant increase in damage to any single tissue of the host. Thus, cancers which are composed of a variety of cell types of differing sensitivity to chemotherapeutic agents should respond maximally to combinations consisting of drugs of dissimilar mechanism of cytotoxic action. Furthermore, repopulation by a drug-insensitive element following elimination of susceptible cell types should be minimized, since the probability that any given cell in a neoplastic population will spontaneously mutate to acquire resistance simultaneously to two or more active agents is given by the product of the individual mutation frequencies for each of the drugs employed alone.[1] For this reason, the effective use of two or more active drugs on the same tumor would appear to have the potential essentially to eliminate the problem of acquired insensitivity through a random mutation selection process. Kinetic approaches have employed drugs basically in two ways: first, to induce a degree of synchrony in the population of neoplastic cells in an effort to enhance their sensitivity to a second cell-cycle active agent, and second, to stimulate tumor cells present in a resting phase, or G_0, to enter the G_1 compartment where they can be effectively attacked with a second agent.

Of more pertinence to the topic of the present report are approaches in which the selection of agents for use in combination chemotherapy is based upon biochemical and pharmacological considerations. To employ the tools of biochemical pharmacology to develop new combination therapies, it is necessary to understand precisely the mechanism by which known antineoplastic agents inhibit the progression of neoplastic disease. Such information allows certain cellular processes in tumors to be delineated as sites of metabolic vulnerability and thereby earmarks these reactions as likely candidates for a targeted therapeutic attack. Thus, rational drug mixtures can be conceived by capitalizing on: (a) knowledge of the biochemical mechanisms of drug cytotoxicity, and (b) the metabolic parameters required to achieve and sustain the drug-induced critical cellular lesions.[2–4]

For a cytotoxic agent to be effective, there are a number of membrane barriers that must be transversed before an effective concentration can be attained at the "target site or sites" within the neoplastic cell. These are largely membranes from tissues of the gastrointestinal tract, blood cells, the cancer cells themselves and those about various intracellular structures. Selectivity of the membranes of neoplastic cells clearly alters the susceptibility of these cells to growth-inhibitory agents. An example of this phenomenon is provided by the report of Kessel *et al.*[5] which presents evidence that the transport of methotrexate by transplanted murine neoplastic cell lines was a determinant of sensitivity; tumors that transported this agent effectively were quite sensitive to its growth-inhibitory properties, whereas resistant cell lines poorly incorporated the drug. A second interesting example is provided by the acquired insensitivity to actinomycin D by L5178Y cells, which achieve resistance by a decreased permeability to this agent. That decreased permeability might be the result of alterations in the composition of cellular membranes and membrane synthetic machinery was provided by the reports of Kessel and Bosmann[6] and Bosmann.[7] Such findings make it conceivable that changes in active transport mechanisms could be achieved by drug-induced modification of glycoprotein and glycolipid membrane components, thereby increasing the degree of uptake of an effective cytotoxic agent against that neoplastic cell. Such alteration may be attained by treatment of neoplastic cells with an active anticancer agent in combination with a detergent or a solvent, with resultant enhanced cellular uptake. An example of this latter mechanism is provided by the work of Yamada *et al.*[8,9] who reported that rodent hepatoma cells pretreated *in vitro* with Tween 80 had increased sensitivity to nitrogen mustard *N*-oxide; the enhanced susceptibility of these tumor cells was correlated with greater uptake of the alkylating agent.

The greatest probability of success with combination therapy employing an agent to alter the transport of a second cytotoxic drug would appear to be in those cases in which the active inhibitory compound is: (a) so poorly transported that ineffective or only partially effective drug levels can be achieved inside cells, and (b) bound intracellularly and, therefore, would not diffuse outward from cells with altered membranes. It remains to be determined whether such an approach can be employed successfully at the clinical level. The finding that neoplastic cells are antigenically different from their normal counterparts, however, makes it theoretically possible that drugs can be found which alter membrane permeability preferentially in malignant cells.

A good candidate drug for attempted modification of transport by a different mechanism appears to be methotrexate. The findings of Hakala[10] and of Goldman[11] indicate that the transport of this folic acid analog into neoplastic cells is a carrier-mediated process which is characterized by different unidirectional influx and efflux mechanisms. Furthermore, the rate of uptake of methotrexate by transplanted tumors is elevated by substances such as dinitrophenol, azide, antimycin A, oligomycin, iodoacetate and anaerobiasis. The azide-induced increase in the rate of influx of this agent was associated with a rise in both the maximum transport velocity and the influx Michaelis constant. In addition, the efflux of methotrexate was slowed by azide. Although it is unlikely that these toxic agents could find clinical usefulness in combination with methotrexate, their activity encourages the design and synthesis of new agents capable of depressing energy stores, which (a) have less toxicity to the host, and (b) may increase the intracellular concentration of the folic acid antimetabolite. Compounds with these characteristics should be useful in combination with methotrexate against tumor cells that have acquired insensitivity to the folic acid antagonist by virtue of either an altered transport mechanism or a rise in the intracellular levels of the target enzyme dihydrofolate reductase. In the latter situation, difficulty derives from an inability to administer to the patient a quantity of methotrexate sufficient to attain intracellular concentrations capable of binding a significant amount of the increased number of molecules of dihydrofolate reductase.[12]

Knowledge of the biochemical mechanism of action of a tumor inhibitory agent on occasion may allow the use of a second compound to provide a gain in therapeutic index by reducing the toxicity of the cytotoxic agent for normal tissue without appreciably decreasing cancerostatic potency. Leucovorin (folinic acid), a precursor of the end product of the methotrexate-inhibited enzyme dihydrofolate reductase, provides an example of this mechanism. The utilization of this combination in sequence in some instances rescues the host but not the tumor from the toxic effects of methotrexate.[13–17]

Perhaps the best experimental illustration of a gain in therapeutic synergy by a drug combination is provided by the use of cytosine arabinoside in admixture with 6-thioguanine. This combination, which has clinical utility in the treatment of acute myelogenous leukemia,[18] functions to protect the host against the lethal toxicity of 6-thioguanine without decreasing effectiveness against the tumor.[19] The biochemical mechanism for the synergism is visualized as being due to incorporation of 6-thioguanine into the DNA of cancer cells, an event postulated to be necessary for the carcinolytic action of 6-thioguanine, while incorporation of the purine analog into the DNA of the normal tissues of the host is prevented by inhibition of DNA synthesis by cytosine arabinoside. Since cytosine arabinoside interferes with the biosynthesis of DNA in neoplastic as well as normal cells, such a mechanism of necessity requires schedule dependency.[20]

Two additional recent reports of host protection with enhanced antitumor activity which appear to have clinical potential involve use of 1,2-bis(3,5-dioxopiperazin-1-yl)-propane in combination with daunomycin[21] and *N*-acetylcysteine plus isophosphamide[22] to gain enhanced therapeutic efficacy.

Enhanced antitumor activity theoretically can be obtained when one agent either: (a) inhibits the enzymatic destruction of an active cytotoxic compound, or (b) delays the excretion of the tumor-inhibitory agent. The use of an agent that decreases the rate of destruction or excretion of an active cytotoxic compound should theoretically be efficacious only in those instances in which an insufficient concentration of the cytotoxic agent is maintained in the environment of the neoplastic cells. This situation might be expected to occur with a drug that is either rapidly excreted or catabolized or is slowly transported into the neoplastic cells. It is clear, however, that in some situations increased toxicity to the host with a decrease in therapeutic index can occur. An example of enhanced therapeutic efficacy by this mechanism is given in the treatment of the L1210 lymphoma with tetrahydrouridine in combination with cytosine arabinoside.[23] In this instance, tetrahydrouridine serves to inhibit the catabolic enzyme pryrimidine nucleoside deaminase, which converts cytosine arabinoside to the inactive compound uridine arabinoside.

Another means of achieving potentiation of inhibition of neoplastic cell growth by drug combinations involves the use of an agent to enhance the intracellular conversion of a drug to its active tumor-inhibitory form. This type of mechanism is provided by the combination of either 6-mercaptopurine or 6-thioguanine with 6-methylmercaptopurine ribonucleoside, a mixture that causes synergistic inhibition of the growth of several transplanted rodent tumors.[24–27] The mechanism by which this is accomplished requires the conversion of 6-methylmercaptopurine ribonucleoside to its nucleotide form by the enzyme adenosine kinase. The resultant analog nucleotide, through inhibition of phosphoribosylpyrophosphate amidotransferase,[28–30] causes the intracellular accumulation of phosphoribosylpyrophosphate not employed for purine nucleotide biosynthesis.[31,32] The spared phosphoribosylpyrophosphate is then utilized in part to increase the quantity of 6-thiopurine converted to its active nucleotide form. In addition, 6-methylmercaptopurine ribonucleotide appears to protect 6-thio-GMP formed from 6-thioguanine by metabolic degradation, perhaps by serving as an alternate substrate for catabolic enzymes.[32]

Modification of tissue storage or protein binding of a carcinostatic agent by a second drug conceivably could alter therapeutic potency. Methotrexate provides an example of a compound that is bound to plasma proteins with about 50 per cent of the drug present in the plasma being bound to albumin;[33,34] such binding in theory limits the effective blood concentration of these drugs. Commonly used weak organic acids such as salicylate displace methotrexate from its plasma albumin binding sites. Although it is most unlikely that displacement of methotrexate by a second drug would influence the therapeutic efficacy of this agent, it is conceivable that a more tightly bound cytotoxic compound could gain enhanced or decreased therapeutic potency through such displacement.

The selection of drugs for use in combination chemotherapy may be made solely on the basis of biochemical considerations. This approach generally envisions the use of two or more agents to attain more complete interference with some metabolic process critical to survival in each susceptible cell of a neoplastic population than can be achieved with any of the drugs employed alone. The mixture of agents can be directed at the same receptor or enzyme, or at different target sites of either close or distant biochemical relationship within the cancer cell. Although the aim of employing two or more chemical agents usually involves the attainment of more complete blockade of a functional process, a variety of responses are possible when two agents act on a single site, provided that the compounds are not bound to the target interdependently and are causing only competitive or noncompetitive inhibition. If both inhibitors are competitive with respect to the same enzymatic molecule, they will both presumably occupy the same binding site and, therefore, compete for this site. Two equally potent competitive inhibitors should, therefore, produce an effect equivalent to the activity of the same number of total molecules of either drug when employed alone; however, if one of these agents is less effective than the other, a degree of antagonism will occur. Two noncompetitive inhibitors presumably react at different areas on the target enzyme potentially to result in either enhancement or antagonism of inhibitory potency. In addition, one agent may be competitive and the other noncompetitive with respect to a given enzymatic substrate; in this case, the drugs react at different loci on the target enzyme and either an enhanced or antagonistic action can be produced.

Two or more chemical agents may bind to the target enzyme interdependently. This implies that the binding of these agents is enhanced by the presence of the other. Such interdependent binding may obviously result in either a more or less effective inhibition of catalytic activity. Finally, two inhibitors may react with each other to form a new species with an altered potency. A theoretical approach to the direction of a multi-inhibitor attack on a single enzyme has been discussed.[4] In a hypothetical model, a therapeutic assault directed against phosphoribosylpyrophosphate amidotransferase, the catalyst for the initial step in the *de novo* biosynthetic pathway for purine nucleotides, was visualized by two agents simultaneously occupying the separate inhibitory regulatory sites on the enzyme molecule for AMP and for GMP or IMP. Since the carcinostatic 6-thiopurines, after activation to the nucleotide level, inhibit the activity of this enzyme by occupation of the IMP–GMP site, it is theoretically possible to enhance the inhibitory potency of the 6-thiopurines against this target by the simultaneous use of an adenine analog capable to being converted to a nucleotide.

Another potential combination directed against a single site may be provided by the metaphase-arresting drugs, colchicine and vinblastine, which mutually potentiate their binding to the microtubule subunit protein.[35]

The most common mechanism of action for two or more drugs in combination is that they act upon different target sites within the neoplastic cells. Within this context, several theoretical approaches to the development of synergistic drug combinations have been proposed. The concept of "sequential blockade" was conceived by Potter;[36] this approach employs two or more inhibitors to interfere with the activities of different enzymes of a limited portion of a multi-enzyme sequence (Fig. 1). The

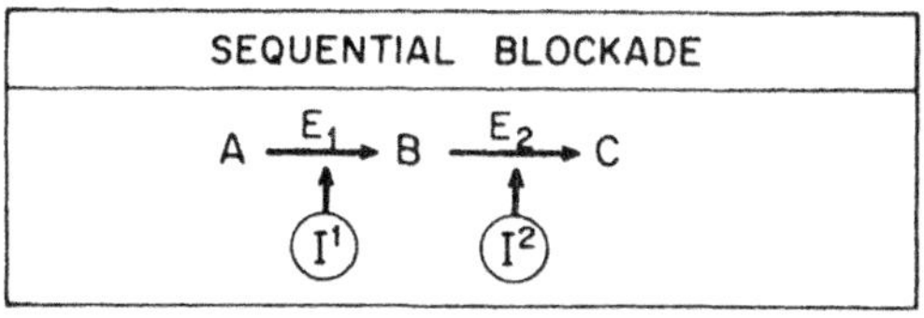

FIG. 1. Schematic mechanism of sequential inhibition (from A. C. Sartorelli, *Cancer Res.* **29**, 2292, 1969).

kinetics of sequential inhibition have been discussed in a number of publications.[37–39] The formation of the end product C in such a sequence is dependent on the slowest reaction or, in a steady state, on the initial step in the metabolic sequence. Interference with the limiting enzymatic reaction results in a decrease in the amount of end product C which is formed; a further decrease in the amount of end product produced does not take place upon addition of a second drug until the quantity of this agent makes the second enzyme rate limiting. The degree of over-all inhibition of the multi-enzyme sequence at this time becomes independent of the inhibitory action of the first compound.[38,39] When noncompetitive or irreversible inhibitors are used, enhanced inhibition of the formation of end product C is impossible; however, with competitive inhibitors, the susceptibility of enzyme E_2, made rate limiting by inhibitor I^2 employed alone, will be decreased in time by the resultant accumulation of intermediate B, which would compete with I^2 to decrease the inhibition at this enzymatic step. In such a situation, inhibition of E_1 by a second drug which does not render this enzymatic step rate limiting would diminish the rate of accumulation of intermediate B and thereby enhance the degree of inhibition of this pathway. These theoretical situations are valid only in a closed system from which the substrates, intermediates and inhibitors cannot escape, and they pertain primarily to steady state conditions. Black,[37] using a mathematical model, has demonstrated that the combined effect of two drugs acting by sequential blockade is synergistic when the enzyme concentration either approximately equals or greatly exceeds that of the inhibitor and the substrate. Although the concentration of inhibitors in most experimental situations would be expected to exceed that of the target enzyme, it seems reasonable to assume that the converse will occur at the onset and termination of inhibition processes, when the concentration of inhibitors at the target enzyme site *in situ* might be expected to be relatively small. In this instance, the duration of interference of a given metabolic sequence might be extended to a degree that prevents the survival of neoplastic cells.

The use of cytosine arabinoside, an inhibitor of DNA polymerase following conversion to the triphosphate level, in combination with either guanazole, hydroxyurea, or 2-formylpyridine thiosemicarbazone, agents which interfere with the activity of ribonucleoside diphosphate reductase, can be considered to be examples of the sequential inhibition of the synthesis of DNA. Such combinations of cytosine arabinoside in admixture with an inhibitor of the enzyme ribonucleoside diphosphate reductase cause synergistic inhibition of the growth of the L1210 lymphoma.[40]

The action of 6-thioguanine on purine nucleotide biosynthesis provides what may be considered to be another example of sequential blockade produced by a single agent used alone.[41] 6-Thioguanine, following conversion to its active inhibitory nucleotide form, interferes with the activities of phosphoribosylpyrophosphate amidotransferase, inosine 5′-phosphate dehydrogenase and ATP:GMP phosphotransferase. Such sequential blockade has been envisioned to produce a marked decrease in the intracellular concentration of guanine nucleotides, which leads to a decrease in the rate of synthesis of RNA and DNA and of the activities of a variety of enzymatic reactions that utilize GTP as a coenzyme. The contribution of sequential blockade of guanine nucleotide biosynthesis by this 6-thiopurine to the ultimate death of the neoplastic cells is unknown.

The theory of "concurrent inhibition," shown in Fig. 2, was suggested by Elion *et al.*[42] Concurrent blockade refers to the action of two or more inhibitors that interfere with alternate metabolic pathways capable of producing a given metabolite critical for cell survival. The rate of formation of end product C from two alternate routes is the sum of the reactions catalyzed by enzymes E_1 and E_2 in Fig. 2. It is difficult to envision how two agents that inhibit alternate metabolic pathways to the same end product create a decrease in the concentration of end product that is greater than the sum of the individual inhibitions produced by each of the two drugs, when the considerations are based solely on the predicted kinetic behavior of isolated enzyme systems. However, since these kinetic considerations ignore the subsequent

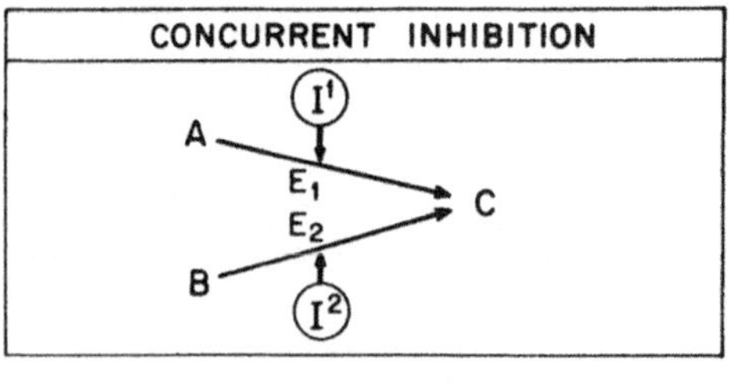

FIG. 2. Schematic mechanism of concurrent inhibition (from A. C. Sartorelli, *Cancer Res.* **29**, 2292, 1969).

metabolic disposition of the end product, they are not necessarily predictive of synergism in the biological sense, which results from a degree of depletion of a metabolite that is incompatible with cell survival. No unequivocal examples of this type of mechanism appear to exist in the literature.

The conceptual attack in both sequential and concurrent blockade is directed at the enzymatic level. The concept of "complementary inhibition"[3,4,43–45] envisions the use of two or more agents to cause damage to selected macromolecular targets (Fig. 3).

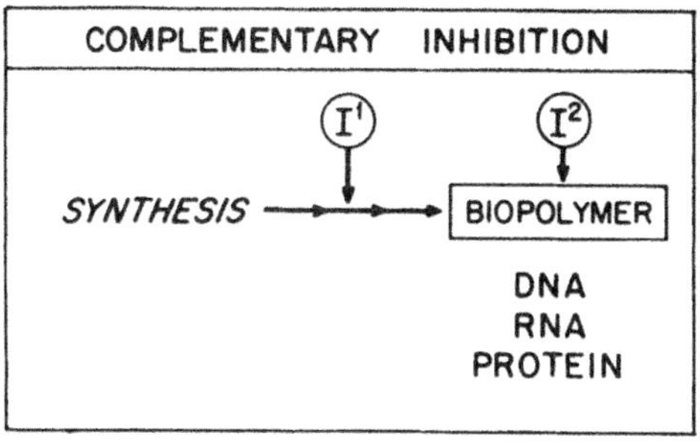

FIG. 3. Schematic mechanism of complementary inhibition (from A. C. Sartorelli, *Cancer Res.* **29**, 2292, 1969).

In this approach, one drug is used to alter the structure of the polymeric target, either directly through interaction or indirectly by modifying intermediary metabolism, in combination with another agent which functions to decrease the availability of the direct precursor molecules by enzymatic inhibition. Complementary therapeutic assault should, thereby, provide more complete inhibition of either the synthesis of biochemical function of the target molecules in neoplastic cells only minimally damaged by either of the chemotherapeutic agents alone, and also delay the cellular repair of drug-induced damage to the targeted macromolecular structures. A number of synergistic drug combinations can be considered to be models of complementary inhibition, with a metabolic assault being directed at the levels of either DNA, RNA or protein (Table 1). At the level of DNA, several examples of complementary inhibition are

TABLE 1. COMPLEMENTARY INHIBITION DIRECTED AT THE LEVEL OF DNA AND RNA

Macromolecule	Therapeutic attack		
	Polymer level	Intermediate	Precursor level
DNA	Nitrogen mustards BCNU, CCNU* Mitomycin C	6-Thioguanine Cytosine arabinoside	5-Fluorouracil Guanazole Hydroxyurea Heterocyclic thiosemicarbazones
RNA	Ribonuclease		Actinomycin D

*Abbreviations used: BCNU, 1,3-bis(2-chloroethyl)-1-nitrosourea; CCNU, 1-(2-chloroethyl)-3-cyclohexyl-1-nitrosourea.

available. Studies employed have primarily utilized nitrogen mustards, nitrosoureas or other alkylating agents to damage DNA templates, that is to function at the polymer level. However, other classes of drugs that bind to DNA, such as the acridines, which distort by intercalation the structure of these molecules and consequently their function as templates in replication and transcription, theoretically should also be potentially useful in admixture with agents capable of creating biochemical lesions in the pathways involved in the fabrication and utilization of the deoxyribonucleoside triphosphate precursors of DNA.[3,43–47] Compounds such as mitomycin C, an antibiotic with the potential to cross-link complementary strands of the DNA double helix,[48,49] uracil mustard, 1,3,-bis(2-chloroethyl)-1-nitrosourea (BCNU) and 1-(2-chloroethyl)-3-cyclohexyl-1-nitrosourea (CCNU), an alkylating agent, and nitrosourea derivatives with similar ability, have caused synergistic inhibition of tumor growth when employed in combination with certain antimetabolites possessing the ability to limit the availability of deoxyribonucleoside triphosphates for replication of DNA. Some of the antimetabolites employed include: (a) 5-fluorouracil, which inhibits thymidylate synthetase after conversion to a deoxyribonucleotide;[50] (b) cytosine arabinoside, which inhibits DNA polymerase following conversion to the triphosphate level;[51,52] and (c) 6-thioguanine, which functions at the nucleotide level to limit the formation of guanine nucleotides by sequential blockade of purine nucleotide biosynthesis.[41] Since 6-thioguanine is incorporated into DNA,[53] it can conceivably also act at this level and, therefore, is one of several agents (i.e. cytosine arabinoside and 5-iodo-2′-deoxyuridine) which may be considered to be of an intermediate nature in that they can act at both the polymer and precursor levels. The conceptual visualization of more complete inhibition of the replication of DNA in neoplastic cells by the use of agents that modify the structure of these macromolecules and thereby interfere with template function in replicative reactions, in combination with drugs which interfere with the synthesis of DNA by limiting the availability of the deoxyribonucleoside triphosphate precursors as the explanation of the potent antitumor activity of such drug mixtures would seem to be an oversimplification, in view of the complexities involved in replicative processes. The use of such a concept, however, has enabled the prediction of several drug combinations with synergistic potency in experimental animal tumor systems.

The concept of complementary inhibition has been employed at the level of RNA using the combination of actinomycin D and ribonuclease which cause synergistic inhibition of the growth of Sarcoma 180.[43] Actinomycin D was theorized to function in this admixture by inhibiting the synthesis of new molecules of RNA, and ribonuclease to destroy those molecules of pre-existing RNA which might be conserved and utilized for cell survival. Measurement of the total RNA content of tumor cells treated with these two agents indicated that the cellular content of RNA was markedly depleted by the combination.[43]

The combination treatment of animal tumors with L-asparaginase and the glutamine antagonist 6-diazo-5-oxo-L-norleucine[54] provides what might be considered an example of complementary inhibition directed against the synthesis of protein. The mixture of these two agents appears to function to inhibit synergistically the growth of transplanted animal tumors by reducing the asparagine pool in neoplastic cells. The L-asparaginase limits the external supply of asparagine to neoplastic cells by reducing blood levels of this amino acid, and the 6-diazo-5-oxo-L-norleucine apparently acts by direct inhibition of asparagine synthetase present in tumor cells or in adjacent normal cells which serve locally to feed malignant cells. This model is complicated by the fact that the glutamine antagonist also reduces intracellular pools of ATP, a substrate of asparagine synthetase, which may further serve to augment the induced deficiency of asparagine. A perhaps clearer example of a directed synergistic attack on the metabolic pool of asparagine is provided by the synergistic combination against animal tumors[55] of L-asparaginase and 5-chloro-4-oxo-2-aminopentanoic acid, a relatively potent inhibitor of asparagine synthetase.[56]

An additional concept (Fig. 4) which might be of use in the development of active antineoplastic agents is exemplified by an attempt to use to therapeutic advantage the transcriptional and translational errors induced by point mutations, caused by agents such as ethyl methanesulfonate and *N*-methyl-*N*′-nitroso-*N*-nitroguanidine, or by the frame shift mutations of the acridines. This concept which might be termed "error amplification" envisions the magnification of genomic lesions by the use of an agent such as 5-fluoro-2′-deoxyuridine to create a deficiency of thymine deoxyribonucleotides. The combination of certain mutagens with drugs that cause a deficiency of thymine deoxyribonucleotides should result in a minimization of metabolic repair with continued synthesis of RNA and protein. This situation could lead to multiple copies of messenger RNA with the potential to miscode. Thus, the consequences of a drug-induced change of a single base or base pair conceivably can be amplified to render cellular repair mechanisms more difficult and presumably reduce cell survival.

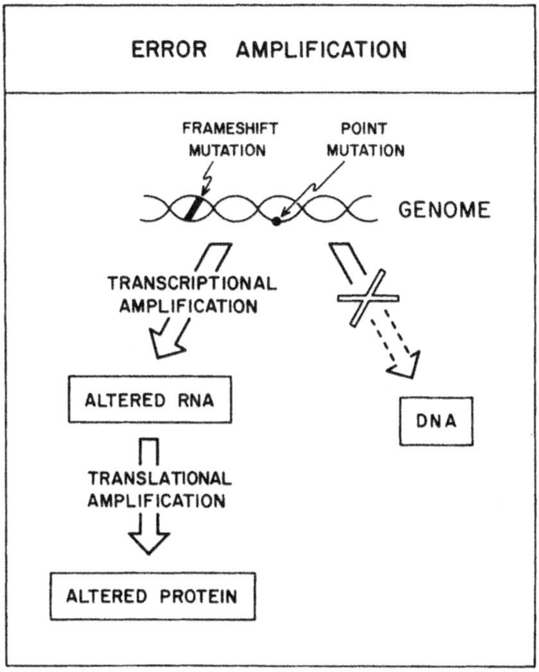

FIG. 4. Schematic mechanism of error amplification.

Although a variety of drug mixtures have produced potent antitumor effects against tumors of man, the use of biochemical and pharmacological approaches to seek new and potent therapies has been little explored and, therefore, has contributed minimally to the therapeutic management of cancer in man. The diversity of alternate metabolic routes which must be interfered with simultaneously in order to alter significantly the economy of the cancer cell argues for the use of combination chemotherapy, as does the knowledge that the selection of drug-resistant variants becomes much lower in the presence of two or more agents with significant inhibitory activity. Therefore, the search for new drug combinations with synergistic potency against tumors without enhanced host toxicity is an important avenue for therapeutic development. The selection of drugs to be employed in combination obviously cannot be carried out on a random basis; drug mixtures can, however, be selected on the basis of biochemical knowledge of the mechanism of action of each agent, as well as from a knowledge of the pharmacological properties which dictate cellular uptake, interaction with target receptors and rates of metabolism and drug clearance. It is important, therefore, that oncologists with biochemical and pharmacological orientation address themselves to an understanding of the parameters of drug action and that these factors be employed in the development of synergistic drug combinations with clinical potential.

REFERENCES

1. E. FREI, III and E. J. FREIREICH, in *Advances in Chemotherapy* (Eds. A. GOLDIN, F. HAWKING and R. J. SCHNITZER), Vol. 2, p. 269. Academic Press, New York (1965).
2. J. M. VENDITTI and A. GOLDIN, in *Advances in Chemotherapy* (Eds. A. GOLDIN and F. HAWKING), Vol. 1, p. 397. Academic Press, New York (1964).
3. A. C. SARTORELLI, in *Progress in Experimental Tumor Research* (Ed. F. HOMBURGER), Vol. 6, p. 228. S. Karger, Basel (1965).
4. A. C. SARTORELLI, *Cancer Res.* **29**, 2292 (1969).
5. D. KESSEL, T. C. HALL, D. W. ROBERTS and I. WODINSKY, *Science, N.Y.* **150**, 752 (1965).
6. D. KESSEL and H. B. BOSMANN, *Cancer Res.* **30**, 2695 (1970).
7. H. B. BOSMANN, *Nature, Lond.* **233**, 566 (1971).
8. T. YAMADA and Y. IWANAMI, *Gann* **53**, 225 (1962).
9. T. YAMADA and T. BABA, *Gann* **54**, 171 (1963).
10. M. T. HAKALA, *Biochim. biophys. Acta* **102**, 210 (1965).
11. I. D. GOLDMAN, *J. biol. Chem.* **244**, 3779 (1969).
12. A. C. SARTORELLI, B. A. BOOTH and J. R. BERTINO, *Archs Biochem. Biophys.* **108**, 53 (1964).
13. J. A. R. MEAD, J. M. VENDITTI, A. W. SCHRECKER, A. GOLDIN and J. C. KERESZTESY, *Biochem. Pharmac.* **12**, 371 (1963).
14. A. GOLDIN, J. M. VENDITTI, I. KLINE and N. MANTEL, *Nature, Lond.* **212**, 1548 (1966).
15. R. D. SULLIVAN, E. MILLER and M. P. SIKES, *Cancer, N.Y.* **12**, 1248 (1959).
16. E. LEFKOWITZ, R. J. PAPAC and J. R. BERTINO, *Cancer Chemother. Rep.* **51**, 305 (1967).
17. W. M. HRYNIUK and J. R. BERTINO, *J. clin. Invest.* **48**, 2140 (1969).
18. T. S. GEE, K.-P. YU, B. T. AUGUSTIN, I. H. KRAKOFF and B. D. CLARKSON, *Cancer, N.Y.* **23**, 1019 (1969).
19. L. H. SCHMIDT, J. A. MONTGOMERY, W. R. LASTER, JR. and F. M. SCHABEL, JR., *Proc. Am. Ass. Cancer Res.* **11**, 70 (1970).
20. G. A. LEPAGE and T. KANEKO, *Cancer Res.* **29**, 2314 (1969).
21. R. J. WOODMAN, I. KLINE and J. M. VENDITTI, *Proc. Am. Ass. Cancer Res.* **13**, 31 (1972).
22. I. KLINE, M. GANG and J. M. VENDITTI, *Proc. Am. Ass. Cancer Res.* **13**, 29 (1972).
23. G. L. NEIL, T. E. MOXLEY and R. C. MANAK, *Cancer Res.* **30**, 2166 (1970).
24. F. M. SCHABEL, JR., W. R. LASTER, JR. and H. E. SKIPPER, *Cancer Chemother. Rep.* **51**, 111 (1967).
25. M. C. WANG, A. I. SIMPSON and A. R. P. PATERSON, *Cancer Chemother. Rep.* **51**, 101 (1967).

26. A. R. P. PATERSON and A. MORIWAKI, *Cancer Res.* **29**, 681 (1969).
27. E. M. SCHOLAR, P. R. BROWN and R. E. PARKS, JR., *Cancer Res.* **32**, 259 (1972).
28. J. F. HENDERSON, *Biochem. Pharmac.* **12**, 551 (1963).
29. J. F. HENDERSON, I. C. CALDWELL and A. R. P. PATERSON, *Cancer Res.* **27**, 1773 (1967).
30. D. L. HILL and L. L. BENNETT, JR., *Biochemistry, N.Y.* **8**, 122 (1969).
31. A. R. P. PATERSON and M. C. WANG, *Cancer Res.* **30**, 2379 (1970).
32. J. A. NELSON and R. E. PARKS, JR., *Cancer Res.* **32**, 2034 (1972).
33. E. S. HENDERSON, R. H. ADAMSON and V. T. OLIVERIO, *Cancer Res.* **25**, 1018 (1965).
34. R. L. DIXON, E. S. HENDERSON and D. P. RALL, *Fedn Proc.* **24**, 454 (1965).
35. W. A. CREASEY, in *Handbook of Experimental Pharmacology* (Eds. A. C. SARTORELLI and D. G. JOHNS), Springer, Berlin (1974).
36. V. R. POTTER, *Proc. Soc. exp. Biol. Med.* **76**, 41 (1951).
37. M. L. BLACK, *J. med. chem.* **6**, 145 (1963).
38. R. E. HANDSCHUMACHER, *Cancer Res.* **25**, 1541 (1965).
39. J. L. WEBB, *Enzyme and Metabolic Inhibitors*, Vol. 1, p. 949. Academic Press, New York (1963).
40. F. M. SCHABEL, JR., W. R. LASTER, JR. and M. W. TRADER, *Proc. Am. Ass. Cancer Res.* **12**, 67 (1971).
41. R. P. MIECH, R. E. PARKS, JR., J. H. ANDERSON, JR. and A. C. SARTORELLI, *Biochem. Pharmac.* **16**, 2221 (1967).
42. G. B. ELION, S. SINGER and G. H. HITCHINGS, *J. biol. Chem.* **208**, 477 (1954).
43. A. C. SARTORELLI, *Nature, Lond.* **203**, 887 (1964).
44. A. C. SARTORELLI and B. A. BOOTH, *Cancer Res.* **25**, 1393 (1965).
45. A. C. SARTORELLI and B. A. BOOTH, *Cancer Res.* **27**, 1614 (1967).
46. F. M. SCHABEL, JR., in *The Proliferation and Spread of Neoplastic Cells*, pp. 379–408. Williams & Wilkins, Baltimore (1968).
47. F. M. SCHABEL, JR., in *Pharmacological Principles in Antitumor Chemotherapy* (Eds. T. C. HALL and K. KARRER), pp. 65–82. Wiener Medizinischen Akademie, Vienna (1968).
48. V N. IYER and W. SZYBALSKI, *Proc. natn. Acad. Sci. U.S.A.* **50**, 355 (1963).
49. I. MATSUMOTO and K. G. LARK, *Expl Cell Res.* **32**, 192 (1963).
50. C. HEIDELBERGER, *Expl Cell Res.* **9**, (suppl.) 462 (1963).
51. J. J. FURTH and S. S. COHEN, *Cancer Res.* **28**, 2061 (1968).
52. A. P. KIMBALL and M. J. WILSON, *Proc. Soc. expl. Biol. Med.* **127**, 429 (1968).
53. G. A. LEPAGE, *Cancer Res.* **20**, 403 (1960).
54. G. S. TARNOWSKI, I. M. MOUNTAIN and C. C. STOCK, *Cancer Res.* **30**, 1118 (1970).
55. J. H. BURCHENAL, B. D. CLARKSON, M. D. DOWLING, JR., T. GEE, M. HOGHBIN and C. T. C. TAN, *Int. Symp. on L-Asparaginase*, pp. 243–251, Paris (1971).
56. T. C. CHOU and R. E. HANDSCHUMACHER, *Biochem. Pharmac.* **21**, 39 (1972).

Pp. 141–150, Supplement Number 2, 1974.
Biochemical Pharmacology. Printed in the U.S.A.

THERAPEUTIC SYNERGISM IN ANIMAL MODELS – INCREASED ANTITUMOR SPECIFICITY RESULTING FROM DIMINISHED TOXICITY FOR THE HOST

JOHN M. VENDITTI and ABRAHAM GOLDIN

Drug Research and Development, Division of Cancer Treatment
National Cancer Institute, Bethesda, Md. 20014, U.S.A.

THERE IS abundant evidence, at both the clinical and preclinical levels, that a combination of antitumor drugs may provide a more effective therapy than the inidividual drugs.[1] This has stimulated further preclinical investigations of new and potentially even more effective combined modalities of treatment. It is the responsibility of the preclinical investigator not only to discover more effective therapies, but also to investigate the optimal conditions for their usage and the underlying mechanisms leading to improved therapy.

In previously published reviews of the combination chemotherapy of neoplasia,[2,3] we made the point that different investigators used varying definitions of drug synergism and that, in many instances, synergism could be demonstrated in accordance with the investigator's definition. Such definitions were often derived from and applied to studies *in vitro* or to studies *in vivo* in which improved therapy was not the principal criterion of effectiveness. Our own view was that, if synergism indicated the cooperative action of agents to produce some beneficial therapeutic effect that could not be achieved with either of the individual drugs, then we should feel free to define the improved therapy as therapeutic synergism.[4,5]

A basic factor that influences the antitumor efficacy of combination therapy and individual drug treatment alike is the limitation imposed by toxicity for the host. For combinations of antitumor drugs, increased selective destruction of tumor cells leading to superior therapeutic results may be attained when the sum of the individual drug effects against the tumor is greater than the sum of their effects against the host. Thus, one advantage of combination chemotherapy may reside in some reduction in the limitation of host toxicity, particularly when the drugs exert their respective cytotoxic actions via different mechanisms. Conceptually, one might expect therapeutic synergism when two antitumor drugs cooperate in a manner such that each retains its full effect against the tumor while their toxicities are less than completely additive, or when each retains its full effect against the tumor while one actually protects the host against the toxicity of the other. Therapeutic synergism might also be attained when an agent without antitumor action *per se* diminishes the host toxicity of an active antitumor drug without diminishing its capacity to destroy tumor cells. The data to be presented were selected to provide a few notable examples of such effects in the treatment of leukemia L1210 in mice. Unless noted otherwise, DBF_1 or CDF_1 hybrid mice were implanted i.p. with 10^5 L1210 cells on Day 0 and treated i.p.‡

In 1968, Schabel *et al.*[6] reported the enhanced effectiveness of daunomycin plus 6-mercaptopurine against leukemia L1210 (Table 1). The inclusion of parallel groups of nonleukemic mice in this experiment contributed importantly to the interpretation of the results. Daunomycin alone was only moderately effective in the leukemic mice and produced a 44 per cent increase in median lifespan over controls (ILS) at each of three daily dosage levels. This moderate activity and the flat dose-response curve are typical for daily treatment of L1210 with daunomycin. It is noteworthy that substantially the same therapeutic effect in leukemic mice was achieved at doses which ranged from nonlethal to frankly lethal. 6-Mercaptopurine (6-MP), the more effective of the individual drugs, elicited a 75 per cent ILS at its optimal antileukemic dose, 70 mg/kg/day. However, this dosage of 6-MP alone was lethal to four of ten normal mice. While there was an atypical inversion in the antileukemic dose response for 6-MP, the drug clearly retained highly significant activity at a number of nonlethal dosage levels. It was estimated, from this and similar experiments, that the *q.d.* × 15 LD_{10} dose for 6-MP was about 60 mg/kg, and for daunomycin about 1.0 mg/kg. The maximum ILS (175 per cent) was observed with the combination of 1.5 mg/kg of daunomycin plus 50 mg/kg of 6-MP, although a number of other combination dosages produced a minimal number of long-term survivors. Each of nine combination dosage

TABLE 1. ENHANCED EFFECTIVENESS OF DAUNOMYCIN (DAU) PLUS 6-MERCAPTOPURINE (6-MP) AGAINST LEUKEMIA L1210*

Daily dose (mg/kg-i.p., days 1–15)		Median survival time L1210 (i.p.)			Normal S/T (day 45)		
Dau	6-MP	Dau (days)	6-MP (days)	Comb. (days)	Dau	6-MP	Comb.
2.0	30	11.5	11.0	17.0	1/10	10/10	4/10
1.5	30	11.5	11.0	19.5	5/10	10/10	10/10
1.0	30	11.5	11.0	17.0	10/10	10/10	10/10
2.0	40	11.5	13.0	16.0	1/10	10/10	0/10
1.5	40	11.5	13.0	19.0(1/10)†	5/10	10/10	10/10
1.0	40	11.5	13.0	19.0(1/10)	10/10	10/10	10/10
1.5	50	11.5	11.5	22.0	5/10	10/10	8/10
1.0	50	11.5	11.5	16.0(1/10)	10/10	10/10	10/10
1.0	60	11.5	12.0	19.0	10/10	10/10	7/10
	70		14.0			6/10	
Controls		(8.0)			(10/10)		

*See Ref. 6.
†Survivors/total.

‡In recent years, the Division of Cancer Treatment (DCT), NCI has placed increased emphasis on studies of combinations of therapeutic modalities. Most of the examples included in this presentation were found in two of DCT's contract laboratories by Dr. F. M. Schabel, Jr. and his colleagues at the Southern Research Institute, Birmingham, Ala., and Dr. I. Kline and his colleagues at Microbiological Associates, Inc., Bethesda, Md.

levels was more effective than any of the individual drug doses. Examination of the normal mouse lethality indicates that, when the 6-MP dosage was at the nonlethal level of 50 mg/kg or less, the combination was not more toxic and, in most cases, was less toxic than daunomycin alone.

The combination of cytosine arabinoside (Ara-C) and 6-thioguanine (6-TG) provides a definitive example in which two antitumor agents cooperate to provide therapeutic synergism by virtue of the ability of one to protect against the host toxicity of the other, with no apparent loss of either's ability to destroy tumor cells. LePage and Kaneko[7] found that, under specific conditions, Ara-C blocked the incorporation of 6-TG into DNA, and they proposed treatment with the combination of Ara-C plus 6-TG as an effective means of reducing toxicity without sacrificing antitumor efficacy. Subsequently, Schmidt *et al.*[8] demonstrated the antileukemic superiority of this combination over the individual drugs against L1210, also under very specific conditions of treatment scheduling; they also demonstrated the ability of Ara-C to protect against the toxicity of 6-TG.

The data summarized in Table 2 show the protection by Ara-C against the lethal toxicity of 6-TG in normal mice. When given *q.* 3 hr × 8 on every fourth day × 4,

TABLE 2. PROTECTION BY CYTOSINE ARABINOSIDE (ARA-C) AGAINST LETHALITY OF 6-THIOGUANINE (6-TG) IN NORMAL MICE*

6-TG (mg/kg/injection†	Ara-C (mg/kg/injection)† 0	0.47	0.94	1.88	3.75	7.5	15
	(No. of survivors/total)						
0	39/40	10/10	10/10	10/10	10/10	10/10	10/10
0.45	7/7	10/10	10/10	10/10	9/9	10/10	9/10
0.90	0/10	9/10	9/10	10/10	10/10	10/10	10/10
1.35	1/10	1/10	9/10	9/9	10/10	8/10	9/10
1.80	0/10	0/10	0/10	3/10	3/10	4/10	0/10

*See Ref. 8.
†Treatment *q.* 3 hr/24 hr days 1, 5, 9, 13.

Ara-C alone was not lethal at doses up to and including 15 mg/kg/injection. This is close to the LD_{10} dose of Ara-C on this treatment schedule. The LD_{10} dose of 6-TG alone on this treatment schedule may be estimated at between 0.45 and 0.90 mg/kg/injection. It is clear that the toxicity of these agents, when combined in this way, is less than additive and that Ara-C at less than LD_{10} doses actually protected against the toxicity of 6-TG. That the combination of Ara-C and 6-TG is therapeutically synergistic against L1210 is shown by results of several experiments, pooled and summarized in Table 3. Inasmuch as Ara-C alone is generally curative when given on this intensive-intermittent treatment schedule to mice with 10^5 L1210 cells implanted i.p., the present study was designed to present a greater challenge to therapy, and 10^6 L1210 cells were injected i.v. on day 0. Under these conditions, untreated mice exhibited a median survival time of 5.0 days, 6-TG alone was only moderately effective, and Ara-C alone was substantially more effective, but neither of the individual drugs was curative. Examination of mortality among parallel groups of

TABLE 3. EFFECTIVENESS OF DIVIDED-INTERMITTENT TREATMENT WITH CYTOSINE ARABINOSIDE (ARA-C) PLUS 6-THIOGUANINE (6-TG) AGAINST LEUKEMIA L1210*

I.P. dose (mg/kg) q3hr/24hr. Days 1,5,9,13			Mice with tumor		Normal mice	
Ara-C	6-TG	ILS (%)	S/T	Pct. Surv.	S/T	Pct. Surv.
22	0	345	1/27	4	28/49	57
15	0	480	0/30	0	47/48	98
10	0	422	0/29	0	46/49	94
6.7	0	327	0/29	0	48/48	100
0	1.0	125	0/20	0	1/30	3
0	0.67	105	0/30	0	29/50	58
0	0.45	60	0/30	0	47/49	96
15	1.0	604	9/18	50	12/20	60
10	1.0	625	6/19	32	11/17	65
15	0.67	606	7/20	35	15/18	83
10	0.67	558	9/29	31	27/29	93
6.7	0.67	550	1/10	10	10/10	100

*See Ref. 8. Tumor inoculum – 10^6 cells, IV.

normal mice indicates that the optimal antileukemic dose of 6-TG alone (1.0 mg/kg/injection), while it may have been very effective against the tumor cells, was lethal to the host. In contrast, when Ara-C (15 mg/kg) and 6-TG (1.0 mg/kg) were given in combination, 12 of 20 normal mice and 9 of 18 leukemic mice survived.

Another example of therapeutic synergism arising from the ability of one antitumor drug to protect against the toxicity of a second is provided by the combination of ICRF-159 plus daunomycin. In attempting to elucidate the mechanisms of untoward cardiac effects attending the clinical use of daunomycin,[9] Herman *et al.*[10] found that daunomycin-induced electrocardiographic abnormalities in the isolated dog heart could be partially reversed by pre-perfusion with the chelating agent Versene (EDTA) or the structurally related ICRF-159 (Fig. 1). Woodman *et al.*[11] showed that both EDTA or ICRF-159 protected mice against the lethal toxicity of daunomycin. Moreover, ICRF-159 was more effective than EDTA in blocking daunomycin toxicity. Table 4 summarizes an experiment in which normal mice and leukemic (L1210) mice were given a single treatment with ICRF-159 and daunomycin, individually and combined. The optimal dose of ICRF-159 alone (400 mg/kg) produced a 67 per cent ILS in leukemic mice, and was lethal to only one of six normal mice. The lowest dose of daunomycin alone (2.5 mg/kg) was not lethal to normal mice but was also not very effective in the leukemic mice. Higher doses of daunomycin alone (5.0 or 10 mg/kg) were lethal to the host. When a nonlethal dose of daunomycin was combined with ICRF-159, increasing dosages of the latter resulted in progressively increased antileukemic efficacy over that achieved with daunomycin alone, presumably due to the antitumor activity of ICRF-159. When ICRF-159 was combined with lethal doses of daunomycin, the former protected against the toxicity of the latter. Again, increasing ICRF-159 dosage resulted in an increase in antileukemic effectiveness. Maximum

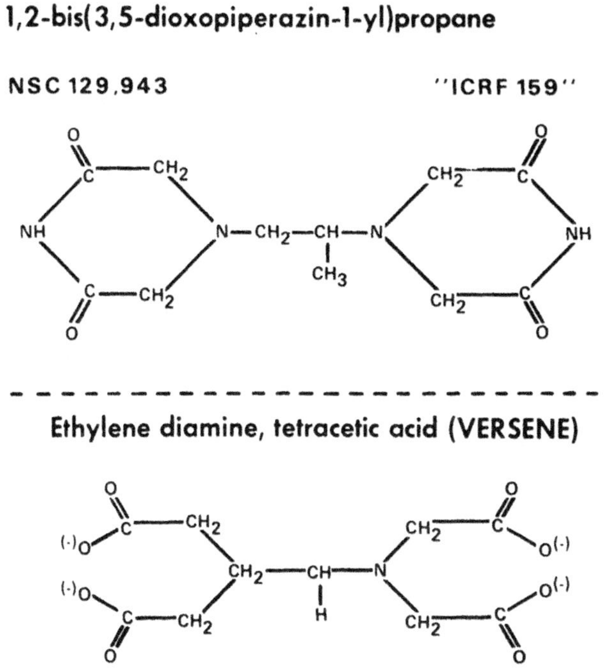

FIG. 1. Structure of ICRF-159 (NSC-129,943) and Versene (EDTA).

TABLE 4. INFLUENCE OF ICRF-159 ON DAUNOMYCIN ANTILEUKEMIC (L1210)* ACTIVITY (ICRF-159 GIVEN 10 MINUTES PRIOR TO DAUNOMYCIN – DAY 1 ONLY)

(mg/kg-I.P.)		L1210	Normal	(mg/kg-I.P.)		L1210	Normal
ICRF-159	Daun.	ILS (%)	S/T Day 60	ICRF-159	Daun.	ILS (%)	S/T Day 60
800	0	0	1/6	400	5.0	67	6/6
400	0	67	5/6	200	5.0	67	6/6
200	0	44	6/6	100	5.0	50	6/6
100	0	11	6/6	0	5.0	17	0/6
400	10	78	4/6	400	2.5	61	5/6
200	10	61	6/6	200	2.5	55	6/6
100	10	44	6/6	100	2.5	44	6/6
0	10	0	0/6	0	2.5	22	6/6

*I.P. tumor.

antileukemic activity (78 per cent ILS) was achieved with the combination dosage of 400 mg/kg of ICRF-159 plus 10 mg/kg of daunomycin, but the efficacy of the combination was not substantially greater than that seen with optimal ICRF-159 treatment alone. Sandberg *et al.*[12] reported that daunomycin activity against L1210 was not remarkably dependent on the treatment schedule. However, it has been shown[13] that the anti-L1210 effectiveness of ICRF-159 was treatment-schedule dependent, intermittent treatment (one treatment every fourth day or treatment every 3 hr on every fourth day) being more effective than a single treatment or daily treatment (Fig. 2). When ICRF-159 and daunomycin were combined against L1210 using intermittent or daily treatment, the therapeutically synergistic quality of the combination became evident (Fig. 3). When treatment was given daily, the optimal combination dosage was approximately twice as effective as the optimal daily dose of ICRF-159 alone and three times more effective than the optimal daily dose of daunomycin alone. The synergistic effect of the combination was most pronounced when treatment was given on every fourth day, 63 per cent of the combination-treated mice surviving for more than 60 days. With the maximally effective *q.* 4 *d.* schedule, the optimal combination dosage included ICRF-159 at its optimal dose when used alone plus daunomycin at a dose which was higher than the optimal dose for daunomycin treatment alone.

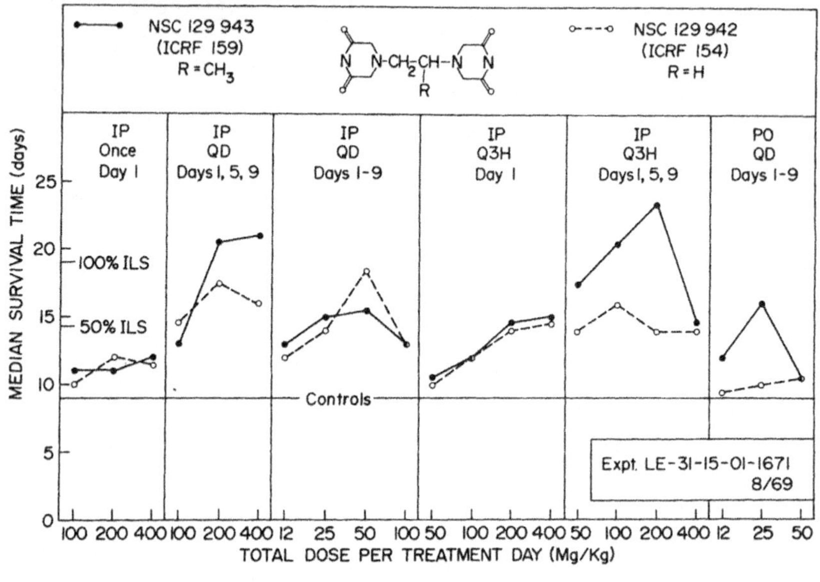

FIG. 2. Influence of treatment schedule on activity of ICRF-159 and ICRF-154 against i.p. inoculated L1210.[13]

The studies of the combinations of Ara-C plus 6-TG and ICRF-159 plus daunomycin are important for a number of reasons. New therapeutically synergistic combinations were identified. They provided clear-cut examples of therapeutic synergism with two antitumor drugs arising from the ability of one to diminish the host toxicity of the other without an apparent diminution in antitumor effectiveness. This, in turn, permitted the administration of more total effective drug before toxicity became limiting. In addition, these studies further emphasized the importance of the treatment schedule as a factor influencing the efficacy of combination chemotherapy. That the treatment schedule may severely influence the effectiveness of a drug combination as well as of an individual drug adds to the complexities of experimental design in the evaluation of combined modalities of treatment. For example, in the

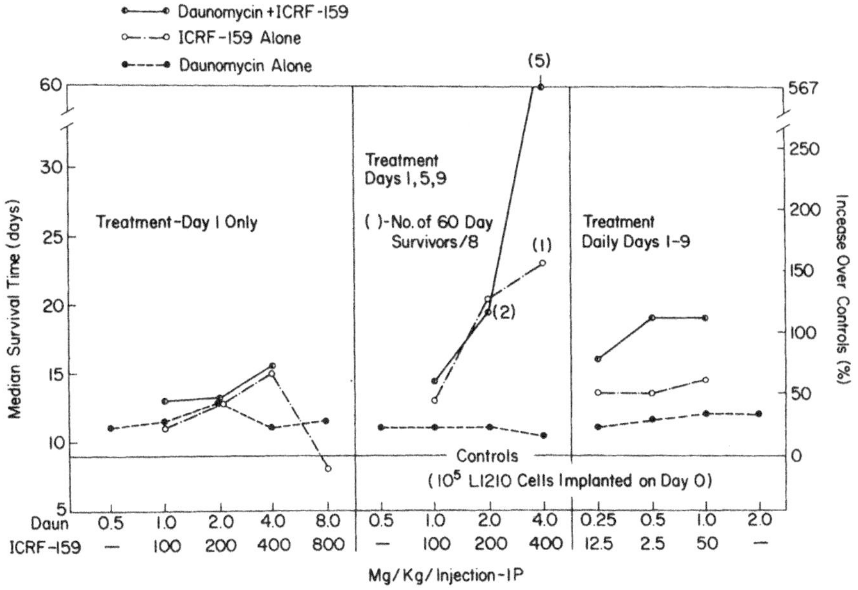

FIG. 3. Influence of treatment schedule on the antileukemic (L1210) effectiveness of combination chemotherapy with daunomycin (NSC-82151) and ICRF-159 (NSC-129,943).

previously discussed ICRF-159 plus daunomycin studies, ICRF-159 was given about 10 min prior to daunomycin. Although therapeutic synergism was evident when multiple treatment schedules were used, it was not observed when treatment was limited to 1 day only. In contrast, Wodinsky *et al.* (personal communication) have found this combination to be highly synergistic against L1210 when treatment was limited to day 1 only when ICRF-159 was administered 4 hr prior to daunomycin. In the latter study, the advantage of the combination was attributable to the ability of ICRF-159 to protect against lethal daunomycin toxicity.

Therapeutic synergism may result from the ability of a therapeutically inactive agent to protect the host specifically from the toxicity of an antitumor drug. One procedure that has been used in an attempt to improve therapeutic efficacy is to treat with a combination of a metabolite plus a corresponding antimetabolite. For example, Goldin *et al.*[14] reported that simultaneous administration of citrovorum factor (CF) plus aminopterin or methotrexate (MTX) to mice with L1210 diminished the therapeutic efficacy of the folic acid antagonists. However, when the CF was delayed for 12 or 24 hr after administration of either aminopterin or MTX, there was an increase in therapeutic efficacy. The advantages of the combinations were attributed to the ability of delayed CF to still protect the host against the toxicity of the antifols after the actions of the latter against the tumor cells appeared to be complete.

In a more recent study,[1] the combination of deoxycytidine plus Ara-C failed to provide a more effective antileukemic (L1210) therapy than treatment with Ara-C alone. In the experiment summarized in Table 5, Ara-C was given daily over a wide range of dosage levels and at varying time intervals after administration of deoxycytidine. The progressive increase in the optimal dose of Ara-C in the combination

TABLE 5. PROTECTION BY DEOXYCYTIDINE AGAINST TOXICITY AND ANTI-LEUKEMIC (L1210) EFFECTIVENESS OF CYTOSINE ARABINOSIDE (ARA-C)*

Ara-C Daily Dose	Ara-C Alone	Time (min) of administration of 320 mg/kg/day Deoxycytidine relative to Ara-C			
		−120	−60	0	+60
(mg/kg)	Median day of death (No. of 90 day survivors/8 mice				
65	12.0 (0)	23.0 (0)	>97.0 (5)	29.0 (0)	18.0 (0)
39	41.0 (2)	>97.0 (5)	33.0 (0)	25.0 (0)	78.5 (2)
23	>97.0 (5)	80.0 (2)	29.0 (0)	23.5 (0)	>97.0 (6)
14	79.5 (3)	44.0 (0)	28.5 (0)	14.0 (0)	54.0 (2)
0	–	Deoxycytidine alone – 10.0 days (No survivors)			
0	–	Untreated controls – 11.0 days (No survivors)			

*SC treatment begun 3 days after SC tumor implantation and continued daily to death or Day 70.

with decreasing time interval between the administration of metabolite and antimetabolite indicates that deoxycytidine was able to protect the mice competitively against the toxicity of Ara-C. However, under the conditions of this experiment, the combination did not result in increased therapeutic efficacy over that achieved with the optimal dose of Ara-C alone. A possible explanation for the apparent reduced effectiveness when deoxycytidine was given immediately prior to Ara-C (Table 5; "0" min) might be the failure to give the antimetabolite at a dosage level sufficiently high to compensate for the protective action of deoxycytidine against the tumor. In any case, from these data it was concluded that the combination of deoxycytidine plus Ara-C resulted in a decrease in toxicity to the host that was offset by an essentially equivalent decrease in toxicity to the tumor.

The combination of *N*-acetylcysteine (NAC) plus isophosphamide (Isoph) does provide an additional example of therapeutic synergism resulting from the ability of an agent devoid of antitumor activity to protect the host but not the tumor against the toxicity of an active antitumor drug. Connors and Elson[15] reported that thiol pretreatment of rats reduced the toxicity of the more chemically reactive nitrogen mustards, and Primack[16] reported that irrigation of bladders of monkeys and dogs with acetylcysteine protected against cyclophosphamide-induced cystitis. Such findings prompted the investigation of the effects of NAC on the toxicity and antileukemic (L1210) effectiveness of cyclophosphamide and the related drug, Isoph.[17] The experiment summarized in Fig. 4 shows the marked therapeutic advantage against L1210 of the combination of NAC plus Isoph over Isoph alone. The optimal dose of Isoph alone (300 mg/kg) produced three 90-day survivors among eight mice. At a higher dose of Isoph alone (500 mg/kg), one animal survived, but most succumbed to drug toxicity as evidenced by a median survival time of 3.5 days. NAC alone at 1500 mg/kg was not toxic and had no antitumor activity. All of the mice that were given 1500 mg/kg of NAC + 500 mg/kg of Isoph survived for more than 90 days (Fig. 4). Whether bladder cystitis contributes to the lethal toxicity of Isoph in the mouse is not known. Clearly, however, NAC protected the mice from Isoph-induced

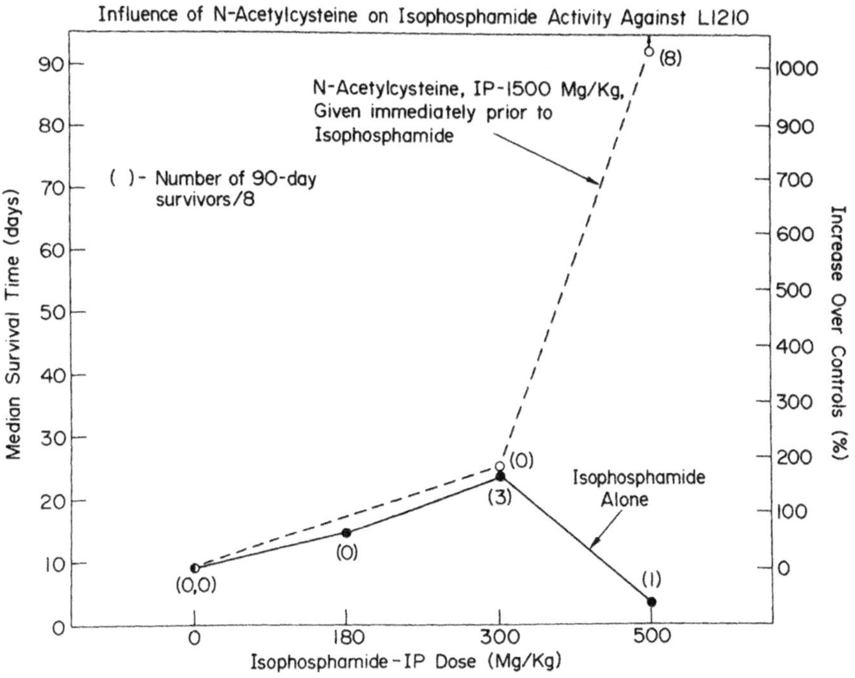

FIG. 4. Influence of *N*-acetylcysteine on isophosphamide activity against L1210.[17] Treatment was given once on the day after i.p. implantation of 10^5 L1210 cells.

lethality, an observation that has been repeatedly confirmed in non-tumor-bearing animals. That such protection against toxicity did not reduce the anti-L1210 activity of Isoph has also been confirmed in a number of experiments. The resulting increase in antileukemic specificity seen with the combination appeared to be due to the ability to give safely a higher dose of the active antitumor drug. Enhancement of the anti-L1210 activity of cyclophosphamide has been observed with prior NAC treatment. However, the therapeutic advantage over treatment with cyclophosphamide alone has not been as clear-cut as the advantage of NAC plus Isoph over Isoph alone.

Conclusion. With an increasing number of drugs emerging as "active" from experimental screens, the possibilities for studies of two, three or more drugs in combination are abundant. Rationales for the selection of drug pairs for experimental conbination studies have been based on a number of approaches, *in vitro, in vivo,* and biochemical. A major rationale for selecting drugs for combination in clinical trials has been dissimilarity of qualitative toxicity or, in the quantitative sense, the appearance of less than additive toxicity. Usually, clinical combinations have included drugs with individually demonstrated effectiveness against the particular malignancy under study. The few examples of therapeutic synergism against mouse leukemia L1210 presented herein affirm the hypothesis that lack of additive toxicity is a reasonable basis for expecting a therapeutic advantage from the combination of antitumor drugs. However, it is also clear that reduction of an antitumor drug's toxicity for the host by administration of a protecting agent, which may or may not have antitumor activity itself, need not be accompanied by an equivalent reduction in toxicity for tumor cells. Moreover, when such is the case, a high degree of therapeutic synergism can be realized.

REFERENCES

1. A. GOLDIN, J. M. VENDITTI and N. MANTEL, in *Handbook for Experimental Pharmacology,* (Eds. A. SARTORELLI and D. JOHNS) Vol. 38. Springer-Heidelberg, in press.
2. A. GOLDIN and N. MANTEL, *Cancer Res.* **17**, 635 (1957).
3. J. M. VENDITTI and A. GOLDIN, in *Advances in Chemotherapy* (Eds. A. GOLDIN and F. HAWKING), Vol. 1, pp. 397–498. Academic Press, New York (1964).
4. A. GOLDIN, J. M. VENDITTI, S. R. HUMPHREYS, D. DENNIS, N. MANTEL and S. W. GREENHOUSE, *J. natn. Cancer Inst.* **16**, 129 (1955).
5. J. M. VENDITTI, S. R. HUMPHREYS, N. MANTEL and A. GOLDIN, *J. natn. Cancer Inst.* **17**, 631 (1956).
6. F. M. SCHABEL, JR., W. R. LASTER, JR. and M. W. TRADER, *Proc. Am. Ass. Cancer Res.* **9**, 62 (1968).
7. G. A. LEPAGE and T. KANEKO, *Cancer Res.* **29**, 2314 (1969).
8. L. H. SCHMIDT, J. A. MONTGOMERY, W. R. LASTER, JR. and F. M. SCHABEL, JR., *Proc. Am. Ass. Cancer Res.* **11**, 70 (1970).
9. R. B. LIVINGSTON and S. K. CARTER, *Single Agents in Cancer Chemotherapy,* p. 367. IFI/Plenum, New York (1970).
10. E. H. HERMAN, R. H. MHATRE, I. P. LEE and V. S. WARAVDEKAR, *Proc. Soc. exp. Biol. Med.* **140**, 234 (1972).
11. R. J. WOODMAN, I. KLINE and J. M. VENDITTI, *Proc. Am. Ass. Cancer Res.* **13**, 31 (1972).
12. J. S. SANDBERG, F. L. HOWSDEN, A. DIMARCO and A. GOLDIN, *Cancer Chemother. Rep.* **54**, 1 (1970).
13. J. M. VENDITTI, *Cancer Chemother. Rep.* **2**, Part 3, 35 (1971).
14. A. GOLDIN, J. M. VENDITTI, S. R. HUMPHREYS, D. DENNIS and N. MANTEL, *Cancer Res.* **15**, 742 (1955).
15. T. A. CONNORS and L. A. ELSON, *Biochem. Pharmac.* **11**, 1221 (1962).
16. A. PRIMACK, *J. natn. Cancer Inst.* **47**, 223 (1971).
17. I. KLINE, R. J. WOODMAN and J. M. VENDITTI, *Proc. Am. Ass. Cancer Res.* **13**, 29 (1972).

Pp. 151—161, Supplement Number 2, 1974.
Biochemical Pharmacology. Printed in the U.S.A.

SCHEDULE-DEPENDENT SYNERGISM AND ANTAGONISM BETWEEN METHOTREXATE AND ASPARAGINASE*

ROBERT L. CAPIZZI

Departments of Medicine and Pharmacology, Yale University School of Medicine
New Haven, Conn. 06510 U.S.A.

IN THE treatment of human acute leukemia[1] and experimental murine leukemia,[2] the results of combination chemotherapy are clearly superior to those obtained from the use of single agents. Not infrequently the components of a combination are selected because of differing host toxicity, with the ultimate result being a greater propensity for the destruction of neoplastic tissue than normal tissue. Other potentially useful methods for enhancing the therapeutic results include the use of an appropriately timed antidote after the cytotoxic agent has been administered, in an attempt to "rescue" normal cells without significantly diminishing the antitumor effects of the primary drug.[3] Drug–drug interactions as a result of specific scheduling and sequencing of drugs in a combination may also be useful. The rationale of such an approach is based on biochemical and biological data derived from preclinical and clinical studies which may suggest a regimen that will achieve opposing effects in the normal and neoplastic tissues of the host. Ideally, such interaction would be therapeutically additive or perhaps synergistic, while at the same time being toxicologically antagonistic. To date this approach has not received extensive clinical attention. The purpose of this paper is to illustrate how such properties might be achieved with the combination of methotrexate (MTX) and asparaginase (asn'ase).

METHODS AND MATERIALS

L5178Y. Initial studies were performed with the L5178Y/asn⁻ murine leukemia in cell culture. These cells are asparagine (asn) auxotrophs[4] and are sensitive to therapy with the enzyme asparaginase.[5] Stock cultures were maintained in continuous exponential growth according to the method of Fischer and Sartorelli.[6] Cells were counted in a model B Coulter counter (Coulter Electronics, Hialeah, Fla.) after dilution in 0.9% NaCl. Ascites cells were diluted in cetrimide solution to lyse the erythrocytes prior to counting. Drugs were diluted in 0.9% NaCl solutions prior to administration.

Stock lines of the L5178Y/asn⁻ were also maintained *in vivo* as an ascites tumor by inoculating 10^6 cells intraperitoneally to new host mice (20–25 g male BDF_1, purchased from Jackson Laboratory, Bar Harbor, Me.) at weekly intervals. All therapy was begun 3 days after tumor implantation and was administered by the i.p. route.

The cytotoxic effects of either drug on the L5178Y/asn⁻ were assayed by the soft agar cloning technique as described by Chu and Fischer[7] or by observing the survival time of leukemic mice.

*Supported in part by American Cancer Society Institutional Grant ACS IN-31-M-3.

Biochemical studies. Since the formation of thymidylate by the methylation of deoxyuridylate is mediated through the folate coenzymes, this reaction can be inhibited by MTX through its effect on the enzyme dihydrofolate reductase.[8] This inhibition can be monitored by studying the effects of MTX on the incorporation of tritiated deoxyuridine (^{3}H-UdR) into DNA.[9]

L5178Y/asn$^-$ cells growing *in vivo* as an ascites tumor or *in vitro* in suspension culture were treated with asn'ase. At various times thereafter, the cells were collected, washed free of drug and 0.3 to 0.75 $\times$ 10^6 cells were resuspended in 1 ml Fischer's medium supplemented with 10% horse serum (FS_{10}). The cell suspensions were placed in 10-ml Ehrlenmeyer flasks at 37° in a Metabolite* shaking water bath. After 30 min of incubation with 10^{-6} M MTX or saline, 3 μCi ^{3}H-UdR (sp. act. 3.1 Ci/m-mole) was added to the incubation mixture. Over the next hr 0.1 ml of the cell suspension was removed at 10-min intervals and immediately added to 3 ml of ice-cold 10% trichloroacetic acid (TCA). The precipitate was then washed three times with 3 ml of 10% TCA. After the third wash, the precipitate was dissolved in 0.2 ml of Nuclear Chicago solubilizer, then quantitatively transferred to a liquid scintillation mixture consisting of PPO, POPOP,† toluene and ethanol. The radioactivity was counted in a Packard Tricarb liquid scintillation counter equipped with automatic external standardization for determining the efficiency of counting. The rate of incorporation of ^{3}H-UdR into DNA was calculated using linear regression analysis, and the final results were expressed as des./min/10^6 blasts/min of incubation. The rate of label incorporation in the presence of MTX was expressed as a percentage of control incorporation, i.e. saline treated, at each time point after the addition of asn'ase.

Human acute lymphoblastic leukemia cells were studied in a similar fashion. Peripheral blood or bone marrow cells diluted with an equal volume of Fischer's medium supplemented with 10% horse serum were spun in a table top clinical centrifuge at 300–500 rev/min for 20–30 min at room temperature. The buffy coat was separated from the packed red cells, centrifuged at 2500 rev/min, then resuspended in FS_{10} to provide a cell titer of 5–10 $\times$ 10^6 blasts/ml. The suspensions were then treated as described above for the L5178Y/asn$^-$.

RESULTS

Confirmation of the asn requirement of the L5178Y is shown in Fig. 1. The rates of cell growth under control and experimental conditions were determined as described above. The cells failed to grow during the first 12 hr in asn-free medium and began to lyse during the second 12 hr. If asn (10 μg/ml) were added to the asn-free cultures at the sixth hr, the cells recovered and growth was restored.

The inhibitory effect of MTX on ^{3}H-UdR incorporation into DNA was affected by prior asn deprivation or asn'ase treatment as is shown in Fig 2. Cells in the exponential phase of growth in fully supplemented medium were centrifuged, washed twice and resuspended in asn-free medium. Control cells were handled in a similar fashion except that they were washed and resuspended in asn-supplemented medium. Inhibition of DNA synthesis produced by 2 $\times$ 10^{-6} M MTX did not vary significantly over a 24-hr

*New Brunswick Scientific, New Brunswick, N.J.
†PPO = 2,5-diphenyloxazole; POPOP = 1,4-bis-[2-(4-methyl-5-phenyloxazolyl)] benzene.

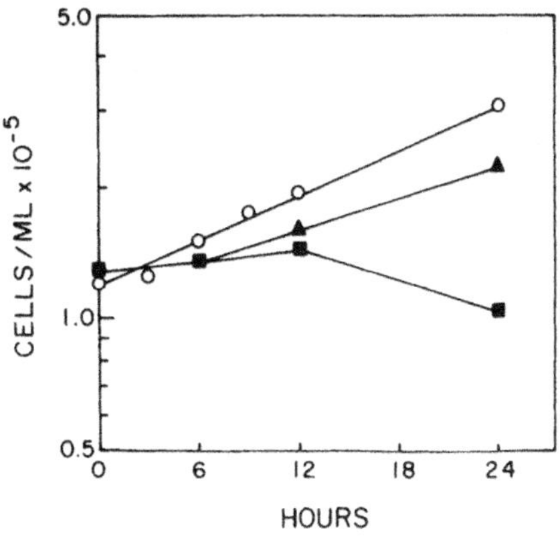

FIG. 1. Effect of the presence or absence of asparagine (asn) on the growth and viability of L5178Y/asn⁻ cells. Key: o——o, cells grown in the presence of 10 μg/ml of asn; ■——■, cells grown in the absence of asn; and ▲——▲, asn, 10 μg/ml, added to medium after 6 hr exposure to asn-less medium.

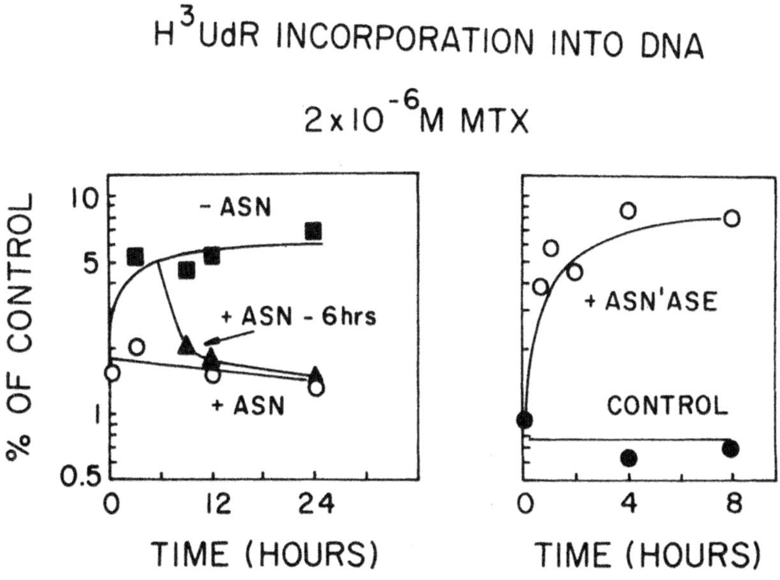

FIG. 2. Effect of the presence or absence of asn or asn'ase on the inhibition of DNA synthesis by MTX. Cells were subjected to similar conditions as in Fig. 1, in addition to exposure to pulses of MTX at the various time points.

period when the cells were grown in fully supplemented medium. However, MTX was much less inhibitory to DNA synthesis in those cells incubated in asn-free medium. This decrease was observed within 3 hr of transfer into asn-free medium and remained unchanged over the 24-hr period of observation. If asn were restored to the culture medium at the sixth hr, MTX-induced inhibition of DNA synthesis was comparable to that achieved in the saline-treated group. Alteration of MTX-induced inhibition of DNA synthesis after pretreatment with asn'ase was qualitatively similar to that observed under asn-less conditions, but the effects occurred earlier and to a greater degree (Fig. 2B).

The cytotoxic effect of MTX was also reduced by asn'ase, as is shown in Fig. 3. Three-hr exposure of the L5178Y/asn⁻ to MTX alone killed 90 per cent of the cells. The simultaneous exposure of the L5178Y/asn⁻ to MTX and a sublethal concentration of asn'ase (0.1 i.u./ml) killed only 40 per cent of the cells. Pretreatment of the cells with asn'ase alone for 3 or 6 hr followed by 3 hr of simultaneous exposure to both asn'ase and MTX allowed almost complete viability, indicating that asn'ase had antagonized the cytotoxic effect of MTX.

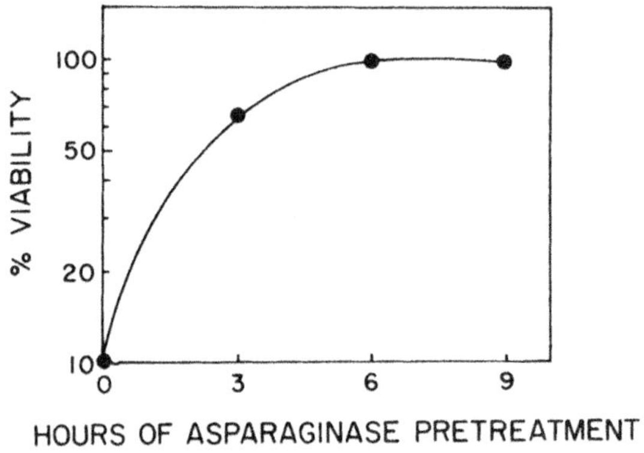

FIG. 3. Effect of concomitant and preceding asn'ase treatment of L5178Y/asn⁻ cells *in vitro* on the cytotoxic effect of MTX. Each time point represents the effect of 3 hr of exposure to 5×10^{-7} M MTX in the presence of increasing exposure to asn'ase (0.1 i.u./ml).

Similar antagonism has also been noted *in vivo*, as is shown in Fig. 4. Mice that had received 10^6 L5178Y/asn⁻ intraperitoneally were treated on the third day after tumor implantation with either MTX or asn'ase alone or the combination. Asn'ase preceded the MTX by 3 hr in those mice treated with both drugs. Beginning 24 hr after therapy (day 4) and extending to day 7, groups of mice were sacrificed by cervical dislocation and the cells were harvested quantitatively by washing the peritoneal cavity with heparinized saline (0.5 unit/ml). Each point represents the mean total cell count of four mice. By day 4 there was a considerable reduction in cell number as a result of one dose of asn'ase, 200 i.u./kg, and/or one dose of MTX, 60 mg/kg. Whereas the cell count depression produced by MTX alone was sustained through day 7, those cells from mice treated with asn'ase alone recovered and resumed growth at a rate

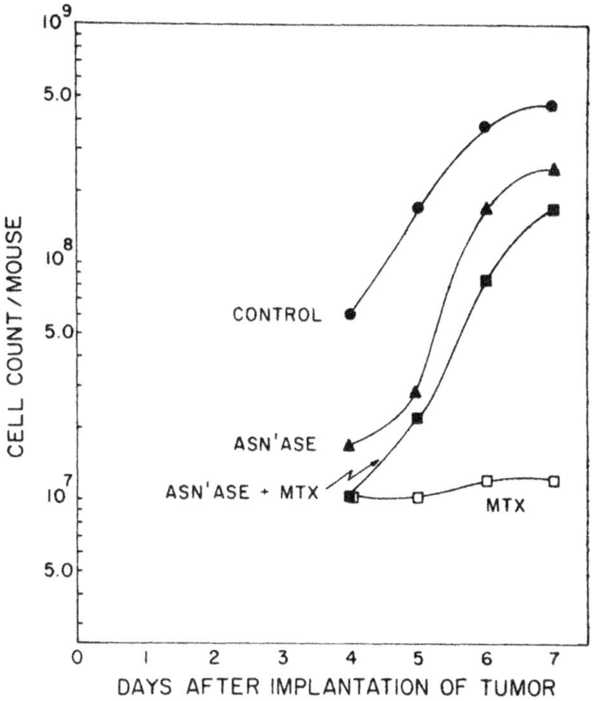

FIG. 4. Effect of asn'ase pretreatment on the cytotoxic effect of MTX *in vivo*. Treatment was administered intraperitoneally on the third day after tumor implantation, and cells were quantitatively harvested from mice over the next 4 days. Control = 0.1 ml of normal saline solution; asn'ase = 200 i.u./kg, MTX = 60 mg/kg; asn'ase and MTX = asn'ase administered 3 hr before MTX.

approaching that of the controls. A similar recovery was seen in those mice treated with the combined regimen of asn'ase and MTX, indicating that asn'ase had significantly antagonized the effect of MTX.

The time–course relationship of asn'ase treatment on MTX effect both biologically and biochemically was explored in several experiments. Mice were inoculated with 10^6 L5178Y/asn$^-$ i.p. and 3 days later were treated with a single i.p. dose of 200 i.u./kg of asn'ase. At various times thereafter, mice were sacrificed, the ascites cells were harvested and the inhibitory effect of MTX on ^{3}H-UdR incorporation into DNA *in vitro* was determined as described above. As is shown in Fig. 5, MTX was less inhibitory of DNA synthesis in cells from the asn'ase-pretreated mice as compared to the inhibition produced in cells from the saline-treated mice. This biochemical antagonism was evident within 1 hr after asn'ase treatment and persisted through the next 24 hr. However, if cells were studied at 48 hr or longer after asn'ase, MTX-induced inhibition of DNA synthesis in the asn'ase-pretreated mice was comparable to that observed in the saline-treated mice.

In an attempt to utilize data such as these in the design of an actual therapeutic protocol, various time points were selected to correlate biochemical indices of drug

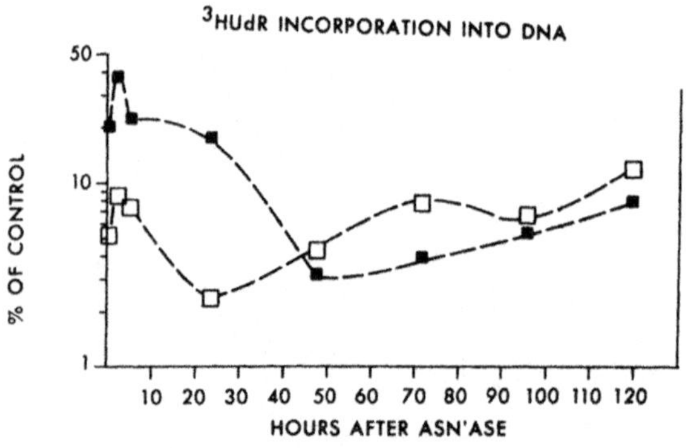

FIG. 5. Effect of asn'ase pretreatment of mice on the inhibition of DNA synthesis by MTX. Leukemic mice were treated with a single dose of asn'ase, 200 i.u./kg, and at various time points thereafter, mice were sacrificed and the L5178Y/asn⁻ cells were harvested and exposed to pulses of MTX (10^{-6} M) *in vitro*.

effect with therapeutic efficacy. Mice were treated with a single dose of asn'ase on the third day after tumor implantation, and MTX was administered either simultaneously or 3, 24, 48, 72 or 96 hr later. Another group of mice received the converse regimen, i.e. MTX followed by asn'ase at various times, or saline, MTX or asn'ase alone on day 3. The results are shown in Fig. 6. The median survival time for mice treated with asn'ase alone was 20 days compared to 15 days for the controls and 18 days for the MTX-treated group. When asn'ase preceded MTX and the interval between the two drugs was 24 hr or less, the results were no better than with either drug alone. However, with an interval of 48 or 72 hr between the two drugs, the results were additive. In contrast, when MTX preceded asn'ase, the interval did not affect the survival time.

Further amplification of these results was sought in a multiple course program in which MTX was administered 24 hr prior to asn'ase and the interval between the preceding asn'ase and succeeding MTX was 7 days. For comparison, the converse regimen, i.e. asn'ase administered 24 hr before MTX and single drug treatment with asn'ase, MTX or saline, was employed. The results of such a program are shown in Fig. 7. The therapeutic effects of the single drugs of of either combination are indicated by the mean survival time (MST). The mice treated with asn'ase or MTX alone survived significantly longer than the saline (NSS)-treated mice (30.8 and 25.9 days vs 15.9 days respectively). Although both combined regimens of MTX and asn'ase produced significant improvements in survival time which were approximately additive, the M and A regimen, i.e. MTX administered prior to asn'ase, caused 55 per cent 90-day survivors, whereas the converse regimen resulted in no long-term survivors. Re-challenge of the cured mice with 10^6 cells produced uniform "tumor takes" with mean survival times comparable to those of the saline-treated group, indicating that the mice were neither innately resistant to the tumor nor did they develop immunological resistance as a result of their surviving the original inoculum.

The enhanced therapeutic effects of the combination may reflect the ability of mice to tolerate larger doses of MTX when it is administered in conjunction with asn'ase.

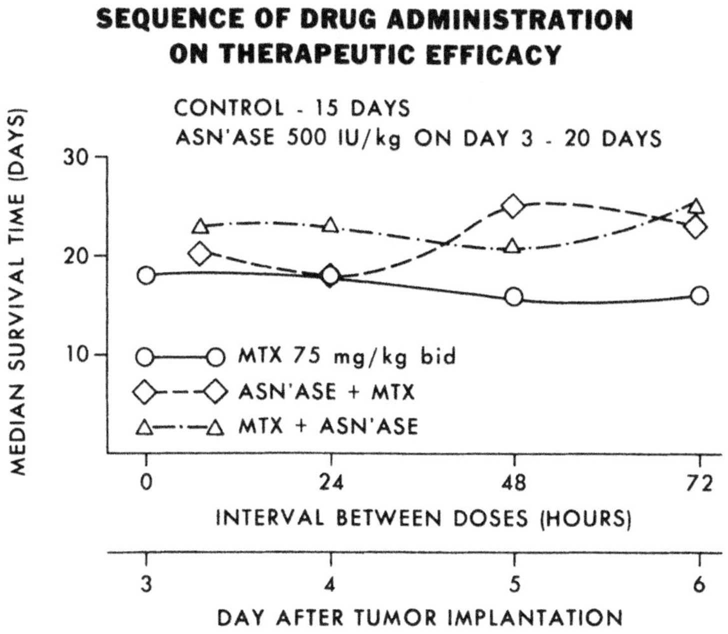

FIG. 6. Leukemic mice were treated with MTX (o——o), asn'ase followed by MTX at various intervals (◇——◇), or MTX followed by asn'ase at various intervals (△——△), and their survival times were observed.

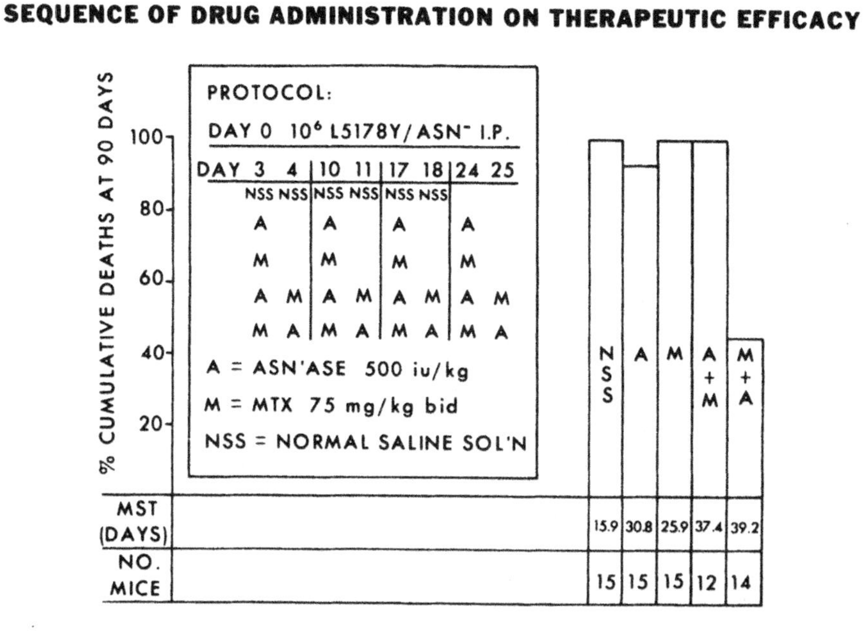

FIG. 7. Leukemic mice were treated according to the protocol shown in the insert. MST = mean survival time for the group.

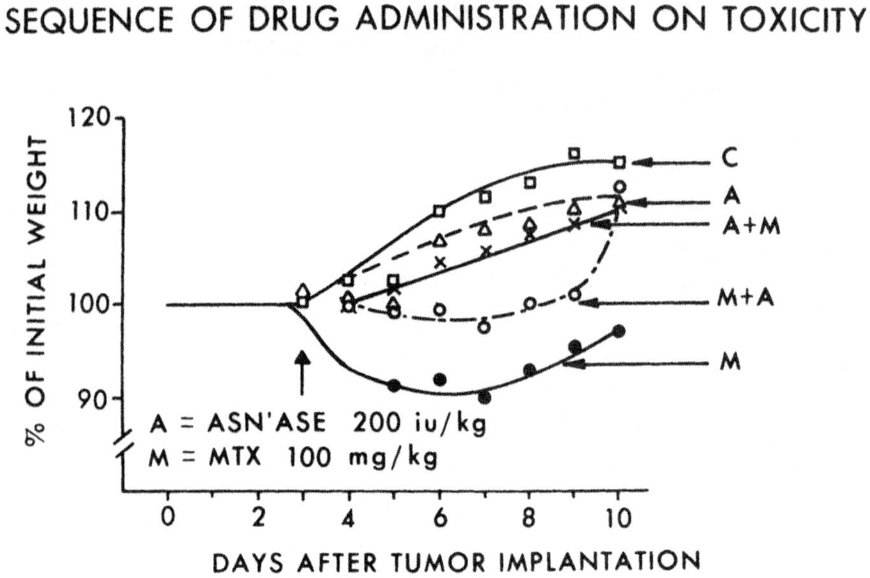

FIG. 8. Mice were inoculated with 10^6 L5178Y/asn⁻ cells and were treated with a single dose of saline (C), MTX, asn'ase or the combination on the third day after tumor implantation. A 3-hr interval was used in those mice treated with the combination.

The percentage of weight loss in a group of animals was used as an index of drug toxicity. The results of such a study are shown in Fig. 8. Leukemic mice treated with saline or asn'ase gained weight as the ascites fluid accumulated; however, a single dose of 100 mg/kg of MTX caused the mice to lose 10 per cent of their body weight. When asn'ase was administered 3 hr before MTX, the weight loss produced by MTX was totally abolished and weight gain was comparable to that of the asn'ase-treated group. Reversing the sequence of the drugs, i.e. administering MTX 3 hr before asn'ase, produced neither gain nor loss of weight. During the period of observation, the mice appeared healthy, with normal skin turgor and no evidence of ascitic fluid.

The results of these preclinical studies suggested an approach for the study and treatment of human leukemia. The inhibitory effect of MTX on ^{3}H-UdR incorporation into the DNA of human leukemia cells was determined before and after a single intravenous dose of asn'ase. If the patient's leukemic cells were sensitive to asn'ase, an initial reduction of MTX effect *in vitro* would be expected. Subsequent assays were performed to establish the time when MTX would be at least as effective as it was initially or possibly more effective in inhibiting ^{3}H-UdR incorporation into DNA. The patient was then treated with a single dose of MTX, followed by a single dose of asn'ase 24 hr later. The original interval of time from asn'ase to MTX treatment was then repeated. Since preclinical data had also indicated a sustained asn'ase-induced antagonism of the toxic effect of MTX, the dose of MTX was gradually increased to the limit of individual patient tolerance.

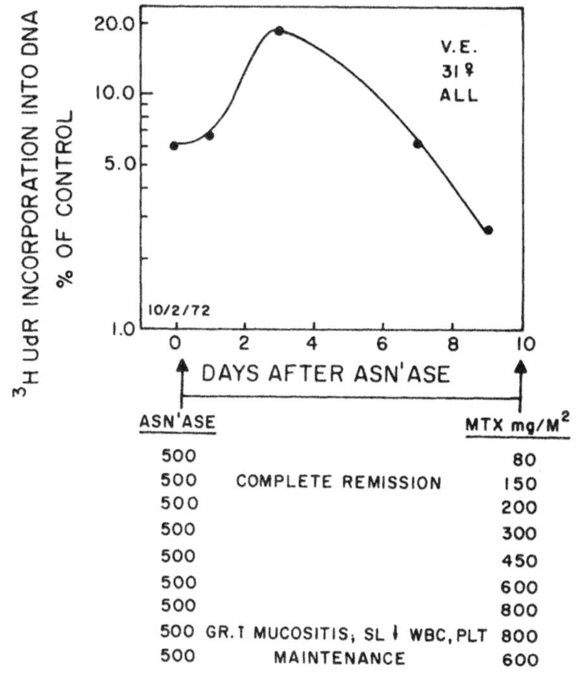

FIG. 9. Effect of asn'ase pretreatment in a patient with acute lymphoblastic leukemia (ALL) on the subsequent inhibitory effect of MTX on DNA synthesis *in vitro*, and her subsequent tolerance to MTX *in vivo*. Biochemical studies were performed after the first dose of asn'ase (i.u./kg). The first dose of MTX was administered 10 days later, and asn'ase was repeated 24 hr after MTX. Thereafter, the interval between asn'ase and each succeeding dose of MTX was 10 days. The asn'ase of a new cycle was administered 24 hr after each dose of MTX.

The results of an initial study are shown in Fig. 9. The patient is a 31-year-old female with acute lymphoblastic leukemia. She had previously relapsed on a combination of drugs which included MTX and had shown signs of MTX toxicity at a dose of 100–130 mg/m^2. The inhibitory effect of MTX on ^{3}H-UdR incorporation into the DNA of bone marrow leukemic cells was assayed before and at various times after the administration of a single i.v. dose of asn'ase. As in the mouse study, the inhibitory effect of MTX was decreased after asn'ase treatment. However, 7 days after asn'ase treatment, sensitivity to MTX was equal to the pretreatment level, and on the ninth day the cells were even more sensitive. Consequently, on the tenth day a single i.v. dose of 80 mg/m^2 of MTX was given, followed by a single dose of 500 i.u. asn'ase/kg 24 hr later. The 10-day cycle was repeated and with each subsequent course she received an increasingly larger dose of MTX. After a second dose of 800 mg/m^2, which for this patient totaled 1.2 g, a slight erythema of her oral mucosa was noted with a 50 per cent decrease in peripheral white count and platelet count. Subsequently, a maintenance dose of MTX at 600 mg/m^2 (900 mg total) was instituted. This dose is approximately five times larger than that which she was previously able to tolerate. The patient continues in remission 9 months after the institution of therapy and has been treated continuously with the combination at 10-day intervals.

DISCUSSION

The observed antagonism between asn'ase and MTX is probably due to the interrelationship between protein and DNA synthesis. Prototype studies for the alteration of MTX activity by asn'ase exist in studies of thymineless death in bacteria. Using an amino acid auxotroph of a thymineless strain of *Escherichia coli* 15, Barner and Cohen[10] found that the simultaneous deprivation of thymine and an essential amino acid (–T–AA medium) allowed characteristic thymineless death for approximately one generation time, but then the rate of thymineless death was markedly impeded. These studies were amplified by Maaloe and Hanawalt,[11] who used a similar thymineless strain of *E. coli* which was also auxotrophic for arginine and uracil. Bacteria did not undergo thymineless death if they were preincubated in medium supplemented with thymine but devoid of arginine and uracil (+T–AU medium). The extent of this resistance to lysis was proportional to the time of preincubation in the +T–AU medium; 90 min of preincubation produced 100 per cent resistance to lysis. After an initial period of DNA synthesis in the +T–AU medium, further increase in cell number and DNA synthesis did not occur. All cells eventually completed one round of DNA replication in the +T–AU medium, and it was concluded that in the absence of protein synthesis a cycle of DNA replication which is in progress goes to completion, but the cells are unable to initiate a new round of DNA replication.[11]

Since the predominant biochemical lesion produced by MTX is inhibition of thymidylate biosynthesis,[8] the cytotoxic result may be analogous to that produced by the thymineless state in bacteria. Further comparability between bacterial systems and mammalian cells is indicated by the observation that the lethal effect of MTX on HeLa and L-cells is antagonized when essential amino acids are eliminated[12,13] or when inhibitors of protein synthesis are added to the medium.[14]

Since a major biochemical effect of asn'ase is the hydrolysis of the amido group of L-asn to form ammonia and aspartic acid,[15,16] the depletion of asn in auxotrophic cell lines causes a very rapid inhibition of protein synthesis[17–20] and subsequently of DNA[20,21] and RNA[20,22] synthesis. It would be reasonable, therefore, to suspect that under certain circumstances of scheduling the combination of asn'ase and MTX would be antagonistic. Several observations may be cited to support this assumption. It has been noted that MTX is more inhibitory in cells actively synthesizing DNA as compared to slow-growing or stationary phase cells.[23] Asn'ase treatment or the elimination of essential amino acids from mammalian cell cultures will prevent or retard DNA replication[20] and cell growth and thus will reduce or nullify the antimetabolic effect of MTX. Since MTX enters the cells by active transport,[24] asn'ase-induced effects on the cell membrane might also cause decreased MTX transport[25] which might, in turn, account for the lessened cytotoxic effect of MTX.

Attenuation of the cytotoxic effects of antineoplastic drugs by concomitant or antecedent protein synthesis inhibition is not limited to MTX. Treatment *in vivo* with inhibitors of protein synthesis (cycloheximide or tenuazonic acid) antagonized the effect of cytosine arabinoside, nitrogen mustard and X-irradiation on the intestinal crypt epithelium of rats but appeared to enhance damage to lymphoid cells.[26]

Similarly, the combination of puromycin and 6-mercaptopurine (6-MP) has been shown to have similar schedule-dependent effects. If puromycin was administered before or concomitantly with 6-MP, the results were no better than those produced by either drug alone. However, synergistic results were observed when puromycin was given after 6-MP.[27]

The clinical results of MTX and asn'ase therapy are consistent with the preclinical observations. The basic reasons for such schedule- and sequence-dependent superiority are not known at the present time, but several possibilities exist. The sequential use of two drugs in intermittent pulses, especially when the drugs may affect different stages in the cell cycle, may effectively synchronize the population such that either or both drugs may be optimally effective. Alternatively, or in addition to the above, it is well established from the present and previous studies[26,28] that the proximate administration of an inhibitor of protein synthesis will attenuate or prevent the gastrointestinal toxicity of MTX. If the therapeutic effect is not antagonized, the administration of a larger dose may permit greater tumor cell kill with a consequent increase in both remission rates and duration without a proportionate increase, and perhaps a decrease, in toxicity.

Acknowledgements – The author wishes to acknowledge the collaboration of Dr. W. P. Summers in the cell culture experiments and the very capable technical assistance of Mr. J. Mullins, Mr. R. Nichols and Mrs. N. Joyce.

REFERENCES

1. E. FREI, III and E. J. FREIREICH, in *Advances in Chemotherapy* (Eds. A. GOLDIN, F. HAWKING and R. J. SCHNITZER), Vol. 2, p. 269. Academic Press, New York (1965).
2. A. GOLDIN, J. S. SANDBERG, E. S. HENDERSON, J. W. NEWMAN, E. FREI, III and J. F. HOLLAND, *Cancer Chemother. Rep.* **55**, 309 (1971).
3. A. GOLDIN, N. MANTEL, S. W. GREENHOUSE, J. M. VENDITTI and S. R. HUMPHREYS, *Cancer Res.* **14**, 43 (1954).
4. E. E. HALEY, G. A. FISCHER and A. D. WELCH, *Cancer Res.* **21**, 532 (1961).
5. D. A. COONEY and R. E. HANDSCHUMACHER, *A. Rev. Pharmac.* **10**, 421 (1970).
6. G. A. FISCHER and A. C. SARTORELLI, *Meth. med. Res.* **10**, 247 (1964).
7. M. Y. CHU and G. A. FISCHER, *Biochem. Pharmac.* **17**, 753 (1968).
8. J. R. BERTINO, *Cancer Res.* **23**, 1286 (1963).
9. W. M. HRYNIUK and J. R. BERTINO, *J. clin. Invest.* **48**, 2140 (1969).
10. H. D. BARNER and S. S. COHEN, *J. Bact.* **74**, 350 (1957).
11. O. MAALOE and P. C. HANAWALT, *J. molec. Biol.* **3**, 144 (1961).
12. R. DEMARS and L. J. HOOPER, *J. exp. Med.* **111**, 559 (1960).
13. J. BORSA and G. F. WHITMORE, *Cancer Res.* **29**, 737 (1969).
14. J. H. KIM, A. G. PEREZ and B. DJORDJEVIC, *Cancer Res.* **28**, 2443 (1968).
15. H. A. CAMPBELL, L. T. MASHBURN, E. A. BOYSE and L. J. OLD, *Biochemistry, N.Y.* **6**, 721 (1967).
16. J. M. ROBERTS, M. D. PRAGER and N. BACHYNSKY, *Cancer Res.* **26**, 2213 (1966).
17. L. H. SOBIN and J. G. KIDD, *Proc. Soc. exp. Biol. Med.* **119**, 325 (1965).
18. J. D. BROOME and J. H. SCHWARTZ, *Biochem. biophys. Acta* **138**, 637 (1967).
19. J. D. BROOME, *J. exp. Med.* **127**, 1055 (1968).
20. K. A. O. ELLEM, A. M. FABRIZIO and L. JACKSON, *Cancer Res.* **30**, 515 (1970).
21. F. F. BECKER and J. D. BROOME, *Science, N.Y.* **156**, 1602 (1967).
22. F. F. BECKER and J. D. BROOME, *Archs Biochem. Biophys.* **130**, 332 (1969).
23. W. M. HRYNIUK, G. A. FISCHER and J. R. BERTINO, *Molec. Pharmac.* **5**, 557 (1969).
24. D. KESSEL, T. C. HALL, D. W. ROBERTS and I. WODINSKY, *Science, N.Y.* **150**, 752 (1965).
25. A. NAHAS and R. L. CAPIZZI, *Proc. Am. Ass. Cancer Res.* **12**, 63 (1971).
26. M. W. LIEBERMAN, R. S. VERBIN, M. LANDAY, H. LIANG, E. FARBER, T. N. LEE and R. STARR, *Cancer Res.* **30**, 942 (1970).
27. D. S. MARTIN, *Cancer Chemother. Rep.* **10**, 57 (1960).
28. L. T. MASHBURN, *Cancer, N.Y.* **28**, 1321 (1971).

Pp. 163—176, Supplement Number 2, 1974.
Biochemical Pharmacology. Printed in the U.S.A.

NEW EXPERIMENTAL DRUG COMBINATIONS WITH POTENTIAL CLINICAL UTILITY*

FRANK M. SCHABEL, JR.

Southern Research Institute, Birmingham, Ala., U.S.A.

CONSISTENT and predictable "cure"† of clinically recognizable (advanced) neoplastic disease in man or animals by a single dose of a single drug has rarely been achieved. I know of no consistent single-dose single-drug "cure" in man, and only two in animals: the "cure" of: (a) Ridgway osteogenic sarcoma in mice with actinomycin D,[1] and (b) a transplantable plasmacytoma in hamsters with cyclophosphamide.[2] Even repeated or sequential treatment of human tumors with a single drug is rarely successful – "cure" of choriocarcinoma with sequential methotrexate[3] and cure of Burkitt's lymphoma with multiple doses of cyclophosphamide[4] being the most consistent.

Combination chemotherapy (two or more drugs), given simultaneously or sequentially, has been more successful than single-drug therapy against leukemias, lymphomas, carcinomas and sarcomas in both man and animals.‡

Since, in the main, single-dose treatment with the best single drugs available fails to "cure," repeated doses are indicated, and once sequential single-drug therapy is begun ultimate failure, due at least in part to the natural selection of a drug-resistant tumor cell population (except in very unusual circumstances, e.g. some cases of choriocarcinoma and Burkitt's lymphoma in man), is the rule.

Since maximal destruction of tumor cells with acceptable lethal toxicity to vital normal cells (selective toxicity for tumor cells) is the aim of the chemotherapist, combination chemotherapy is indicated and has had the most success, both in experimental and clinical cancer chemotherapy reported to date. The principles for selection of candidates for combination chemotherapy listed in Table 1 are indicated and have been successfully applied.

Despite my references above to "success" and "cure," the vast bulk of clinically recognized malignant disease of man and animals beyond the "curative" ability of the surgeon and/or the radiologist is still clearly beyond the available "curative" ability of the chemotherapist. Searches for new anticancer drugs continue throughout the world, and those of us committed to the development of effective anticancer agents believe, based on the medical history of the past 30 years, that better anticancer drugs will be found, but I, for one, do not expect that a single drug curative for all tumors will be

*The previously unpublished work at Southern Research Insitute reported in this paper was supported by Contract NIH-71-2098 from the Division of Cancer Treatment, NCI, NIH, Department of Health, Education and Welfare.

†By "cure," I mean destruction of a large enough fraction of a viable tumor cell population so that the cells surviving treatment can never re-establish the clinically recognizable disease.

‡The principles and results of combination chemotherapy against malignant tumors, both in experimental animals and in man, have been recently reviewed by Frei[5] and by Goldin *et al.*[6]

TABLE 1. PRINCIPLES FOR SELECTION OF CANDIDATE DRUGS FOR COMBINATION CHEMOTHERAPY OF TUMORS

1. Each drug used in combination should be active against the target tumor when used alone.
2. Drugs used in combination should be qualitatively different in toxicity for vital normal cells and have different biochemical mechanisms of action against tumor cells.
3. Tumor cells resistant to one drug in the combination should not be cross-resistant to the other drug(s).

found. It is clearly indicated, while we search for new drugs, that we should continue to improve the effectiveness of currently available drugs by any and all means, including the search for more effective drug combinations. A number of recent observations in both experimental and clinical cancer chemotherapy suggest that improved combination chemotherapy may be developed in studies with: (1) anticancer drugs which bind to or intercalate with DNA in combination with one or more drugs from other classes of anticancer agents, and (2) combinations of two or more alkylating agents with anticancer activity.

Drugs which bind to or intercalate with DNA in combination with other anticancer agents

Gottlieb *et al.*[7] have reported that adriamycin (14-hydroxyl-daunorubicin, NSC-123127), which binds to DNA, and 5-(3,3-dimethyl-1-triazeno)imidazole-4-carboxamide, NSC-45388 (DIC) (Fig. 1), both of which are effective when used alone, appear to be significantly better when used in combination in treating a wide variety of metastatic sarcomas in man. Gottlieb and Luce, during the course of these clinical studies, informed us of their progress with this drug combination. We used it against some experimental tumors and observed therapeutic potentiation* against subcutaneously implanted B16 melanoma, Lewis lung carcinoma and leukemia L1210 in BDF_1 mice, and against early passage adenocarcinoma of the breast in C3H mice.[8] The B16 melanoma, Lewis lung carcinoma and C3H adenocarcinoma of the breast are considered by experimental cancer chemotherapists to be relatively resistant to anticancer drug treatment. The therapeutic potentiation of adriamycin plus DIC against leukemia L1210 has been independently observed in other laboratories.[7] The observed therapeutic potentiation of adriamycin plus DIC in these experimental systems confirms and supports the clinical observations and, in addition, supports the indication for studying the combination against both carcinomas and lymphomas in man.

Compounds which bind to or intercalate with DNA have, in my opinion, great promise for use in developing more effective drug combinations. Drugs known to have anticancer activity against tumors in man or animals or in both, and which have been reported to bind to or intercalate with DNA (excluding the recognized alkylating agents) are listed in Table 2.

The indication for searching for anticancer drug combinations containing DNA binders is clear, based on clinical success to date with adriamycin plus DIC in sarcomas

*Therapeutic potentiation: a greater therapeutic effect against the tumor by sublethal ($\leq LD_{10}$) doses of the two drugs in combination than can be obtained by sublethal doses of either drug when used alone.

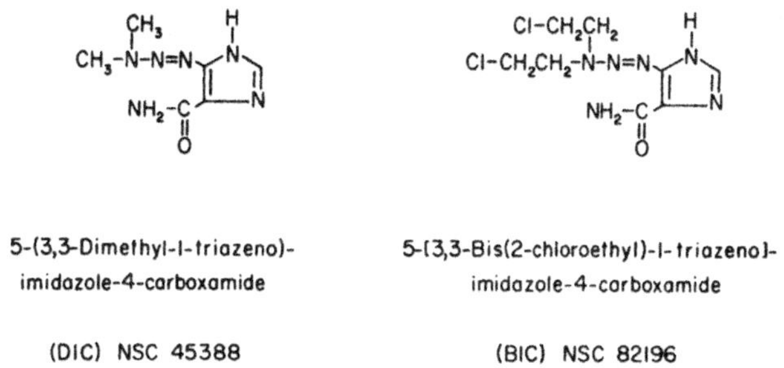

FIG. 1. Structure of DIC and BIC.

TABLE 2. ANTICANCER AGENTS WHICH BIND TO OR INTERCALATE WITH DNA (EXCLUDING RECOGNIZED ALKYLATING AGENTS)

Drug	References*
Actinomycin D	9,16
Daunomycin, adriamycin (Nogalomycin)	9,16
Mithramycin (Chromomycin, Olivamycin)	9
Bleomycin (reacts with DNA to cause removal of bases)	10–14
Anthramycin	9
Camptothecin	15,16
Miracil D	9
cis-diamminedichloroplatinum (II)	17–22
Ellipticine	16
Phthalanilides	23

*This listing is not exhaustive, but includes reviews.

in man[7] and leukemias and carcinomas in animals,[7,8] and with adriamycin or daunomycin plus 1,2-bis(3,5-dioxopiperazin-1-yl)propane (ICRF-159) against L1210.[6] In addition, cure rates of choriocarcinoma in man have been significantly improved by sequential addition of actinomycin D to methotrexate treatment.[24]

If *cis*-diamminedichloroplatinum (II) (*cis*-Pt-II) can be considered to be representative of DNA binders* (Table 2) which may be used to advantage in combination with other anticancer agents, the prospects for the development of therapeutically potentiating drug combinations using DNA binders are great. A number of reports of therapeutic potentiation against leukemia L1210 of combinations of *cis*-Pt-II have appeared and these are listed in Table 3.

We have studied the combination of *cis*-Pt-II plus 5-FU in some depth in the L1210 system and have quantitated the tumor cell kill *in vivo* (Table 4). Therapeutic potentiation of the two drugs in combination is marked and readily reproducible. "Cure" of

*The possibility that *cis*-Pt-II may be acting bifunctionally to cross-link adjacent nucleophilic centers through covalent binding, and thus be reacting like an alkylating agent, has been suggested.[20]

TABLE 3. COMBINATIONS OF *cis*-PT-II WITH OTHER AGENTS REPORTED TO BE THERAPEUTICALLY POTENTIATING AGAINST LEUKEMIA L1210

cis-Pt-II with	Reference
Cyclophosphamide	25–28
Isophosphamide	26,28
5[3,3-bis(2-chloroethyl)-1-triazeno]imidazole-4-carboxamide (BIC)	26,28
Phosphoramide mustard	26
Methotrexate	25–28
5-Azacytidine	26
1-β-D-Arabinofuranosylcytosine (Ara-C)	26,28
ICRF-159	26,28
5-Fluorouracil (5-FU)	25–28
6-Thioguanine (6-TG)	25,27
Vincristine	25,27
Vinblastine	25,27
Campothecin	26
Emetine	28

mice bearing 10^4 or more viable L1210 cells with either drug alone is rarely if ever accomplished. In these studies, increased tumor cell kill by the drug combination was seen in dying mice, and significant cure rates were obtained in mice bearing $>10^5$ viable tumor cells, and some cures were obtained in mice bearing $>10^6$ viable tumor cells.

I hold no brief for *cis*-Pt-II as an outstandingly promising new anticancer agent, either when used alone or in combination with other anticancer agents. Its severe nephrotoxicity in man[29] is well recognized and may be self-limiting with this agent. I have used *cis*-Pt-II as an example, indicating the possibility that DNA binders in combination with other classes of anticancer agents, including alkylating agents, antifols, purine and pyrimidine analogs, mitotic inhibitors, DNA polymerase inhibitors, and other DNA binders, may be a promising area for cancer chemotherapists to investigate.

At least some anticancer agents which are DNA binders probably bind to tumor cells at all phases of the cell cycle, including G_0. Both actinomycin D and daunomycin have been reported to kill $>10^6$ resting L1210 cells *in vitro* (as determined by bioassay in mice) at drug concentrations approximating estimated attainable blood levels *in vivo.*[30] Adriamycin has been reported to be schedule dependent against leukemia L1210 in mice,[31] but currently developing clinical observations suggest that small frequent doses of adriamycin have no clinical advantage over larger doses at 2- to 3-week intervals in treating some adriamycin-sensitive human tumors.*

Theoretically, DNA binders or intercalators gain entry to susceptible tumor cells and attach to the DNA, irrespective of whether or not the cells are in cycle, and when the cells try to replicate their DNA and divide, they self-destruct. If this be true, one might expect high single-dose or sequential therapy at long intervals to be optimal.

We have been studying the effect of some DNA binders on Ridgway osteogenic sarcoma (ROS) in AKR mice. In 1966, Schwartz *et al.*[1] reported that a single dose of actinomycin D would cause total regression and "cure" of ROS when the drug was

*J. A. Gottlieb, personal communication.

TABLE 4. THERAPEUTIC POTENTIATION AGAINST L1210 WITH *cis*-PT-II PLUS 5-FU*

		cis-Pt-II		5-FU		*cis*-Pt-II plus 5-FU		
Expt. No.	Implant	(T/C)	Log reduction	(T/C)	Log reduction	(T/C)	Log reduction	60-Day Survivors/total
413	10^6; i.p.	$1.2 \times 10^7/2.0 \times 10^8$	1.2	$8.5 \times 10^4/2.0 \times 10^8$	3.4	$1.6/2.0 \times 10^8$	8.1	2/10
413	10^5; i.p.	$8.5 \times 10^3/3.5 \times 10^7$	3.6	$1.0 \times 10^5/3.5 \times 10^7$	2.5	$0.5/3.5 \times 10^7$	7.8	6/10
418	10^6; i.p.	$1.1 \times 10^7/3.0 \times 10^8$	1.4	$7.6 \times 10^3/3.0 \times 10^8$	4.6	$1.5 \times 10^3/3.0 \times 10^8$	5.3	1/10
418	10^5; i.p.	$5.1 \times 10^5/3.5 \times 10^7$	1.8	$2.0 \times 10^4/3.5 \times 10^7$	3.2	$1.6/3.5 \times 10^7$	7.3	2/10
430	10^5; i.p.	$1.8 \times 10^2/8.5 \times 10^7$	5.7	$1.2 \times 10^4/8.5 \times 10^7$	3.9	$0.8/8.5 \times 10^7$	8.0	4/9
Average log reduction			2.7		3.5		7.3	
Median log reduction			1.8		3.4		7.8	

*Optimal dose $\leq LD_{10}$; therapy, i.p.; *q. d.* 2–6 days; L1210 cells present at end of therapy.

given during the third week after tumor implant, and the tumor was about 1 g in size. We have readily confirmed this activity of actinomycin D against advanced ROS and have also observed marked activity of adriamycin against advanced ROS. In Fig. 2, we have plotted the response of 800-mg tumors to actinomycin D, adriamycin and DIC. Actinomycin D, at a single dose of 0.5 mg/kg, i.p., caused total regression and cure of these large tumors. We have failed to cure similar tumors with actinomycin D on a *q.d.* 1–7 day schedule up to the LD_{10} dose. We also failed to "cure" with adriamycin on a *q.d.* 1–7 day schedule (Fig. 2), but work in progress suggests that adriamycin, like actinomycin D, is more effective with single-dose treatment than on chronic daily therapy. It is probably apparent that we carried out this study to see if therapeutic potentiation against ROS could be shown with adriamycin plus DIC. We failed to show therapeutic potentiation, but advanced ROS does not respond to DIC (Fig. 2), and the first principle in Table 1 may be invoked by way of explanation.

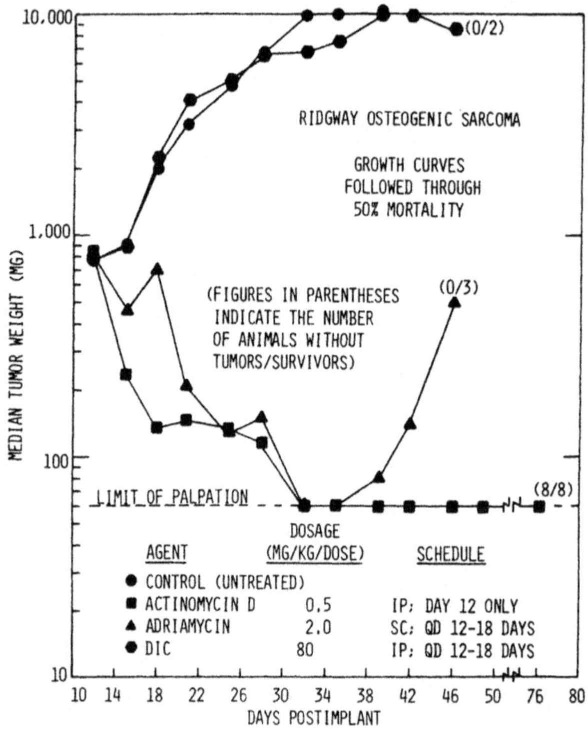

FIG. 2. Response of established ridgway osteogenic sarcoma to actinomycin D, adriamycin and DIC.

The tumor regression data plotted in Fig. 2 support the concept that at least some DNA binders with anticancer activity (actinomycin D and adriamycin) kill tumor cells at all stages in the cell cycle. The growth of ROS seems to obey the classical Gompertzian function (Fig. 2). If this be true, the growth fraction or the labeling index probably was far less than 1, and many viable cells were not in active cell replication (many cells in G_0) when treatment was given. Still, a single dose of actinomycin D of 0.5 mg/kg was able to provide a drug concentration to the viable cells farthest from the vascular bed sufficient to result in binding to the DNA of enough actinomycin D to provide a cytocidal residual when the tumor cells attempted replication.

All DNA binders do not have this effect on ROS. We have failed to show any effect of bleomycin on advanced (800 mg) ROS in mice.

The above observations suggest to me that some anticancer agents that bind to or intercalate with DNA (actinomycin D and adriamycin as examples) may kill tumor cells by interfering with vital DNA replication but without the requirement for treatment during S-phase as with cycle-stage-specific drugs such as 1-β-D-arabinofuranosylcytosine (Ara-C). If they also are therapeutically potentiating with one or more of a broad spectrum of anticancer drugs (*cis*-Pt-II as an example), we may anticipate practically useful drug combinations less restricted by temporal requirements for effective application than those we are currently using.

Combinations of alkylating agents

Modern cancer chemotherapy began with alkylating agents. They have been shown to have broad spectrum activity against experimental tumors in laboratory animals[32] and tumors in man.[33] Alkylating agents are highly reactive compounds and for a time were considered to be relatively nonspecific in inhibiting vital biological functions in both normal and neoplastic cells, and therefore showed little selective toxicity for tumor cells over vital normal cells. As studies with alkylating agents have continued, it has become clear that there are marked differences between alkylating agents as anticancer drugs, both in biological mechanism of action and in selective toxicity for tumor cells, and they continue to hold high promise for development of additional practical utility as anticancer agents.

The first report of therapeutic potentiation by two alkylating agents in combination was that of Valeriote *et al.*,[34] who reported that the combination of cyclophosphamide plus 1,3-bis(2-chloroethyl)-1-nitrosourea (BCNU) (Fig. 3) was therapeutically potentiating against a transplant line of AKR lymphoma. We easily confirmed these observations against Valeriote's passage line of AKR lymphoma, against a similar passage line of AKR lymphoma that we had isolated, and against leukemia L1210.[35] Valeriote *et al.*[34] also reported therapeutic potentiation of BCNU in combination with each of two cyclophosphamide analogs (*N,N,N'*-tris-(2-chloroethyl)-*N',O*-propylphosphoric acid ester-diamide and *N*-(2-chloroethyl)-*N'*-(2-chloroethyl)-*N'O*-propylphosphoric acid ester-diamide) and in combination with 5-[3,3-bis(2-chloroethyl)-1-triazeno] imidazole-4-carboxamide (BIC) (see Fig. 1).

We and others continued to evaluate combinations of cyclophosphamide plus nitrosourea against other experimental tumors, and results of these studies are summarized in Table 5. Therapeutic potentiation has been shown against a number of tumors in mice. The combination of cyclophosphamide plus 1-(2-chloroethyl)-3-(*trans*-4-methylcyclohexyl)-1-nitrosourea (MeCCNU) (Fig. 3) has been shown to have curative therapeutic potentiation against advanced Lewis lung carcinoma[37] and advanced KHT fibrosarcoma[36] in mice. Wheeler[38] has recently reviewed chemical, biochemical and biological activity of the alkylating agents with anticancer activity. He was aware of

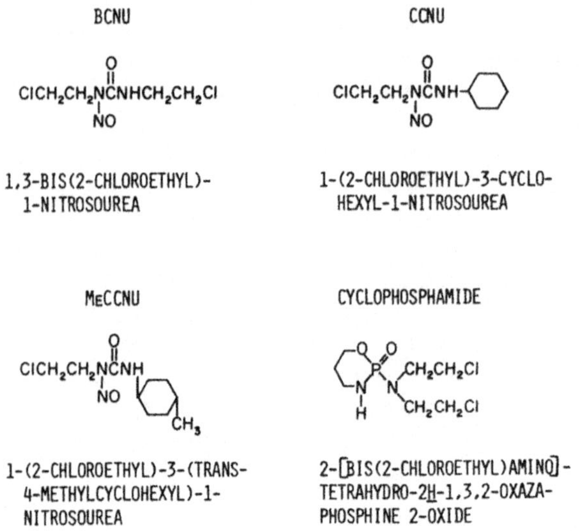

FIG. 3. Structure of BCNU, MeCCNU, CCNU and cyclophosphamide.

TABLE 5. THERAPEUTIC POTENTIATION OF CYCLOPHOSPHAMIDE PLUS A NITROSOUREA AGAINST ANIMAL TUMORS

Tumor	Cyclophosphamide in combination with	Endpoint	Therapeutic potentiation	Reference
Passage AKR lymphoma	BCNU	Lifespan and cure	+	34
Leukemia L1210	BCNU	Lifespan and cure	+	35
Leukemia P1534	BCNU	Lifespan and cure	+	*
KHT fibrosarcoma	BCNU	Lifespan and cure	+	36
Lewis lung carcinoma	MeCCNU	Lifespan and cure	+	37
Sarcoma 180	MeCCNU	Tumor inhibition	–	*
Adenocarcinoma 755	MeCCNU	Tumor inhibition	–	*
B16 melanoma	MeCCNU	Tumor inhibition	+	*
C3H mammary adenocarcinoma	MeCCNU	Tumor inhibition	+	*

*Southern Research Institute, unpublished observations.

the results listed in Table 5, and he suggested that further evaluation of two-drug combinations of alkylating agents was indicated. We studied two-drug combinations consisting of cyclophosphamide or melphalan (L-sarcolysin), a nitrosourea – BCNU, 1-(2-chloroethyl)-3-cyclohexyl-1-nitrosourea (CCNU) or MeCCNU – and either BIC or DIC in mice with generalized leukemia L1210 (implanted i.v.). A detailed report of this study will be presented elsewhere, but two observations are pertinent to this discussion: (1) marked therapeutic potentiation of CCNU + BIC against generalized L1210 was seen, confirming the observation of Valeriote *et al.*[34] against passage AKR lymphoma; and (2) greater than additive toxicity of CCNU + DIC, without therapeutic potentiation, was observed.

The responses of generalized L1210 to CCNU, BIC and CCNU plus BIC are shown in Fig. 4–6. These data were taken from experiments in which BDF_1 mice were implanted i.v. with 10^7 L1210 cells and single-dose treatment with the individual drugs (Figs. 4 and 5) or the combination of CCNU + BIC (Fig. 6) was given i.p. 48 hr later. The fractions of L1210 cells surviving treatment were based on increases in lifespan in dying animals and long-term survivors ("cures").[39] Therapeutic response in these figures was limited to $\leqslant LD_{10}$ doses in normal (non-tumor-bearing) BDF_1 internal toxicity controls. In the studies with CCNU + BIC combinations (Fig. 6) approximately equal fractions of the single-dose LD_{10} of each drug were used in the combinations (e.g. 0.5 LD_{10} of CCNU + 0.5 LD_{10} of BIC = 1.0 LD_{10} of combination).

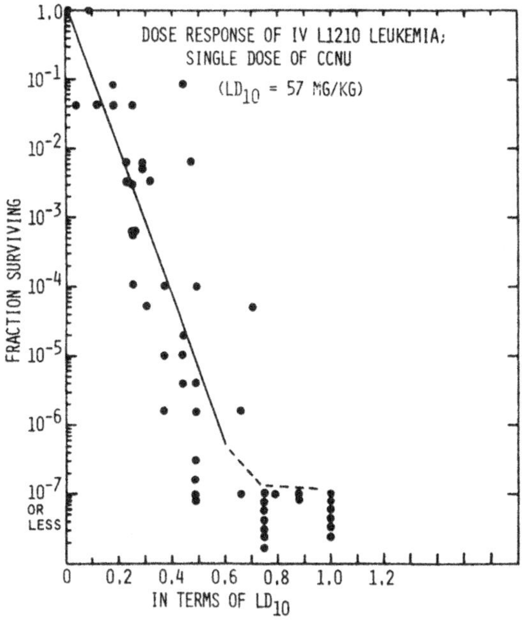

FIG. 4. Response of L1210 leukemia to a single dose of CCNU.

It will be noted that 0.5 to 1.0 × the LD_{10} of CCNU or BIC was required for a 7-log tumor cell kill (Figs. 4 and 5), while a $\geqslant$ 7-$\log_{10}$ cell kill of the two drugs in combination was consistent down to 0.3 LD_{10} of the combination. This observation may be of great practical importance.

Generally, alkylating agents must be given at close to the LD_{10} dose in animals and at close to maximum acceptable doses in man to obtain significant and practically useful tumor response (cell kill).[40] At these doses, recovery of vital normal cells from drug toxicity is often extended (e.g. often greater than 3 weeks in laboratory animals and man with the nitrosoureas) and, during the period of recovery from toxicity to the vital normal cells, the tumor cells surviving drug treatment continue to grow at a rate greater than that prior to drug treatment. Significant tumor cell kill ($\geqslant 7 \log_{10}$) with relatively small fractions of the LD_{10} dose of the effective alkylating agent combina-

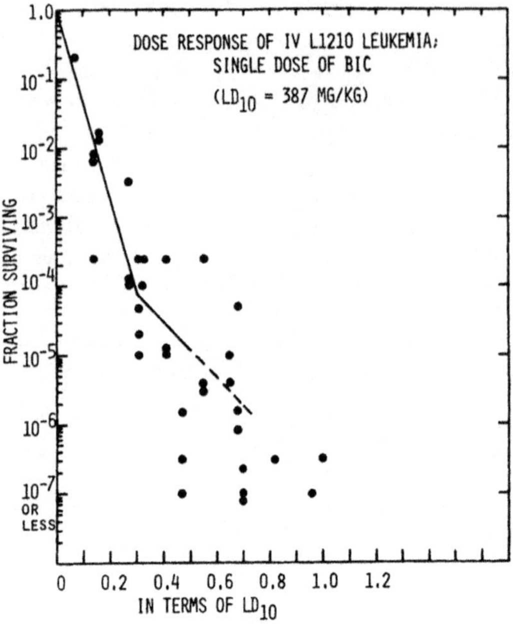

FIG. 5. Response of L1210 leukemia to a single dose of BIC.

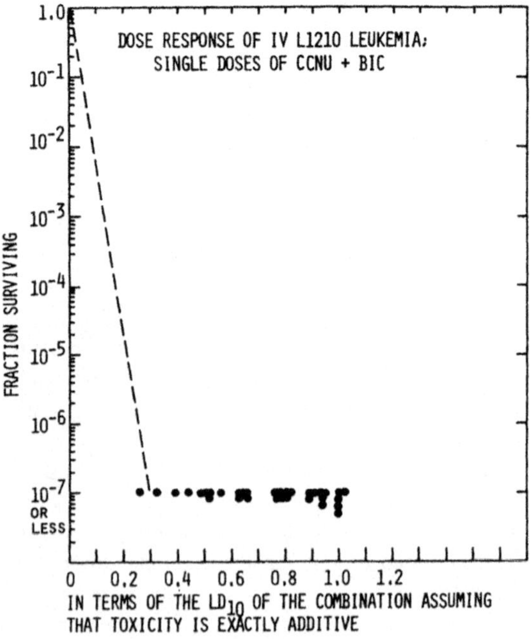

FIG. 6. Response of L1210 leukemia to a single dose of CCNU + BIC.

TABLE 6. TOXICITY OF COMBINATIONS OF BIC + CCNU IN NORMAL BDF[1] MICE*

Individual doses (fraction of single-dose LD_{10}) (mg/kg/dose) CCNU + BIC	Sum of fractions of single-dose LD_{10} values: Per Dose	Total	Schedule	Mortality† (survivors/total)	Maximum Mean wt loss (g)
12(0.2) + 120(0.3)	**0.5**	**2.0**	*q.7d.* X 4	**8/10**	4
12(0.2) + 80(0.2)	0.4	1.6	*q.7d.* X 4	10/10	3
12(0.2) + 53(0.14)	0.34	1.4	*q.7d.* X 4	10/10	3
8(0.14) + 270(0.7)	**0.84**	**3.4**	*q.7d.* X 4	**7/10**	5
8(0.14) + 180(0.5)	0.64	2.6	*q.7d.* X 4	10/10	4
8(0.14) + 120(0.3)	0.44	1.8	*q.7d.* X 4	9/10	3
8(0.14) + 80(0.2)	0.34	1.4	*q.7d.* X 4	10/10	3
12(0.2) + 180(0.5)	**0.7**	**2.8**	*q.4d.* X 4	**0/10**	8
12(0.2) + 120(0.3)	0.5	2.0	*q.4d.* X 4	9/10	5
12(0.2) + 80(0.2)	0.4	1.6	*q.4d.* X 4	10/10	6
8(0.14) + 180(0.5)	**0.64**	**2.6**	*q.4d.* X 4	**7/10**	5
8(0.14) + 120(0.3)	0.44	1.8	*q.4d.* X 4	9/10	5
8(0.14) + 80(0.2)	0.34	1.4	*q.4d.* X 4	10/10	3

*Historical single-dose LD_{10}: BIC = 387 mg/kg; CCNU = 57 mg/kg.
†>Forty-five days post-therapy.

tions has great promise for improved cancer chemotherapy, if these combination drug doses can be given at shorter intervals.

We have investigated the doses of CCNU + BIC that can be given to mice on a *q.* 4 *d.* X 4 and *q.* 4 *d.* X 7 schedule (Table 6). All treatments were given i.p., single dose. A number of combination drug doses killing ⩾7 $\log_{10}$ of L1210 cells *in vivo* (⩾ 0.3 combination drug LD_{10}) (Fig. 6) can be given *q.* 4 *d.* X 4 or *q.* 7 *d.* X 4 without exceeding the LD_{10} in normal mice (Table 6).

In similar studies with the combinations of BIC + BCNU and BIC + MeCCNU, essentially the same therapeutic potentiation was observed. We have not conducted similar toxicity studies with BIC + BCNU or BIC + CCNU.

While DIC probably is acting as an alkylating agent,[38] we failed to see therapeutic potentiation with DIC + CCNU against generalized L1210. In fact, these two drugs in simulatneous combinations are more than additive in toxicity in non-tumor-bearing mice (Fig. 7). This observation may be of some further interest, since the combination of DIC + BCNU has recently been reported not to be therapeutically potentiating against malignant melanoma in man.[41]

I hold no brief for BIC plus one or another of the nitrosoureas as combination drug panaceas for curing cancer in animals or man. BIC is a difficult drug to apply clinically, and therapeutic responses in man have not been promising to this time.* The promise of the observed therapeutic potentiation of this combination is that other alkylating agent combinations with similar high therapeutic activity at low fractions of doses with hazardous toxicity or long normal cell recovery times may be found. If such should occur, one of the most serious limitations to alkylating agent cancer chemotherapy (long intervals between effective sequential doses) will be overcome.

*S. K. Carter, personal communication.

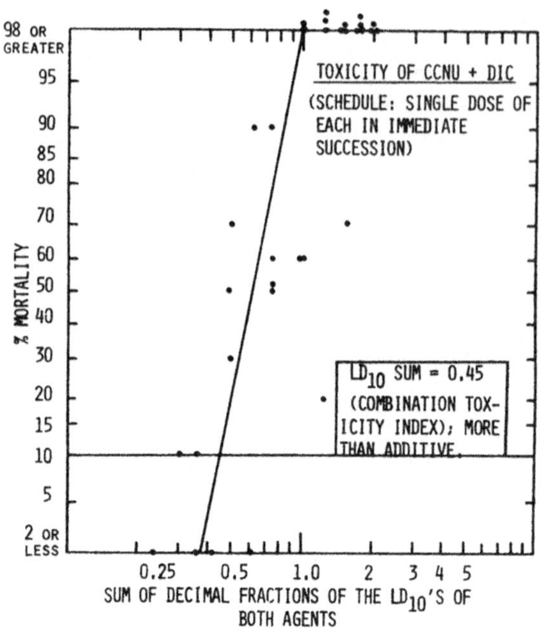

FIG. 7. Effect of simultaneous combination of DIC and CCNU in non-tumor-bearing mice.

The observed sensitivity and cross-resistance of alkylating agent-resistant lines of tumor cells to other alkylating agents are both complex and confusing.[42] L1210 cells resistant to BCNU are sensitive to cyclophosphamide;[43] Lewis lung carcinoma cells resistant to MeCCNU are sensitive to cyclophosphamide;* a hamster plasmacytoma resistant to BCNU is cross-resistant to cyclophosphamide and triethylenemelamine;* L1210 cells resistant to DIC are sensitive to cyclophosphamide, BCNU, CCNU and BIC;[44] L1210 cells resistant to BIC are cross-resistant to BCNU, CCNU and DIC,[45] and some plasma cell myelomas of man, naturally resistant to melphalan, are sensitive to cyclophosphamide.[46] There is no clear evidence that cross-resistance among alkylating agents is self-limiting in considering them for combination chemotherapy, but if possible, clearly demonstrated cross-resistance should be avoided.

SUMMARY

The drug combination of adriamycin plus 5-(3,3-dimethyl-1-triazeno)imidazole-4-carboxamide (DIC) is more active than either drug alone against at least four murine tumors, including several that are relatively insenstitive to drug treatment. Previously reported clinical trials indicate that the combination of adriamycin plus DIC shows therapeutic advantage over either drug alone against at least ten different metastatic sarcomas in man.

Adriamycin acts by binding to DNA. There are at least ten other antitumor drugs with major chemical structural differences which either bind to or intercalate with

*Southern Research Insitute, unpublished data.

DNA. Several of these have broad spectrum antitumor activity when used alone, and in addition, some are known to show therapeutic advantage when used in combination with a wide variety of other anticancer agents (representing most of the chemical and biological classes of known anticancer agents) against a number of different tumors in experimental animals and man. Further, some anticancer agents that bind to DNA (actinomycin D and adriamycin, at least) appear to kill leukemia L1210 and Ridgway osteogenic sarcoma cells whether or not they are in active cellular proliferation. These observations suggest that searches for new drug combinations with therapeutic advantage over those presently known be made among active compounds that bind to or intercalate with tumor cell DNA plus active compounds of other chemical and biological classes.

The combination of 1-(2-chloroethyl)-3-cyclohexyl-1-nitrosourea (CCNU) plus 5-[3,3-bis(2-chloroethyl)-1-triazeno]imidazole-4-carboxamide (BIC) has been shown to retain high cytotoxic specificity for leukemia L1210 cells at relatively low and nontoxic doses for vital normal cells. These observations suggest that therapeutically effective alkylating agent combinations with low toxicity and short recovery times for vital normal cells may be found by further studies of other combinations of active alkylating agents.

REFERENCES

1. H. S. SCHWARTZ, J. E. SODERGREN, S. S. STERNBERG and F. S. PHILIPS, *Cancer Res.* **26**, 1873 (1966).
2. D. P. GRISWOLD, JR., F. M. SCHABEL, JR., W. S. WILCOX, L. SIMPSON-HERREN and H. E. SKIPPER, *Cancer Chemother. Rep.* **52**, 345 (1968).
3. M. C. LI, *Ann. intern. Med.* **74**, 102 (1971).
4. J. L. ZIEGLER, L. FASS, S. K. KYALWAZI and P. P. CARBONE, *Cancer, N.Y.* **26**, 474 (1970).
5. E. FREI, III, *Cancer Res.* **32**, 2593 (1972).
6. A. GOLDIN, J. M. VENDITTI and N. MANTEL, in *Handbook of Pharmacology* (Eds. A. C. SARTORELLI and D. G. JOHNS), Vol. 1, Springer, Berlin (1973), in press.
7. J. A. GOTTLIEB, L. H. BAKER, J. M. QUAGLIANA, J. K. LUCE, J. P. WHITECAR, JR., J. G. SINKOVICS, S. E. RIVKIN, R. BROWNLEE and E. FREI, III, *Cancer, N.Y.* **30**, 1632 (1972).
8. D. P. GRISWOLD, W. R. LASTER, JR. and F. M. SCHABEL, JR., *Am. Ass. Cancer Res.* **14**, 15 (1973).
9. B. A. NEWTON, in *Advances in Pharmacology and Chemotherapy* (Eds. S. GARRATTINI, A. GOLDIN, F. HAWKING and I. J. KOPIN), Vol. 8 pp. 149–84. Academic Press, New York (1970).
10. H. SUZUKI, K. NAGAI, H. YAMAKI, N. TANAKA and H. UMEZAWA, *J. Antibiot., Tokyo* **XXII**, 446 (1969).
11. K. NAGAI, H. SUZUKI, N. TANAKA and H. UMEZAWA, *J. Antibiot., Tokyo* **XXII**, 569 (1969).
12. K. NAGAI, H. SUZUKI, N. TANAKA and H. UMEZAWA, *J. Antibiot.., Tokyo* **XXII**, 624 (1969).
13. C. W. HAIDLE, *Molec. Pharmac.* **7**, 645 (1971).
14. C. W. HAIDLE, K. K. WEISS and M. T. KUO, *Molec. Pharmac.* **8**, 531 (1972).
15. S. B. HORWITZ, C. CHANG and A. P. GROLLMAN, *Molec. Pharmac.* **7**, 632 (1971).
16. H. E. KANN, JR. and K. W. KOHN, *Molec. Pharmac.* **8**, 551 (1972).
17. J. A. HOWLE and G. R. GALE, *Biochem. Pharmac.* **19**, 2757 (1970).
18. H. C. HARDER and B. ROSENBERG, *Int. J. Cancer* **6**, 207 (1970).
19. G. R. GALE, J. A. HOWLE and E. M. WALKER, JR., *Cancer Res.* **31**, 950 (1971).
20. J. A. HOWLE, H. S. THOMPSON, A. E. STONE and G. R. GALE, *Proc. Soc. exp. Biol. Med.* **137**, 820 (1971).
21. P. HORÁČEK and J. DROBNÍK, *Biochim. biophys. Acta* **254**, 341 (1971).
22. J. A. HOWLE, G. R. GALE and A. B. SMITH, *Biochem. Pharmac.* **21**, 1465 (1972).

23. L. L. BENNETT, JR., in *Progress in Experimental Tumor Research* (Ed. F. HOMBURGER), Vol. 7, pp. 259–325. S. Karger, Basel (1965).
24. G. G. ROSS, L. L. STOLBACH and R. HERTZ, *Cancer Res.* **22**, 1015 (1962).
25. R. J. SPEER, S. LAPIS, H. RIDGWAY, T. D. MYERS and J. M. HILL, *Wadley med. Bull.* **1**, 103 (1971).
26. R. J. WOODMAN, A. E. SIRICA, M. GANG, I. KLINE and J. M. VENDITTI, *Chemotherapy* **18**, 169 (1973).
27. R. J. SPEER, S. LAPIS, H. RIDGWAY, T. D. MYERS and J. M. HILL, in *Advances in Antimicrobial and Antineoplastic Chemotherapy*, Vol. 2 (Eds. M. SEMONSKÝ, M. HEJZLAR and S. MASÁK), *Proc. Seventh Int. Congr. Chemother.* p. 253–254, University Park Press, Baltimore (1972).
28. J. M. VENDITTI, in *Advances in Antimicrobial and Antineoplastic Chemotherapy*, Vol. 2 (Eds. M. SEMONSKY, M. HEJZLAR and S. MASAK), *Proc. Seventh Int. Congr. Chemother.* p. 233–234, University Park Press, Baltimore (1972).
29. A. H. ROSSOF, R. E. SLAYTON and C. P. PERLIA, *Cancer, N.Y.* **30**, 1451 (1972).
30. L. J. WILKOFF, H. H. LLOYD and E. A. DULMADGE, *Chemotherapy* **16**, 44 (1971).
31. J. M. VENDITTI, *Cancer Chemother. Rep.* **2**, 35 (1971).
32. L. H. SCHMIDT, R. FRADKIN, R. SULLIVAN and A. FLOWERS, *Cancer Chemother. Rep.* (suppl.) **2**, 1 (1965).
33. R. B. LIVINGSTON and S. K. CARTER (Eds.) *Single Agents in Cancer Chemotherapy*, p. 1–405 IFI/Plenum, New York (1970).
34. F. A. VALERIOTE, W. R. BRUCE and B. E. MEEKER, *J. natn. Cancer Inst.* **40**, 935 (1968).
35. F. M. SCHABEL, JR., in *Proc. Fifth Int. Congr. Chemother., Symp. B-10, Cancer Chemother.* (Eds. T. C. HALL and K. KARRER), p. 65–82. Verlag der Wiener Medizinischen Akademia, Vienna (1968).
36. H. S. LIN and W. R. BRUCE, *Series Hemat.* **5**, 89 (1972).
37. J. G. MAYO, W. R. LASTER, JR., C. M. ANDREWS and F. M. SCHABEL, JR., *Cancer Chemother. Rep.* **56**, 183 (1972).
38. G. P. WHEELER, in *Cancer Medicine* (Eds. HOLLAND and FREI), p. 791–806. Lea & Febiger, Philadelphia (1973).
39. H. E. SKIPPER, F. M. SCHABEL, JR. and W. S. WILCOX, *Cancer Chemother. Rep.* **35**, 1 (1964).
40. H. E. SKIPPER, F. M. SCHABEL, JR., L. B. MELLETT, J. A. MONTGOMERY, L. J. WILKOFF, H. H. LLOYD and R. W. BROCKMAN, *Cancer Chemother. Rep.* **54**, 431 (1970).
41. M. E. COSTANZA, L. NATHANSON, R. LENHARD, J. WOLTER, J. COLSKY, R. A. OBERFIELD and A. SCHILLING, *Cancer, N.Y.* **30**, 1457 (1972).
42. H. E. SKIPPER, D. J. HUTCHISON, F. M. SCHABEL, JR., L. H. SCHMIDT, A. GOLDIN, R. W. BROCKMAN, J. M. VENDITTI and I. WODINSKY, *Cancer Chemother. Rep.* **56**, 493 (1972).
43. S. K. CARTER, F. M. SCHABEL, JR., L. E. BRODER and T. P. JOHNSON, in *Advances in Cancer Research* (Eds. G. KLEIN and S. WEINHOUSE), Vol. 16, pp. 273–332. Academic Press, New York (1972).
44. I. KLINE, R. J. WOODMAN, M. GANG and J. M. VENDITTI, *Cancer Chemother. Rep.* **55**, 9 (1971).
45. D. D. TYRER, I. KLINE, M. GANG, A. GOLDIN and J. M. VENDITTI, *Cancer Chemother. Rep.* **53**, 229 (1969).
46. D. E. BERGSAGEL, D. H. COWAN and R. HASSELBACK, *Can. med. Ass. J.* **107**, 851 (1972).

Pp. 177—182, Supplement Number 2, 1974.
Biochemical Pharmacology. Printed in the U.S.A.

NEW COMBINATIONS IN THE TREATMENT OF LUNG CANCER*

GERALD P. BODEY,† ROBERT LIVINGSTON and JEFFREY GOTTLIEB

Department of Developmental Therapeutics, The University of Texas M. D. Anderson Hospital and Tumor Institute at Houston, Houston, Texas 77025, U. S. A.

LUNG CANCER is the most common malignant disease in men, and the death rate has increased over 10-fold during the past 30 years. Less than 10 per cent of unselected patients with lung cancer survive 5 years. Even in patients undergoing presumptive curative surgery, the 5-year survival is only 25 per cent. Among patients dying within 1 month after presumed curative surgery, 26 per cent had residual disease or metastases at autopsy.[1] Consequently, other modalities of therapy are needed if long-term survival is to be accomplished in this disease.

A wide variety of chemotherapeutic agents have been studied in patients with extensive lung cancer. Few of these agents have had any impact on the disease process. Those drugs which have induced partial remissions have seldom been effective for more than a few months. Consequently, many chemotherapists have become somewhat pessimistic about the treatment of this common malignant disease.

Several developments in recent years have influenced the design of our protocols for the treatment of lung cancer. The development of an experimental animal tumor model, the Lewis lung carcinoma, has provided significant preclinical evaluations of new agents and combinations. Studies of tumor cell kinetics have increased our understanding of mechanisms of drug activity and suggested more effective therapeutic schedules. New antitumor agents such as bleomycin and nitrosourea derivatives have been discovered. Lastly, the concept of combination chemotherapy has expanded our horizons and already has led to substantial improvement in the control of several malignant diseases.[2,3]

Vincristine has not been studied extensively as single agent therapy of lung cancer. In a recent collation of the literature, a partial response rate of 17 per cent was determined among 29 patients entered on various studies (Table 1).[4] Cyclophosphamide has been used extensively in lung cancer, both as adjuvant therapy in surgical patients and as single agent therapy in patients with extensive disease. A variety of regimens have been employed and results have been very variable. In a collated series of 340 patients, the partial response rate was 28 per cent.[4]

Initial reports in the Japanese literature suggested that bleomycin was moderately effective in patients with extensive bronchogenic carcinoma. During a phase II study of this drug conducted by the Southwest Cancer Chemotherapy Study Group, 68 patients

*Supported in part by Grant CA 05831 and CA 03754 from the National Cancer Institute, National Institutes of Health, U.S. Public Health Service, Bethesda, Md. 20014.

†Scholar of the Leukemia Society of America, Inc.

TABLE 1. THERAPEUTIC REGIMENS IN LUNG CANCER

Regimen	Entered	Adequate trial	Partial response/ adequate trial (%)
Vincristine*	29		17
Bleomycin	68	60	5
Cyclophosphamide*	340		28
Methyl CCNU	114	81	20
Bleomycin + vincristine	17	15	27
Methyl CCNU + cyclophosphamide	20	19	16
COMB No. 1	24	21	43
COMB No. 2	13	12	83
Total COMB	37	33	57

*Referred to in Ref. 4 as "patients entered."

with lung cancer were studied.[5] Bleomycin was administered either intravenously or intramuscularly at a dose of 10 mg/m^2 of body surface area semiweekly. Only three responses were observed among the 60 patients who received an adequate trial (Table 2). Patients were considered to have had an adequate trial if they received 2 weeks of therapy. They were considered to have had a partial response if there was greater than a 50 per cent reduction in the two widest diameters of all measurable tumor masses during chemotherapy without appearance of any new lesions.

TABLE 2. BLEOMYCIN IN BRONCHOGENIC CARCINOMA

	Cell type of bronchogenic carcinoma			
	Epidermoid	Adenoca	Oat cell	Total
Entered	35	9	24	68
Complete remission	0	1	0	1
Partial response	1	1	0	2

Using advanced Lewis lung carcinoma in rodents, Mayo *et al.*[6] demonstrated that 1-(2-chloroethyl)-3-(*trans*-4-methylcyclohexyl)-1-nitrosourea (methyl CCNU), a new oral nitrosourea, was considerably more effective than other nitrosoureas or other conventional chemotherapeutic agents. For example, 7 days after tumor implant, surgical removal of the implant resulted in no long-term survivors, cyclophosphamide in 1 per cent, but methyl CCNU in 34 per cent long-term survivors. However, the latter drug was not effective in disease of longer duration. In studies of methyl CCNU conducted by the Southwest Cancer Chemotherapy Study Group, 114 patients with lung cancer were included.* The drug was administered orally at a dose of 150–200 mg/m^2 every

*J. Gottlieb, unpublished observations.

6 weeks. Eighty-one of these patients received an adequate trial, which was considered to be survival for 6 weeks (Table 3). Fifteen patients achieved a partial response, and one patient with epidermoid carcinoma achieved a complete remission. Major toxicity included nausea, vomiting and myelosuppression.

TABLE 3. METHYL CCNU IN LUNG CANCER

	Cell type of lung cancer				
	Epidermoid	Adenoca	Oat cell	Alveolar	Total
Entered	56	27	26	5	114
Adequate trial	41	19	17	4	81
Partial response	9	3	2	2	16
Response/entered (%)	16	11	8	40	14
Response/adequate trial (%)	22	16	12	50	20

None of these agents used alone produced encouraging results in bronchogenic carcinoma. However, recent studies *in vitro* using Chinese hamster ovarian cells have demonstrated that 50 per cent of asynchronous cells are killed by 12 μg/ml of bleomycin at 30 min.[7] The remaining cells were more resistant, and only an additional 25 per cent were killed by concentrations up to 100 μg/ml. Further studies with synchronized cells revealed that bleomycin was more effective against cells in G_2 of the cell cycle, but especially against cells in mitosis. At a concentration of 50 μg/ml, only 2 per cent of cells in mitosis survived. At a concentration of 1 μg/ml, bleomycin killed 60 per cent of cells in mitosis and 50 per cent in G_2, but less than 10 per cent of cells in other phases of the cell cycle. Vincristine causes an accumulation of cells in mitosis, probably through damage to a mitotic spindle precursor in late S or G_2 of the cell cycle. This effect of vincristine reaches a maximum at 6–12 hr after administration in human bone marrow.[8] The related vinca alkaloid, vinblastine, has a similar stathmokinetic effect against squamous cell carcinomas.[9] This information suggested that the two drugs might be used effectively in combination. When tested in the Lewis lung tumor, vincristine was inactive, but prior treatment with vincristine enhanced the antitumor activity of bleomycin.*

Seventeen patients with lung cancer were treated with vincristine and bleomycin.[10] Vincristine was administered intravenously at a dose of 1 mg (0.75 mg for patients over 50 years old), followed 6 hr later by bleomycin, 20 mg/m^2 intramuscularly (maximum dose 35 mg). The regimen was given semiweekly for 6 weeks, after which time patients were evaluated for antitumor response and placed on other therapy. This change in therapy was necessitated by the potentially fatal pulmonary toxicity of bleomycin at total doses exceeding 300 mg. Seventeen patients with lung cancer were entered on this preliminary study, and 15 received an adequate trial (2 weeks of therapy). Four patients achieved partial responses, representing a 27 per cent response

*F. M. Schabel, Jr., unpublished observations.

rate among patients receiving an adequate trial (Table 1). One of five patients with epidermoid, one of one with oat cell and two of nine with adenocarcinoma responded. Major toxicity from this regimen included nausea, vomiting, skin changes, alopecia and neuropathy. No unexpected toxicity occurred as a result of the use of these two drugs in combination. Although this was only a small study, the results appeared to be more encouraging than with either bleomycin or vincristine alone. Since neither of these agents has substantial myelosuppressive toxicity, it was anticipated that they could be added to myelosuppressive regimens without necessitating a reduction in dosage of these agents.

While these clinical studies were in progress, Mayo *et al.*[6] demonstrated that the combination of methyl CCNU and cyclophosphamide was highly synergistic against Lewis lung carcinoma. For example, 16 days after subcutaneous tumor implant, when metastatic disease was present, if the implant was removed surgically, the combination of methyl CCNU and cyclophosphamide produced 55 per cent long-term survivors, whereas either drug alone, or the combination without local surgery, was ineffective.

Twenty patients with lung cancer were entered on a study of the combination of methyl CCNU and cyclophosphamide and 19 received an adequate trial (Table 1). Three patients achieved a partial response (one of six epidermoid, one of two oat cell and one of eleven adenocarcinoma). Methyl CCNU was administered orally at a dose of 100–250 mg/m^2 and cyclophosphamide was administered intravenously at a dose of 800–1000 mg/m^2.[11] Both drugs were repeated at 6-week intervals. Toxicity was manifested mainly by nausea, vomiting and myelosuppression. Myelosuppression usually occurred early and was felt to be largely due to cyclophosphamide. Secondary falls in blood counts due to methyl CCNU did occur, however, most often after multiple courses of therapy, and were usually less severe than the early myelosuppression caused by the cyclophosphamide.

After these initial studies, a four-drug regimen was developed consisting of vincristine, bleomycin, cyclophosphamide and methyl CCNU. This combination (COMB) is especially advantageous because the drugs have largely independent toxicities and each can be administered at optimum dose. In the original schedule (COMB No. 1), cyclophosphamide was given intravenously at a dose of 1 g/m^2 and methyl CCNU was given orally at a dose of 100 mg/m^2 on day 1. The following day, 0.75–1 mg vincristine was administered intravenously, and 6 hr later 30 mg bleomycin was administered intravenously. The latter two drugs were given twice weekly for 6 weeks, and the former two drugs were given once every 6 weeks. At the present time, 24 patients with lung cancer have been assigned to this regimen and 21 have received an adequate trial (Tables 1 and 4). Nine patients (43%) have achieved a partial response, including all five patients with oat cell carcinoma and three of six with epidermoid carcinoma.

Since pulmonary toxicity prevents the administration of total doses of bleomycin in excess of 300 mg, the dosage regimen of COMB was revised to permit the administration of this drug for longer than a 6-week period. Consequently, the dose of bleomycin was reduced to 15 mg given intravenously twice weekly for 12 weeks, again with 0.75–1.0 mg vincristine 6 hr before each dose of bleomycin. It was also decided to administer the cyclophosphamide and methyl CCNU every 4 weeks, since most patients had recovered from the myelosuppressive toxicity by that time. The dosage of cyclophosphamide was reduced to 800 mg/m^2 and the dose of methyl CCNU was

TABLE 4. COMB THERAPY IN LUNG CANCER

	Cell type of lung cancer			
	Epidermoid	Adenoca	Oat cell	Total
COMB No. 1				
Entered	8	11	5	24
Adequate trial	6	10	5	21
Partial response	3	1	5	9
Response/entered (%)	38	9	100	38
Response/adequate trial (%)	50	10	100	44
COMB No. 2				
Entered	6	2	5	13
Adequate trial	6	1	5	12
Partial response	5	0	5	10
Response/entered (%)	83	0	100	77
Response/adequate trial (%)	83	0	100	83
Total				
Entered	14	13	10	37
Adequate trial	12	11	10	33
Partial response	8	1	10	19
Response/entered (%)	57	8	100	51
Response/adequate trial (%)	67	9	100	58

maintained at 100 mg/m^2 every 4 weeks. Thirteen patients have received this drug regimen (COMB No. 2) and 12 have received an adequate trial. Ten achieved partial responses (83 per cent). All five patients with oat cell, and five of six with epidermoid carcinomas responded (Table 4).

A total of 33 patients have received an adequate trial on the COMB regimens at the present time and 19 have responded (58 per cent). Especially impressive is the 100 per cent response rate for the ten patients with oat cell carcinoma. Eight of 12 patients (67 per cent) with epidermoid carcinomas also have responded. Unfortunately, patients with adenocarcinomas have not responded favorably to this regimen.

Toxicity data have been obtained from 48 patients who received either COMB regimen for a variety of tumors. The median lowest neutrophil count was 0.3/mm^3 for COMB No. 1 and 0.6/mm^3 for COMB No. 2. Only five patients developed platelet counts less than 50,000/mm^3. Virtually all patients developed peripheral neuropathy, anorexia and skin toxicity. Eleven patients developed proven or probable pulmonary toxicity from bleomycin which was clinically significant in four and probably contributed to death in two patients.

Certainly these early studies suggest that COMB is effective against oat cell and epidermoid carcinoma of the lung. It appears that lower doses of bleomycin for longer periods are superior to higher doses for a shorter duration. These studies also indicate the important interplay between basic scientific research and clinical investigation.

REFERENCES

1. G. A. HIGGINS and G. W. BEEBE, *Archs Surg. Lond.* **94**, 539 (1967).
2. E. J. FREIREICH, E. S. HENDERSON, M. K. KARON and E. FREI, III, in *Proliferation and Spread of Neoplastic Cells*, pp. 441–53. Williams & Wilkins (1968).
3. V. T. DEVITA, JR., A. SERPICK and P. P. CARBONE, *Ann. intern. Med.* **73**, 881 (1970).
4. P. P. CARBONE, J. K. FROST, A. R. FEINSTEIN, G. A. HIGGINS, JR. and O. S. SELAWRY, *Ann. intern. Med.* **73**, 1003 (1970).
5. E. FREIREICH, J. LUCE and J. GOTTLIEB, *Proc. Int. Symp. on Bleomycin*, Rio de Janeiro, Brazil (November 1971) in press.
6. J. G. MAYO, W. R. LASTER, JR., C. M. ANDREWS and F. M. SCHABEL, JR., *Cancer Chemother. Rep.* **56**, 183 (1972).
7. S. BARRANCO and R. HUMPHREY, *Cancer Res.* **31**, 1218 (1971).
8. E. FREI, III, J. WHANG, R. B. SCOGGINS, E. J. VANSCOTT, D. P. RALL and M. BEN, *Cancer Res.* **24**, 1918 (1964).
9. J. MEYER and R. DONALDSON, *Archs Path.* **87**, 479 (1969).
10. R. B. LIVINGSTON, G. P. BODEY, J. A. GOTTLIEB and E. FREI, III, *Cancer Chemother. Rep.*, in press.
11. G. P. BODEY, J. A. GOTTLIEB, R. LIVINGSTON and E. FREI, III, *Cancer Chemother. Rep.*, in press.

Pp. 183–192, Supplement Number 2, 1974.
Biochemical Pharmacology. Printed in the U.S.A.

CHEMOTHERAPY OF METASTATIC SARCOMAS USING COMBINATIONS WITH ADRIAMYCIN*,†

JEFFREY A. GOTTLIEB, LAURENCE H. BAKER, ROBERT M. O'BRYAN, JAMES K. LUCE, JOSEPH G. SINKOVICS and JOSEPH M. QUAGLIANA

Developmental Therapeutics, M. D. Anderson Hospital, Tumor Institute at Houston
Houston, Texas 77025, U.S.A.

ALTHOUGH scattered reports in the literature indicate that the different sarcomas are responsive to chemotherapeutic agents, principally cyclophosphamide, actinomycin D and/or vincristine, relatively few series of significant numbers of patients treated with a similar therapeutic regimen have appeared. While combining reports from the articles that have appeared may be subject to a considerable number of inaccuracies, such data suggest that the remission rate for patients with metastatic sarcomas has rarely exceeded 20 per cent in the past, with most of these remissions incomplete and short-lasting, and thus of relatively little clinical benefit to the patient.[1,2]

Recently, several phase II studies in sarcomas performed by the Southwest Cancer Chemotherapy Study Group and M. D. Anderson Hospital showed impressive preliminary activity. These studies involved two new agents, namely the antitumor antibiotic, adriamycin, and the synthetically synthetized purine analog, dimethyl triazeno imidazole carboxamide (DIC). As shown in Table 1, our data and data from other centers suggested that the activity of these two agents, when used alone, was substantial and that a combination regimen involving adriamycin and DIC might be worth pursuing.

Concurrent with these clincial efforts, several important preclinical studies were also being undertaken. These investigations, which were performed independently at the National Cancer Institute and at Southern Research Institute, showed that adriamycin and DIC could be combined in near full dosage with the efficacy of the combination at least additive, and not associated with an increase in toxicity. Thus the lifespan of mice bearing L1210 leukemia treated with the combination was significantly longer than that of animals treated with either agent alone, and similar results were seen in a number of solid tumor systems including B16 melanoma and C3H adenocarcinoma.[4,‡]

Spurred on by these studies and by our own observations at M. D. Anderson, that the combination appeared better than the single drug studies, a broad phase II study combining adriamycin and DIC in the treatment of metastatic sarcomas was begun in the Southwest Group in July of 1971. The regimen used for that study is shown in Table 2. Adriamycin at a dose of 60 mg/m^2 was given intravenously on day 1, with DIC at a dose of 250 mg/m^2 given intravenously on days 1–5 with an appropriate

*This work was supported by Grants No. CA 03754, CA 07177-09, CA 08096, CA 13238, CA 10379-06 and CA 04915 from the National Cancer Institute.
†This work is drawn from data from four protocols of the Southwest Cancer Cheomtherapy Study Group: Protocols No. 434, 442, 445 and 7210.
‡F. M. Schabel, Jr., personal communication.

TABLE 1. LITERATURE SUMMARY OF RESPONSES IN SARCOMAS TO ADRIAMYCIN OR DIC*

	Adriamycin		DIC	
Diagnosis	No. patients	CR/PR†	No. patients	CR/PR
Sarcoma, unspecified and misc.	37	–/5	7	–/–
Osteogenic sarcoma	35	2/8	6	–/1
Ewing's sarcoma	20	–/12	2	–/–
Rhabdomyosarcoma	16	–/2	13	–/2
Chondrosarcoma	8	–/1	1	–/–
Fibrosarcoma	5	–/3	11	–/1
Liposarcoma	4	–/2	2	–/–
Leimyosarcoma		–/–	24	1/5
Synovial cell sarcoma	3	1/2	1	–/–
	131	3/35 (29%)	67	1/9 (15%)

*From Gottlieb *et al.*[3]
†CR = complete remission; PR = partial remission.

TABLE 2. COMBINATION CHEMOTHERAPY REGIMENS WITH ADRIAMYCIN IN SARCOMAS

	Adriamycin and DIC (SWG No. 445)
Adequate marrow reserve	
Adriamycin	60 mg/m^2 i.v. *d*1 only
DIC	250 mg/m^2 i.v. *d*1 to 5
Inadequate marrow reserve	
Adriamycin	45 mg/m^2 i.v. *d*1 only
DIC	200 mg/m^2 i.v. *d*1 to 5
	Vincristine, adriamycin and DIC (SWG No. 7210)
Add vincristine	1.0 mg/m^2 (top dose 1.5 mg) *d*1 and 5

decrease for patients with extensive prior therapy. In a subsequent study which was begun in September of 1972, vincristine was added and administered on the first and fifth day, as is shown in Table 2. The entire regimen was repeated every 3 weeks. To prevent the known cardiotoxicity of high cumulative doses of adriamycin, the total dose of adriamycin was limited to 550 mg/m^2.[5] Once this dose was reached, the patients continued on DIC alone, and in the case of the three-drug study on vincristine as well.

The doses of adriamycin and DIC in this regimen are approximately full dose, i.e. the dose used when the drugs are used alone. Although it was empiric observations that led to the initial thoughts of combining adriamycin and DIC, there are several theoretical reasons why these drugs should be effective in the sarcomas. These tumors may often have low proliferative fractions with numerous cells presumably in the G_0 state or at least not affected by extensive trials in the past with cell cycle sensitive agents.[2] Adriamycin is capable of killing cells regardless of their cell cycle stage, although it may be slightly more effective against cells in mitosis and in S.[6,7] Relatively similar characteristics have been observed with DIC, that is, it too can kill nonproliferating tumor cells, although its period of major efficacy may be in the late G_2 phase.[8] This possibly suggests a sequential killing effect in that cells escaping the slight superiority of adriamycin in the S phase would still have to face the slight superiority of DIC in the G_2 phase and adriamycin again in mitosis.

The empiric addition of vincristine also took into consideration the kinetic and pharmacologic behavior of adriamycin. It has been shown by Benjamin *et al.*[9] that adriamycin has a long plasma half-life, in excess of 25 hr.[10] Several other investigators have shown in experimental animal tumor systems that, after vincristine produces a mitotic arrest, the cells released are partially synchronized, in that a subsequent wave of S has been observed.[10] As the concentration of adriamycin slowly decreases in the plasma, the mitotic arrest and the second wave of S produced by the administration of vincristine may increase the cell-killing ability of these low levels of adriamycin because of the previously mentioned superiority of that drug against these stages of the cell cycle. Statistical tests to see if vincristine is actually improving the efficacy of the two drugs cannot yet be applied.

RESULTS AND DISCUSSION

Table 3 shows the current status of these two studies. The adriamycin–DIC regimen (the Southwest Group's protocol No. 445) has accumulated 234 patients plus 20 more patients who have not yet been evaluated. The three-drug regimen with vincristine (SWG No. 7210) has 45 patients. Since it was subsequently shown that the median interval from the start of therapy until response was approximately 2 months, 39

TABLE 3. ADRIAMYCIN COMBINATIONS IN SARCOMAS

	Adriamycin and DIC (SWG No. 445)		Vincristine, adriamycin and DIC (SWG No. 7210)	
Entered		234		45
Inevaluable		34		5
Early death (< 3 wks)	16		4	
< 1 Course completed	18		1	
Evaluable		200		40
CR		22		2
PR		63		17
All responses/entered		85/234 (36%)		19/45 (42%)
All responses/evaluable		85/200 (42.5%)		19/40 (48.5%)
		20 more too early		79 more too early

patients were considered inevaluable. Twenty of these died from rapidly progressing malignancy before completing a single course within the first 3 weeks of ths study. An additional 19 failed to complete a single course. This group provided some information because, while a number of them were lost to follow-up, the remainder are largely patients removed from study because of their inability to accept therapy. What was impressive in analyzing these patients was the disproportionate number that were young (in the 15–20 year group). They either discontinued therapy on their own or convinced their physician to take them off study. This refractoriness of teenagers to accept therapy has been noted in other diseases and must be considered when designing protocols aimed at this age group.

Considering only the two-drug study with adriamycin and DIC, there were 85 responders, including 22 complete responders, for an over-all complete and partial response rate of 36 per cent, considering everyone who received even 1 day of therapy, and 42.5 per cent for the 200 evaluable patients. The three-drug study in which vincristine was added shows a 42.5 per cent response rate considering all patients and a 48.5 per cent response considering only the 40 evaluable patients. Table 3 shows that most of the patients on this last study have not been evaluated and explains why statistical tests to see if vincristine is adding to the response rate have not yet been applied.

Table 4 shows the response rate by diagnosis of patients treated with the two-drug and three-drug regimens. The combined results shown in the third column indicate a relatively uniform response rate in the various types of sarcomas, with a few notable exceptions. Thus no patient with chondrosarcoma has achieved a greater than 50 per cent decrease in his tumor mass. While several of these patients had progressive disease prior to starting therapy, which subsequently stabilized, and a number had impressive subjective responses, no patients with chondrosarcoma have had significant decreases in the bulk of their tumor. The only other tumor with significant accrual which seems to

TABLE 4. COMPLETE AND PARTIAL RESPONSE RATE IN 240 EVALUABLE PATIENTS

Diagnosis	Adriamycin and DIC (A-DIC) SWG No. 445	Fincristine, adriamycin, DIC (VA-DIC) SWG No. 7210	Combined
Angiosarcoma	3/8*	0/1	3/9 (33%)
Chondrosarcoma	0/9	0/1	0/10
Ewing's sarcoma	1/2		1/2 (50%)
Fibrosarcoma	11/23	3/6	14/29 (48%)
Leiomyosarcoma	17/36	5/10	22/46 (48%)
Liposarcoma	5/16	2/4	7/20 (35%)
Mesothelioma	4/9	0/2	4/11 (36%)
Neurofibrosarcoma	10/22		10/22 (45%)
Osteogenic sarcoma	13/31	1/5	14/36 (39%)
Rhabdomyosarcoma	7/17	2/3	9/20 (45%)
Synovial cell sarcoma	5/8		5/8 (63%)
Undifferentiated sarcoma	9/19	6/8	15/27 (56%)
Totals	85/200 (42%)	19/40 (48%)	104/240 (43.4%)

*CR and PR/evaluable patients.

be lagging behind is the liposarcoma group. The rest of the tumors, including fibrosarcoma, leiomyosarcoma, neurofibrosarcoma, osteogenic sarcoma, rhabdomyosarcoma and undifferentiated sarcoma, all have similar response rates of approxiamtely 40–50 per cent. A few of the less common tumor types also seem to have a similar response rate, but their numbers are too small to be certain. In addition to partial remissions, complete remissions have been seen in all the cell tumor types listed, except chondrosarcoma, and in the relatively infrequent tumors in this series, the Ewing's sarcoma, mesothelioma and synovial cell sarcoma (Table 5). The similarity in the response rate seen here suggests that sarcomas, once metastatic, may be viewed as a single disease with regard to chemotherapy with the exceptions mentioned above.

TABLE 5. COMPLETE RESPONSES WITH ADRIAMYCIN AND DIC (SWG NO. 445) AND VINCRISTINE, ADRIAMYCIN AND DIC (SWG NO. 7210)

Diagnosis	No. of patients
Angiosarcoma	1
Fibrosarcoma	3
Leiomyosarcoma	6
Liposarcoma	2
Neurofibrosarcoma	3
Osteogenic	3
Rhabdomyosarcoma	3
Undifferentiated	3
Total	24

It is interesting to speculate why chondrosarcoma is so refractory. Recent investigations with tumor angiogenesis factor by Folkman[11] have noted that, of all tumors, the chondrosarcoma requires the least number of blood vessels to sustain it. It is tempting to postualte that the waste materials of cell metabolism are neatly packaged in the cartilaginous matrix, and thus do not require blood vessels to carry these wastes away. This inadequancy of blood supply may lead to poor perfusion of the tumor with the chemotherapeutic agents, and thus account for the poor response noted.

Table 6 shows the duration of the responses in the two-drug, adriamycin and DIC study. Of the 22 complete responders, 19 patients remain in remission for a median duration which is now nearly 1 year. For the partial remissions, the duration is now almost one-half year with 40 per cent of these patients still responding. These data suggest that the remissions achieved with this two-drug combination are superior not only to reported regimens with other agents but also to the single-drug studies with adriamycin and DIC in which the median duration of response was less than 4 months. For the 11 per cent of patients achieving complete remission, the durations of response are especially gratifying. Most of these patients have resumed completely normal activity, receiving maintenance therapy with DIC alone at approximately monthly intervals. A number have now had all therapy discontinued.

Table 7 shows a breakdown of the response rate by sex. In the two-drug combination, the response rate for women was 50 per cent; for men it was only 36 per cent.

TABLE 6. DURATION OF RESPONSE IN 85 RESPONDERS TO ADRIAMYCIN AND DIC

	Median (mos)	Range (mos)	No. still in remission
CR	9+	2+ – 18+	19/22 (86%)
PR	5+	1 – 18+	25/63 (40%)
All responders	6+	1 – 18+	44/85 (52%)

TABLE 7. RESPONSE BY SEX

	Female	Male
Adriamycin + DIC (SWG No. 445)	47/93 (50%)*	38/107 (36%)
Vincristine, adriamycin, DIC (SWG No. 7210)	11/18 (61%)	8/22 (36%)
Combined	58/111 (52%)	46/129 (36%)

*CR and PR/evaluable patients (% response).

In the three-drug study, the response rate for women was 61 per cent and for men again 36 per cent. While not yet statistically significant, an improved response rate has also been previously observed in women receiving DIC for malignant melanoma,[12] and the possible superiority of DIC-containing regimens for women with sarcomas must be considered. This sex variation will be carefully scrutinized as the numbers in this study become larger. We are also attempting to verify this sex difference in laboratory animals.

The response by the site of the primary tumor is shown in Table 8. The rate of response in this table is only for the two-drug combination and is listed in order of decreasing response rate from left to right. Thus it can be seen that an over-all response rate of approxiamtely 40–50 per cent is seen in all the common primary sites, with two exceptions. Patients whose disease started in the pelvis and trunk and patients whose disease began in the gastrointestinal tract appear to have significantly lower response rates than those whose disease starts elsewhere. In addition to providing a response rate by the site of the primary tumor, Table 8 also gives the incidence of primary locations in these metastatic sarcomas. Thus, of 200 patients, 70, or 35 per cent had limb primaries.

Table 9 shows the response by the site of metastatic lesion. Subcutaneous and skin metastases appear somewhat more responsive that the bone and liver metastases, but over-all the response rate appears quite similar. The lone exception appears to be the relatively infrequently encountered CNS metastases, which had lower response rates than those with the other locations. Since it is known that adriamycin and DIC

TABLE 8. RESPONSE BY SITE OF PRIMARY IN 200 PATIENTS RECEIVING ADRIAMYCIN AND DIC

		Primary sites						
	No. of patients	H and N	G U and uterus	Retroper.	Unknown and misc.	Limb	Pelvis and trunk	GI tract
Angiosarcoma	8	1/2*		0/1	2/3	0/2		
Chondrosarcoma	9				0/1	0/3	0/5	
Ewing's sarcoma	2	1/1					0/1	
Fibrosarcoma	23	2/3		2/3	1/1	5/11	1/5	
Leiomyosarcoma	36		6/12	7/9	3/4			1/11
Liposarcoma	16	1/1		0/3	1/4	3/8		
Mesothelioma	9			1/3†	3/6‡			
Neurofibrosarcoma	22	2/3		1/2	1/4	5/11		1/2
Osteogenic sarcoma	31	1/2			1/1	7/20§	4/8	
Rhabdomyosarcoma	17	2/4		1/2	1/3	2/7		1/1
Synovial cell sarcoma	8	1/3				4/5		
Undifferentiated sarcoma	19		3/5	1/3	4/8	1/3		
Totals		11/19	9/17	13/26	17/35	27/70	5/19	3/14
Response rate		(58%)	(53%)	(50%)	(49%)	(39%)	(26%)	(21%)

*CR and PR/evaluable.
†Peritoneum.
‡Pleura.
§All leg.

TABLE 9. RESPONSE BY SITE OF METASTASES IN 200 PATIENTS RECEIVING ADRIAMYCIN AND DIC

		Metastatic sites						
	No. of patients	Misc.	Nodes, skin and subcutaneous	Lung	Soft tissue	Liver	Bone	CNS
Angiosarcoma	8		0/2	2/4*	0/2		2/3	
Chondrosarcoma	9	0/1	0/2	0/7	0/1		0/4	0/1
Ewing's sarcoma	2			1/1			1/2	0/1
Fibrosarcoma	23		2/3	6/15	5/7	1/2	1/5	1/1
Leiomyosarcoma	36	0/1	2/3	11/22	4/10	5/16	2/6	0/1
Liposarcoma	16		2/3	2/9	3/8	1/3	0/1	0/2
Mesothelioma	9	1/1	1/1	3/6	2/3	2/3		
Neurofibrosarcoma	22		1/3	6/14	4/8	0/1	2/3	
Osteogenic sarcoma	31	1/1	2/4	12/27	0/1	2/5		
Rhabdomyosarcoma	17		1/2	6/9	0/4	1/2	2/2	0/1
Synovial cell sarcoma	8	1/1	2/2	4/7	1/1			
Undifferentiated sarcoma	19		3/4	7/13	2/5	1/2	0/3	
Totals		3/5	16/29	60/134	21/50	13/34	10/29	1/7
Response rate		(60%)	(55%)	(45%)	(42%)	(38%)	(34%)	(14%)

*CR and PR/evaluable patients. Many patients had more than one type of metastases.

penetrate the blood–brain barrier poorly, and thus have very low levels in the cerebrospinal fluid,[13,14] this observation is not unexpected. Again these data provide important information regarding the incidence of metastatic locations in the sarcoma patients. Thus, of the 200 patients involved in this study, 134 (67 per cent) had pulmonary metastases.

Toxicity is summarized in Table 10. The production of acceptable myelosuppression was built into the protocol and was therefore expected. The recovery from myelosuppression (which was predominantly granulocytopenia) has been by the third week in all but approximately 10 per cent of the patients, thus readily permitting an every 3-week schedule. The other toxicities have been relatively inconsequential, and have been discussed in detail in our previous publications on this protocol.[3,15]

TABLE 10. TOXICITY

Toxic effect	Incidence (%)
Nausea and vomiting	100
Alopecia	100
Myelosuppression	86
Stomatitis	15
EKG abnormalities	7
Neurotoxicity	7
Fever	6
Other (hepatic, skin, phlebitis, confusion, eosinophilia)	5

Comparison of responding and non-responding patients showed that the former tended to have slightly less previous therapy and thus tolerated more vigorous therapy, i.e. received higher doses of both drugs. However, there was no significant difference in the degree of myelosuppression produced in the two groups. It was also interesting to note that the age distribution of the responders was virtually identical to that of the non-responders.

CONCLUSION

We are encouraged by these studies because it seems clear that the response rate in this particularly tragic disease is improving with combination chemotherapy. Starting with single drug responses below 30 per cent, we are now approaching a 50 per cent response rate with out three-drug combination. Where to from here can logically be asked. We have recently begun a four-drug combination in which cyclophosphamide has also been added. Approximately 20 patients are on this regimen. While the results are still too early to analyze, several very impressive complete remissions have already occurred on this four-drug combination. We are also currently adding immunotherapy to our protocol in two different ways. For patients who were on the two-drug studies discussed here, we are adding immunotherapy as part of their maintenance regimen. For patients who are beginning the four-drug combination with cyclophosphamide, vincristine, adriamycin and DIC, we are randomly allocating one-half of the patients (stratified by sex and some less responsive diagnoses) to receive BCG scarification from the start of their therapy. It is our hope that the immunotherapy will not only improve the per cent achieving response, but also will prolong the duration of response and subsequently of survival of patients with metastatic sarcomas.

REFERENCES

1. E. M. JACOBS, *Cancer, N.Y.* **25**, 324 (1970).
2. R. LIVINGSTON and S. CARTER, *Single Agents in Cancer Chemotherapy,* IFI/Plenum, New York (1970).
3. J. A. GOTTLIEB, L. H. BAKER, J. M. QUAGLIANA, J. K. LUCE, J. P. WHITECAR, JR., J. G. SINKOVICS, S. E. RIVKIN, R. BROWNLEE and E. FREI, III, *Cancer, N.Y.* **30**, 1632 (1972).
4. A. GOLDIN, *Int. Symp. Adriamycin,* pp. 64–74. Springer, New York (1972).
5. E. A. LEFRAK, J. PITHA, S. ROSENHEIM and J. A. GOTTLIEB, *Cancer, N.Y.* **32**, 302 (1973).
6. S. C. BARRANCO, E. W. GERNER, K. H. BURK and R. M. HUMPHREY, *Cancer Res.* **33**, 11 (1973).
7. B. DREWINKO and J. A. GOTTLIEB, *Cancer Res.* **33**, 1141 (1973).
8. S. SHIRAKAWA and E. FREI, III, *Cancer Res.* **29**, 1944 (1969).
9. R. S. BENJAMIN, D. H. HUFFMAN, P. H. WIERNIK and N. R. BACHUR, *Fourteenth Int. Cong. Hematology,* abstr. 508. Sao Paulo, Brazil (July, 1972).
10. H. O. KLEIN, K. J. LENNARTZ, R. GROSS, M. EDER and R. FISCHER, *Dt. med. Wschr.* **97**, 1273 (1972).
11. J. FOLKMAN, *Ann. Surg.* **175**, 409 (1972).
12. L. NATHANSON, J. WOLTER, J. HORTON, J. COLSKY, B. I. SHNIDER and A. SCHILLING, *Clin. Pharmac. Ther.* **12**, 955 (1971).
13. D. DIFRONZO, R. A. GAMBETTA and L. LENAZ, *Revue Étud. clin. biol.* **16**, 572 (1971).
14. T. L. LOO, J. K. LUCE, J. H. JARDINE and E. FREI, III, *Cancer Res.* **28**, 2448 (1968).
15. J. A. GOTTLIEB, *Cancer Bull.* **25**, 2 (1973).

Pp. 193–206, Supplement Number 2, 1974.
Biochemical Pharmacology. Printed in the U.S.A.

BLEOMYCIN AND PHLEOMYCIN - RECEPTIVITY OF TARGET SITES

PAUL PIETSCH and ASSIA MURRAY

Division of Optometry, Indiana University, Bloomington, Ind. 47401, U.S.A.

PHLEOMYCIN and bleomycin can do a number of things to viruses, cells, DNA and replicative RNA both *in vitro* and *in vivo*. Under fortuitous conditions, they block replication in a highly selective manner. It is revealing, though, to watch these antibiotics affect sensitive but growing bacteria. Take *Bacillus subtilus*, for example. Confronted with phleomycin-909 at many times the lethal dose, the cells, nonetheless, continue to multiply, replicate DNA and increase the turbidity of the beer at a normal rate, for a generation time before arrest finally begins to set in.[1]

These extremely sensitive bacilli dramatize a fundamental facet of the phleomycin–bleomycin problem, namely the shifting nature of the target. *B. subtilis* is not singular in this regard. In fact, except for cell-free conditions, we know of no situation where the receptors present a static, passive target. A guess is that the phasic nature of receptivity accounts for the survival of *Streptomyces vertilillus*, the organism that produces phleomycin–bleomycin antibiotics.

We see the shadow of the fickle receptors in reports from the clinic on bleomycin where the results of therapy have ranged from spectacular to discouraging, depending on the tumor, the study and even the particular patient (*cf.* Refs. 2–4).

Our activities have been aimed at understanding receptiveness to the phleomycins and bleomycins – what receptivity means in molecular terms, in terms of the fate of cells, when receptivity takes place, and how to assess and predict its future occurrence. We have just recently made some preliminary progress on the latter.

General Properties

First let us discuss a few things about this family of antibiotics. Phleomycin and bleomycin are overlapping heterogeneous subclasses of a family that may embrace zorbamycin and YA-56.[5] Phleomycin and bleomycin differ in the relative proportions of certain compounds and toxic impurities. The kind of material in a sample depends on the particular strain of *S. verticillus* and also on the growth medium.[6] A typical sample usually contains a dozen or more fractions, identified in the literature by letters and subscripts. Takita *et al.*[7] have shown phleomycins D_2 and F to be the same compounds as bleomycin B_2 and B_4. These workers found, too, that acid hydrolysis converts phleomycin D_1 to D_2, i.e. bleomycin. This fits with data of Pietsch and Eng.[8] The point is that phleomycin and bleomycin contribute to a single molecular pharmacological subject. Some batches of phleomycin contain dangerous kidney toxins, thus making them unsuitable for the clinic. The warning implied in "phleomycin" justifies two names.

The analytical picture is still somewhat murky. The materials are water soluble, chelate copper, average in molecular weight somewhere around 1400–1500 and show broad ultraviolet absorption bands around 245 and 290 nm. Complete structures are still in doubt, but some eight or more monomeric components have been identified in certain phleomycins and bleomycins. They most likely comprise a glycopeptide.[7]

It seems unlikely that a single specific mechanism or one type of receptor will account for everything phleomycin and bleomycin can do. At one time or another, they have arrested synthesis of DNA or viral RNA in a selective manner,[9,10] have blocked the entry of cells into mitosis or meiosis[11,12] without arresting replication, have broken chromosomes,[13] and have interfered with polymerases.[14] A review of the literature[15] indicates that there are many specific actions of the bleomycins and phleomycins, each dependent upon sufficient amounts of the correct substituent, upon different specific receptors, and upon different rhythms of receptivity. Yet the actions relate to one or another particular facet of the growth cycle.

The literature contains many contradictions, claims and counterclaims. Much of the conflict can be reconciled by the simple fact that not all investigators use the same materials. But the problem is more fundamental, for not only do receptors change, but the changes themselves also vary in different populations of cells – even in the same individual animal.

Consider the results of Pietsch and Clapper[1] who investigated acute inhibition of DNA synthesis by phleomycin in mouse rhabdomyosarcoma and spleen: where intraperitoneal injections of phleomycin reduced tritiated thymidine incorporation into the tumor by some 50 per cent, the effect on the spleen was only some 2 per cent. These workers also found phleomycin associated with DNA extracted from rhabdomyosarcoma and spleen; it was in the same relative proportions as the inhibition of replication. Pietsch and McCollister[16] likewise observed different degrees of acute inhibition of DNA synthesis in a number of different mouse tissues and transplanted tumors: regenerating muscle, spleen, testes, myeloid and lymphatic leukemias, melanoma and adenocarcinoma. Responses varied from none in leukemias to 90 per cent in early muscle regeneration. At first Pietsch and McCollister believed the differences must have arisen from variations in population dynamics; but they found otherwise when they tested the question in regenerating muscle at different developmental stages.

In the wounded muscle of a mouse, new fibers appear on the histological scene 4 days after injury. During the preceding days, there occur three waves of DNA replication. The first and third are acutely responsive to phleomycin but nevertheless show quantitative differences. Pietsch and McCollister[16] inflicted wounds at different times in right and left tibialis anterior muscles, timing injury so that waves I and III would occur simultaneously. They also performed experiments with both wounds at wave I during the challenge on the premiss that if phleomycin affected the two stages of development in the same way, the wounds should vary together, and replication ratios should remain constant with or without the antibiotic. But if the response is a true variational change, then ratios for DNA synthesis, too, should vary in response to phleomycin. The results showed that with both sides in the same wave at the challenge, ratios for treated and untreated did hold constant. However, the ratios were appreciably different when the waves were of different age (Table 1).

Thus, even internal changes within the same type of cells can alter receptivity. There seem to be other examples in the literature. For instance, Iwata and Consigli,[17]

TABLE 1. VARIATIONAL CHANGES IN THE ACUTE EFFECTS OF PHLEOMYCIN ON DIFFERENT WAVES OF REPLICATION DURING REGENERATION IN MOUSE SKELETAL MUSCLE*

	Untreated	Phleomycin	Significance level
	(Ratio ± S. D.)		(%)
Wave I/ Wave I'	0.83 ± 0.3	0.87 ± 0.3	Not significant
Wave I/ Wave III	0.38 ± 0.2	0.64 ± 0.2	99.99

*Data from Pietsch and McCollister.[16]

working with cultured mouse embryo cells, found DNA synthesis completely inhibited after 10 hr, although infected with polyoma virus were still synthesizing DNA, albeit at a reduced rate. Clearly the receptor is a changing target.

What about permeability? Might it account for differences? These antibiotics pass into animal and bacterial cells with consummate ease. Pietsch *et al.*[18] monitored the fate of phleomycin *in vivo*, using neutron activation analysis of urine for copper, and confirming their results by means of bacteriological assay. In the mouse, phleomycin passed from peritoneal cavity to blood, to all organs and into the urine quickly and with the same simple kinetics as filtration through dialysis tubine. The half-life of a 20 mg/kg body weight dose in the mouse was 22 min. In other words, effective doses cannot be spaced very far apart, nor would increasing dosage levels improve therapy if receptivity were at a low point.

In 1969, Pietsch and Corbett (unpublished) attempted to formulate methods that might optimize treatment schedules for rhythms of receptivity. They worked with C1498 myeloid leukemia in C57BL/6J host mice. Dividing animals into subgroups, they varied the time of day of treatment over a period of 4 days but held the total dose constant. They carried out a large number of experiments, starting with a given parent tumor. One group would always outlive the others by significant even incredible amounts. But, harmonic analysis of death rate in earlier experiments consistently failed to predict just which of the groups would outlive the others. The experiments tell us little more than what we already know: that these is such a thing as an optimal schedule. Initial conditions, however, would appear to be important factors in the subsequent rhythm of receptivity. They would also appear to create problems that cannot be resolved by strictly *a priori* methods.

What seemed to be required, if bleomycin were ever to achieve its full potentialities, was a practical means of examining biopsy material directly and deciding on an individual basis just when antibiotic binds to the target cells.

Locating antibiotic with mercury

Recall that phleomycin–bleomycin antibiotics chelate copper. There are some four to six metal binding sites per molecule.[19] Furthermore, divalent mercuric ions rapidly occupy those sites or quickly replace cupric ions if they happen to be present. Mercury is exceedingly electron opaque. For example, after pretreating DNA fibers with phleomycin *in vitro*, subsequent dialysis against mercuric chloride procedures opacities of the correct size, distribution and density to be clusters of antibiotic molecules.[20,21] Might the simple procedure of staining with mercuric chloride yield a practical way of locating antibiotic in the cell?

We knew in advance that mercury might deposit on DNA or elsewhere, but not in the very heavy concentrations one would anticipate if phleomycin were bound in the cell. At any rate, we decided to try mercuric chloride staining. We conducted our experiments with Bristol Laboritories lot A9331-909 copper phleomycin. Its infrared characteristics may be found in Pietsch and Eng.[8] The lot is very similar analytically to bleomycin. Because of the extreme sensitivity of wave I in regenerating mouse muscle, we concentrated most of our attention here. We also examined spleens. Our experiments were conducted on 30-g Swiss Webster male mice with puncture wounds in the tibialis anterior muscles. Forty-three hr later, animals received 1.0 mg phleomycin dissolved in saline and injected intraperitoneally. We sacrificed the mice 3 hr after the challenge by cervical dislocation and dissected the tissue while blood still flowed throughout the legs. We fixed tissues for 2 hr in cold 1% OsO_4 buffered to pH 7.4 with Millonig phosphate buffer, dehydrated in ethanol and embedded in Spurr Epoxy resin. Tissues were sectioned on an LKB III ultrotome with a diamond knife. Sections, on grids, were treated in three different ways. For routine staining, grids were floated on a drop of saturated aqueous uranyl acetate for 30 min. For mercuric chloride staining, grids were floated on a drop of 1.0 mM $HgCl_2$ for 15 min. Unstained, control grids were floated on a drop of distilled water for 15 min. All grids were washed ten times each in three changes of filtered, glass-distilled water. Observations were carried out on an HU11A electron microscope.

Figure 1 shows the appearance of mononucleated cells after routine uranyl acetate staining. The specimen came from the wounded muscle of an untreated control mouse.

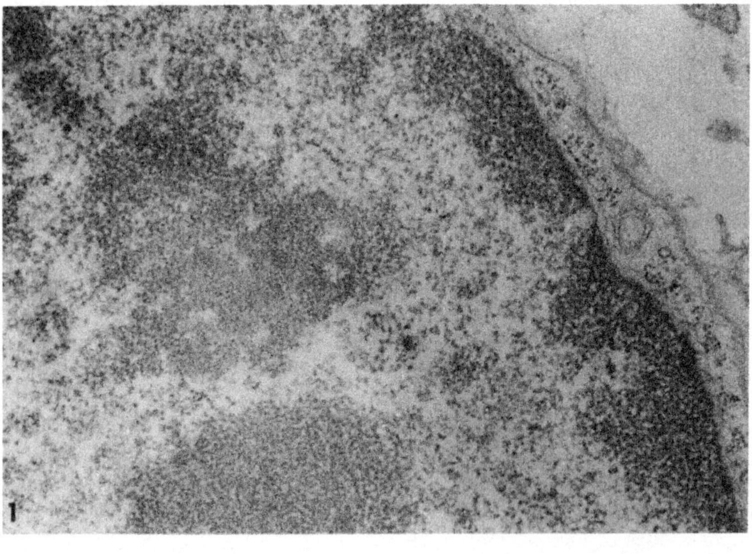

FIG. 1. Mononucleated cell from the muscle wound of an untreated control mouse; stain: uranyl acetate (× 20,400).

Its principal value is to highlight general morphological details. Figure 2 is a section from the same untreated control wound as in Fig. 1. This specimen was not stained with uranyl acetate but was reacted with mercuric chloride. The cell showed no electron opacities that would indicate the presence of mercury bound to cell structures.[22] Still, in some cells from untreated control wounds, we did find some evidence of mercury binding. Figure 3 shows such a case. Mercury spots may be seen there on a strand of nucleic acid-like material resting on the cell. The strand has the circular contour of a microbial chromosome and may have come from an exploded bacterium. At any rate, using the spots on the strand as a criterion, it is possible to find occasional foci of mercury scattered in small numbers and in apparent random order in the nucleus and cytoplasm. There is also a piece of dirt in the photograph. An out-of-focus fringe serves to distinguish such artifacts from bound mercury in the same focal plane as cell structures.

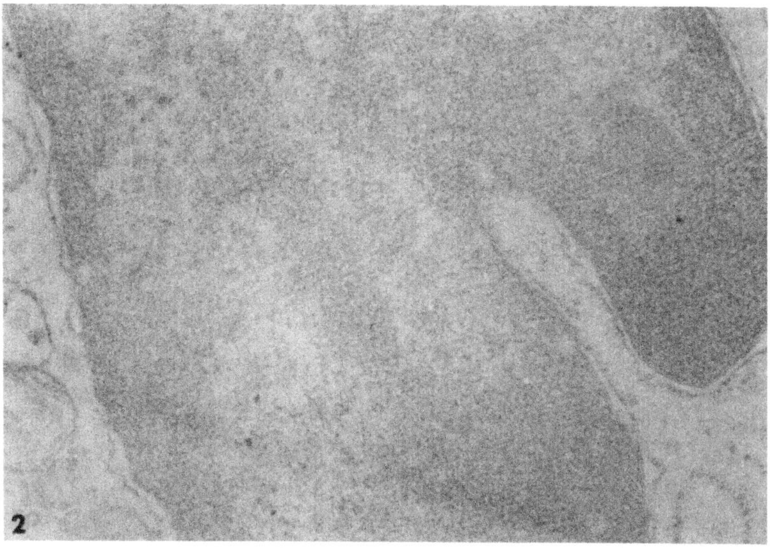

FIG. 2. Another cell from the same untreated control animal as in Fig. 1; stain: mercuric chloride. No mercury spots associated with any structure (× 20,400).

Figure 4 shows a mononucleated cell from a phleomycin-treated specimen after uranyl acetate staining but without mercuric chloride. The general appearance is much like Fig. 1. Figure 5 shows a similar, phleomycin-treated specimen with neither uranyl acetate nor mercuric chloride staining.

Figure 6 is a low power electron micrograph of a cell from the muscle wound of a phleomycin-treated mouse. This specimen was stained with mercuric chloride. The heavy metal is so concentrated here that our first impression was that we were viewing dirt. However, at higher magnification (Fig. 7) it is clear that the mercury spots are intimately associated with structures. Spots are densely packed, especially on chromatin; but not all chromatin contains mercury, and spots are completely absent from amorphous regions of the nucleus. Mercury did occur in the cytoplasm, particu-

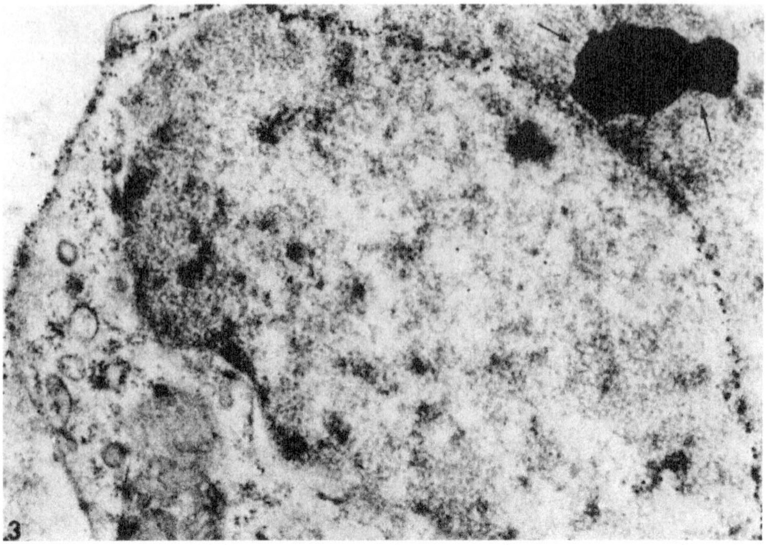

FIG. 3. A third cell from the wound of an untreated control animal; stain: mercuric chloride. Mercury spots appear on a strand of material superimposed on the cell. A few opacities may be found scattered in small numbers in the nucleus and cytoplasm. The large black spot (arrows) is a piece of dirt (X 20,400).

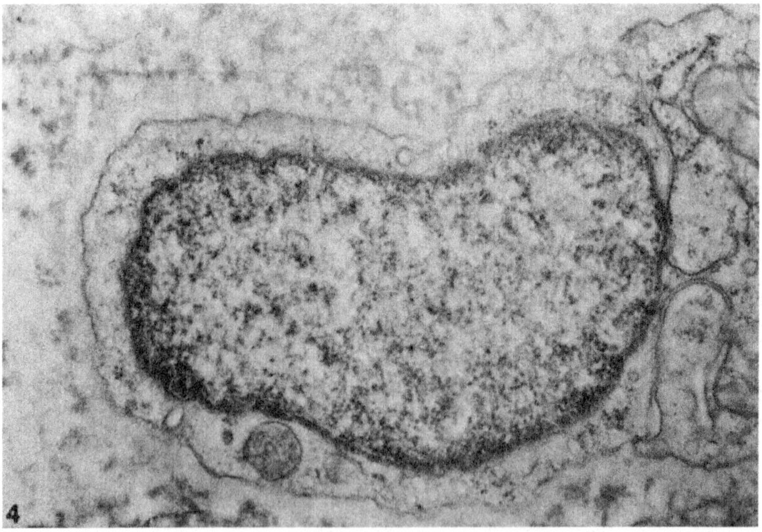

FIG. 4. Mononucleated cell from the muscle wound of a phleomycin-treated mouse; stain: uranyl acetate (X 20,400).

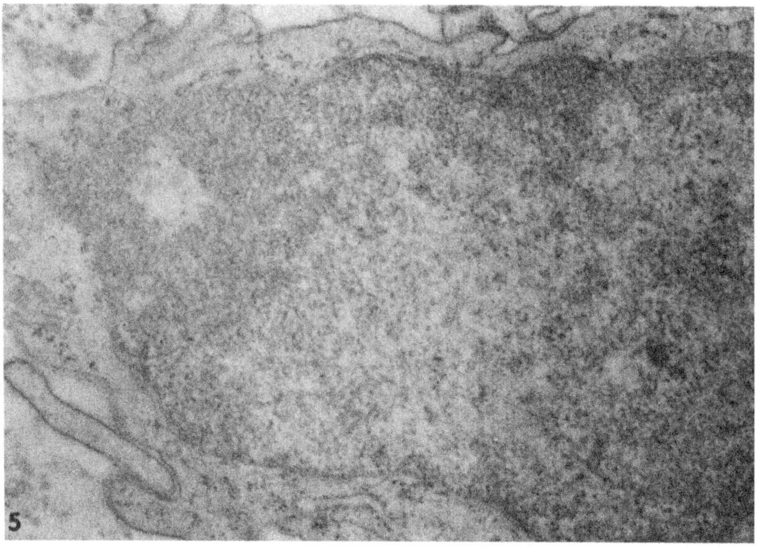

FIG. 5. Unstained cell from the muscle wound of a phleomycin-treated animal (× 20,400).

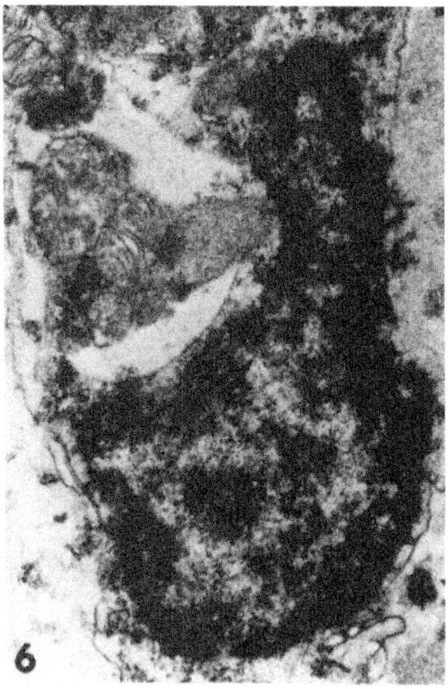

FIG. 6. Mononucleated cell from the muscle wound of a phleomycin-treated mouse; stain: mercuric chloride (× 11,500). (See Fig. 7).

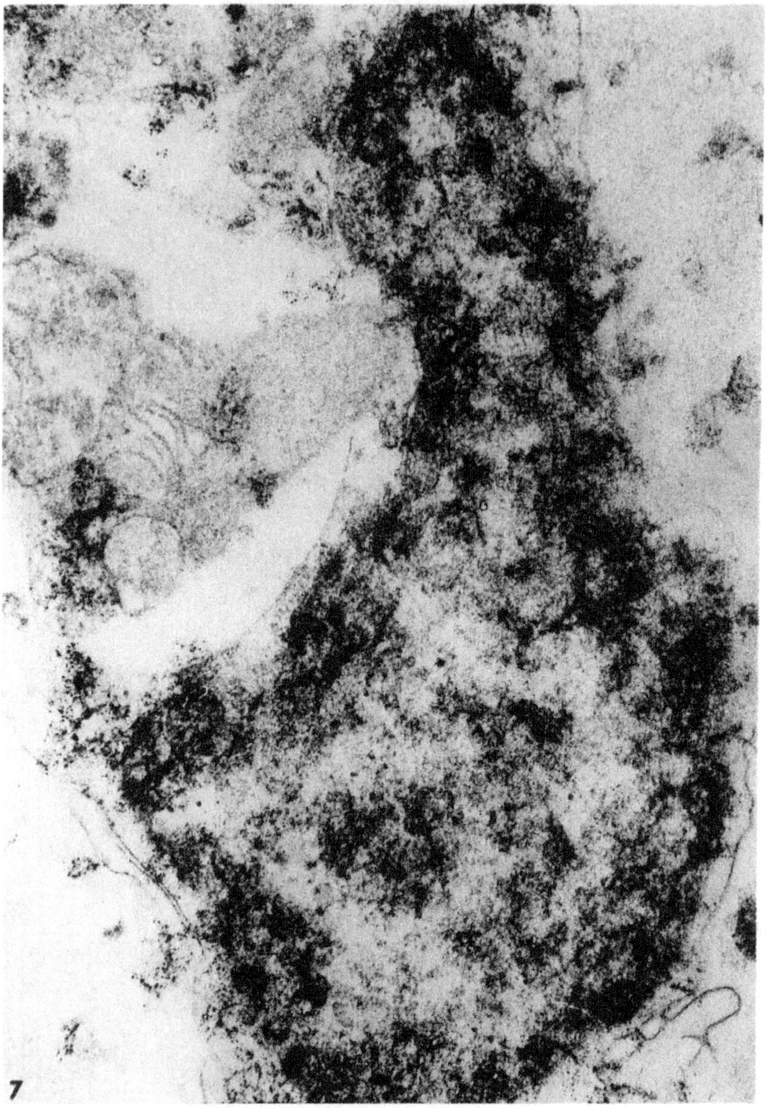

7

FIG. 7. Higher magnification of Fig. 6. Heavy deposits of mercury occur in and may be seen in lesser amounts in structures of the cytoplasm. Note the tendency for mercury to be most concentrated where the chromatin is condensed. However, not all chromatin has mercury spots associated with it. Thus, concentration is not merely due to increase in nuclear material. No mercury is evident in amorphous regions of the nucleus (× 32,000).

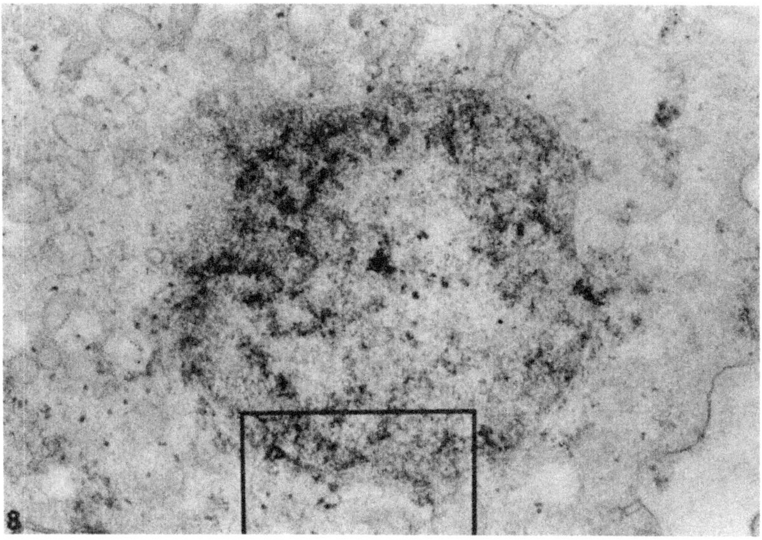

FIG. 8. Another example of a mononucleated cell from the same wound as in Fig. 6. Mercury deposits, while quite conspicuous, are not as heavy as in the previous case. The spots do, however, form highly discrete markings on RNP granules in the cytoplasm. Spots follow the contours of membranes and are totally absent from spaces *per se*. Also, as in the nucleus, not all portions of the same structures contain mercury spots (X 20,400).

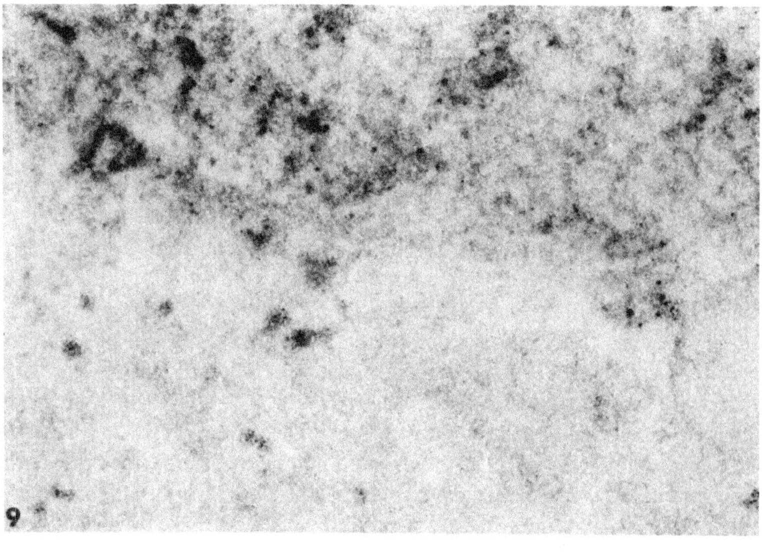

FIG. 9. Higher magnification of the framed area in Fig. 8 (X 108,000).

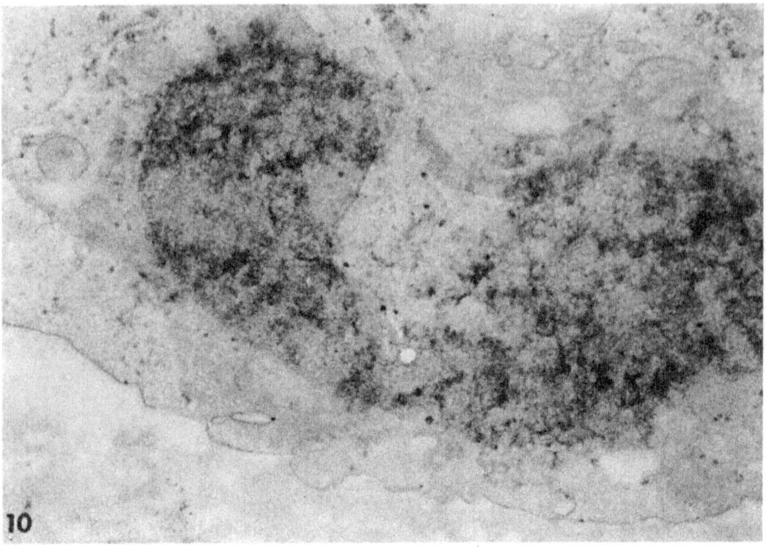

FIG. 10. Lymphoid cell from a muscle wound of a phleomycin-treated animal. The cell was in the general neighborhood of those in Figs. 6–9; stain: mercuric chloride (× 20,400).

larly in certain discrete foci of the rough endoplasmic reticulum (*cf.* Figs. 8 and 9). There, the spots lie on ribonucleoprotein (RNP) granules and are absent from intervening spaces. Still not all RNP granules show spots. In fact, inspection of Figs. 8 and 9 will reveal nests of stained and unstained RNP granules lying side by side.

We have also encountered spots that appear to be passing through the nuclear and the cytoplasmic membranes. In a fixed preparation it is obviously impossible to stipulate direction of the movement. But whatever mercury does associate with, it appears to be on the move, as we would expect of phleomycin.

Figure 10 is a lymphoid cell from the muscle wound of a phleomycin-treated animal. Compare it with the cell in Fig. 11, from the grid. The latter is a typical mononucleated cell of the sort implicated in muscle regeneration.[23,24] Notice how much more dense the mercury is in its nucleus as compared with the lymphoid cell. Pietsch and McCollister[16] observed that phleomycin injected into mice coincident with the advent of these cells virtually eliminated the later actomyosin synthesis associated with regeneration. The heaviest labeling we encountered in any cells was in the mononucleated type from phleomycin-treated wounds. In other words, mercury staining corresponds with where we would anticipate most phleomycin to be bound.

There is another correlation with previous evidence. Occasionally, we encountered a mononucleated cell with distinctly less mercury than was the rule. (Compare the density in the nuclei in Figs. 8 and 11.) These cells lay in nearby regions of the same wound. Yet the mercury spots in Fig. 11 are almost double the density of those in Fig. 8, even though the latter cell did bind the metal. This, too, is what we would expect on the basis of a rhythmic receptivity, i.e. difference among individuals of the same population.

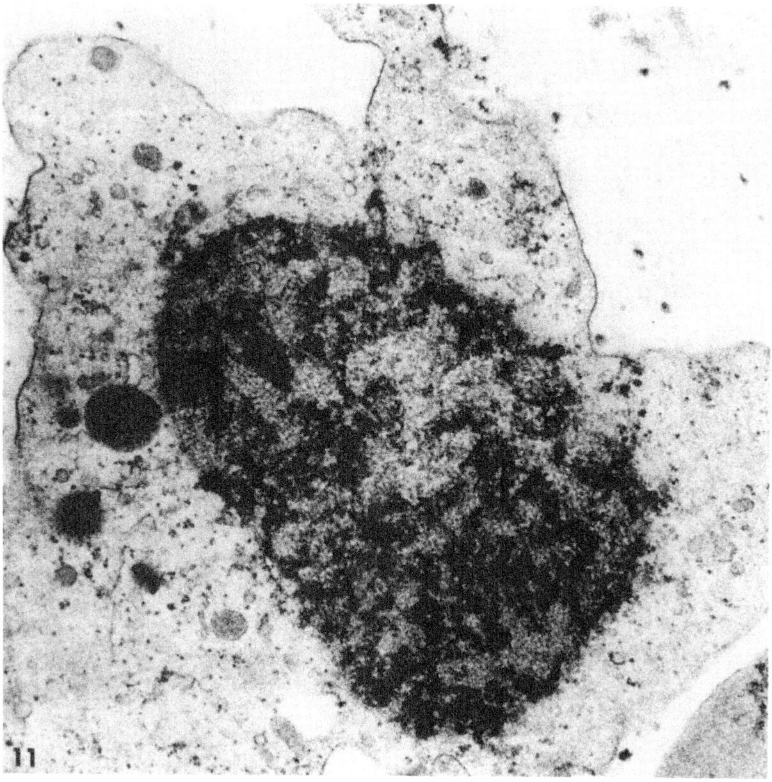

FIG. 11. Mononucleated cell near lymphoid cell of Fig. 10; stain: mercuric chloride. Cells of this type have been implicated in muscle regeneration. Also, phleomycin administered at this time inhibits the regenerative process. The heaviest depositions of mercury were in the nuclei of cells in this class (× 20,400).

Mouse spleen, in contrast with wounded muscle, shows a low grade acute response to *ad hoc* administration of phleomycin.[1,16] Following the argument developed in the preceding paragraph, we would expect to see many cells from this organ with little to no mercury. Indeed, our expectations were vindicated. Figure 12 shows a splenic cell that took considerable searching to find. There are mercury spots distributed throughout most of its nucleus, on what appear to be prophase chromosomes just condensing, and in the rough endoplasmic reticulum of the cytoplasm. Many of this cell's neighbors showed either no mercury or only a limited number of spots. Such a cell may be seen in Fig. 13. Most of its chromatin and cytoplasm are free of mercury. Yet in the upper left of the figure it is possible to see a distinct nest in the chromatin at the nuclear membrane. (Fig. 14 shows this framed region.) The nest seems to be confluent with a grouping of spots on the immediately adjacent segment of rough endoplasmic reticulum.

In summary then, mercury staining followed the distribution of phleomycin we would have predicted from previous data.

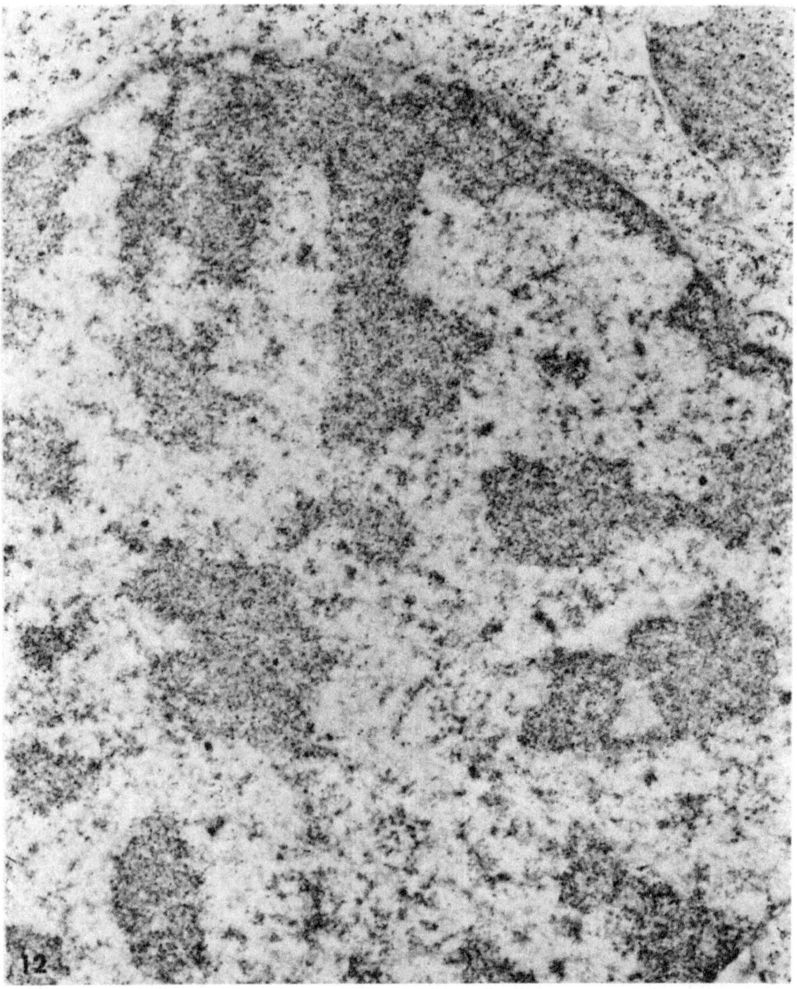

FIG. 12. Nucleus of a splenic cell from a phleomycin-treated mouse; stain: mercuric chloride. The cell is in early prophase. Mercury is bound to chromatin and endoplasmic retuculum (× 20,400).

How might mercury staining be used in bleomycin therapy?

Bleomycin will never achieve its full potentialities in chemotherapy without methods of predicting receptivity. It seems abundantly clear, comparing laboratory and clinical findings, that such predictions will have to be carried out case by case. Thus, therapy would have to be tailored to the individual. There do exist computer methods for the necessary harmonic analysis,[25] but the limiting factor remains the empirical data to decide when the targets maximally cycle into a receptive period. We suggest that these data may be harvested from biopsy material, stained with mercuric chloride, examined by electron microscopy and expressed in terms of percentage of heavily

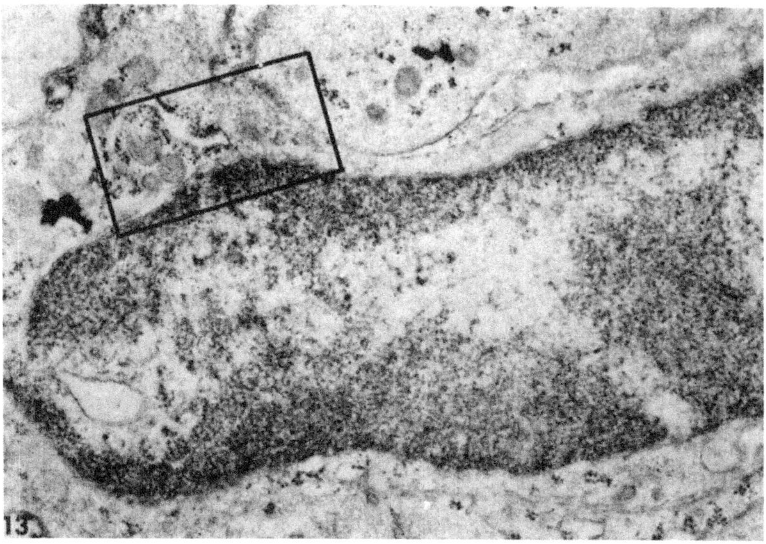

FIG. 13. Another splenic cell from the same specimen as in Fig. 11. A moderately dense concentration of mercury spots may be seen in the framed area. Trace the formation of spots toward the cytoplasm and observe mercury associated with the adjacent segment of endoplasmic reticulum (see also Fig. 14). The rest of the nucleus contains little or no mercury (× 20,400).

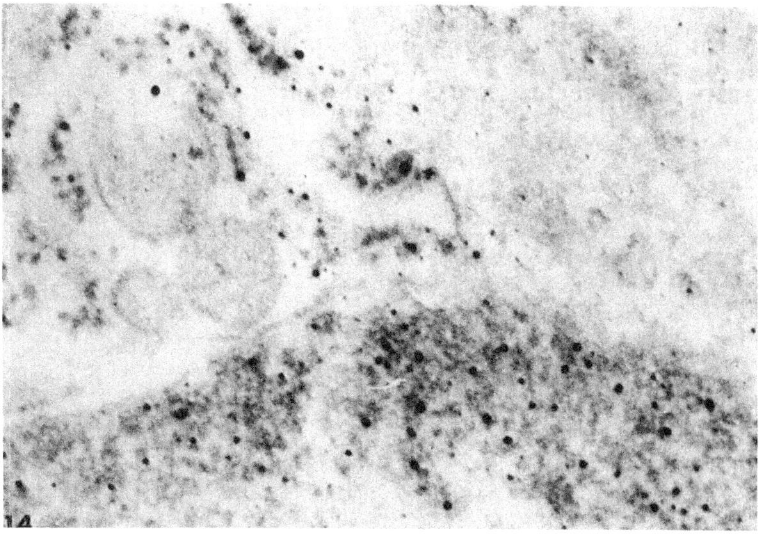

FIG. 14. Framed region from Fig. 13 (× 108,800).

labeled cells as a function of time administration. Since cell types vary in their rhythms of receptivity, inspection of biopsy material from normal tissues might provide data to design a schedule that would catch the tumor at a high point and miss the peaks for other cells. But the principal consideration is to predict the tumor's moments of receptivity, for to miss these periods is to render no therapy at all.

Acknowledgement – We wish to thank Dr. Raymond G. Murray, Dept. of Anatomy and Physiology, Indiana University, for the generous use of his equipment and supplies, Herschel Lentz, Division of Biology, Indiana University, for the use of an expertly maintained electron microscope and Dave Ort of our own department for photography.

REFERENCES

1. P. PIETSCH and G. CLAPPER, *Cytobios* **1**, 145 (1969)
2. T. ICHIKAWA, I. NAKANO and I. HIROKAWA, *J. Urol.* **102**, 699 (1969).
3. G. BONADONNA *et al.*, *Eur. J. Cancer* **8**, 205 (1972).
4. K. E. HALNAN *et al.*, *Br. med. J.* **4**, 635 (1972).
5. Y. ITO *et al.*, *J. Antibiot., Tokyo* (Ser. A) **24**, 727 (1971).
6. H. UMEZAWA, Y. SHUHARA, T. TAKITA and K. MAEDA, *J. Antibiot., Tokyo* (Ser. A), **19**, 210 (1966).
7. T. TAKITA *et al.*, *J. Antibiot., Tokyo* (Ser. A) **25**, 197 (1972).
8. P. PIETSCH and R. ENG, *Microbios* **1**, 213 (1969).
9. N. TANAKA, H. YAMAGUCHI and H. UMEZAWA, *Biochem. biophys. Res. Commun.* **10**, 171 (1963).
10. T. KUNIMOTO, M. HORI and H. UMEZAWA, *J. Antibiot., Tokyo* (Ser. A) **20**, 277 (1967).
11. K. KAJIWARA, U. M. KIM and G. C. MUELLER, *Cancer Res.* **26**, 233 (1966).
12. Y. HOTTA and H. STERN, *Cancer Res.* **29**, 1699 (1969).
13. E. MATTINGLY, *Mutation Res.* **4**, 51 (1967).
14. A. FALASCHI and A. KORNBERG, *Fedn Proc.* Part 1, **23**, 940 (1964).
15. P. PIETSCH, in *Handbuch der experimentellen Pharmakologie. Antineoplastic and Immunosuppressive Agents* (Eds. A. C. SARTORELLI and D. JOHNS), Vol. XXXVII. Springer, Berlin, in press.
16. P. PIETSCH and S. B. MCCOLLISTER, *Nature, Lond.* **208**, 1170 (1965).
17. A. IWATA and R. H. CONSIGLI, *J. Virol.* **7**, 29 (1971).
18. P. PIETSCH, C. CORBETT, D. W. BRIDEN and G. JEWETT, *Physiol. Chem. Physics* **1**, 232 (1969).
19. P. PIETSCH and H. GARRETT, *Cytobios* **1**, 7 (1969).
20. P. PIETSCH and H. GARRETT, *Nature, Lond.* **219**, 488 (1968).
21. P. PIETSCH and C. CORBETT, *Nature, Lond.* **219**, 933 (1968).
22. L. W. CHANG and H. A. HARTMANN, *Expl Neurol.* **35**, 122 (1972).
23. J. W. LASH, H. HOLTZER and H. SWIFT, *Anat. Rec.* **128**, 679 (1950).
24. P. PIETSCH, *Anat. Rec.* **139**, 167 (1961).
25. W. J. DIXON, *Biomedical Computer Programs*, University of California Press, Berkeley (1968).

Pp. 207—216, Supplement Number 2, 1974.
Biochemical Pharmacology. Printed in the U.S.A.

ADRIAMYCIN-DAUNORUBICIN CELLULAR PHARMACODYNAMICS

NICHOLAS R. BACHUR

Biochemistry Section, Baltimore Cancer Research Center, National Cancer Institute
National Institutes of Health, Baltimore, Md. 21211, U. S. A.

AMONG THE newer cancer chemotherapeutic agents, two which have generated an optimism are the anthracycline aminoglycosides, daunorubicin and adriamycin. Since the discovery of daunorubicin 10 years ago[1] and adriamycin 4 years ago,[2] investigators have shown that these substances have antitumor activity in both animals[3,4] and humans.[5,6] Daunorubicin is the most effective single agent for remission induction in acute lymphoblastic and acute myeloblastic leukemia, but adriamycin affects solid tumors to a greater extent.

Chemically these compounds are anthracycline quinone glycosides (Fig. 1) of the amino sugar daunosamine. The only structural difference between daunorubicin and adriamycin is an additional hydroxyl group at position 14 of adriamycin. Although both compounds are water soluble, adriamycin is more polar than daunorubicin because of the additional hydroxyl group.

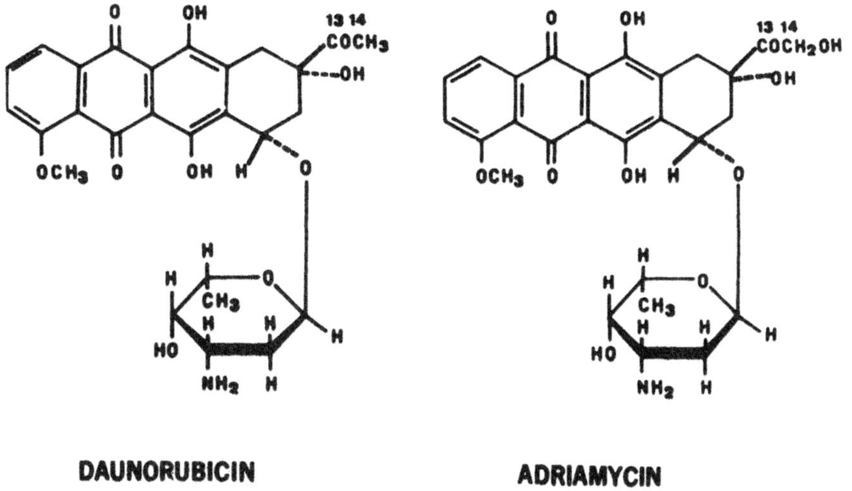

FIG. 1. Structural formulae of daunorubicin and adriamycin.

Both drugs avidly bind to nucleic acids,[7,8] and a number of investigators have described the disruption of DNA and RNA synthesis by daunorubicin and adriamycin in several biological test systems.[9—11] The binding to nucleic acids and the consequent inhibition of nucleic acid synthesis are accepted as the effector mechanism of the drugs.

Recently after measuring X-ray chrystallographic diffraction patterns of DNA–daunorubicin complexes, Pigram *et al.*[12] proposed a specific intercalation of daunorubicin into the DNA double helix (Fig. 2). The planar anthracycline nucleus slips between the stacked bases of the helix and distorts that macromolecule, thereby interfering with the biochemical processing of the DNA. Stabilization of the intercalation complex is obtained by the attractive forces between the positively charged amino group of the antibiotic sugar, daunosamine and the negative phosphate group of the DNA sugar backbone. Since these structural chacteristics are the same for daunorubicin and adriamycin, their intercalation and binding should be similar. The one region of structural difference located on the fourth ring lies outside of the intercalation interaction in the large groove of the DNA. Despite the similarity in binding, however, important differences between the compounds are seen *in vivo*.

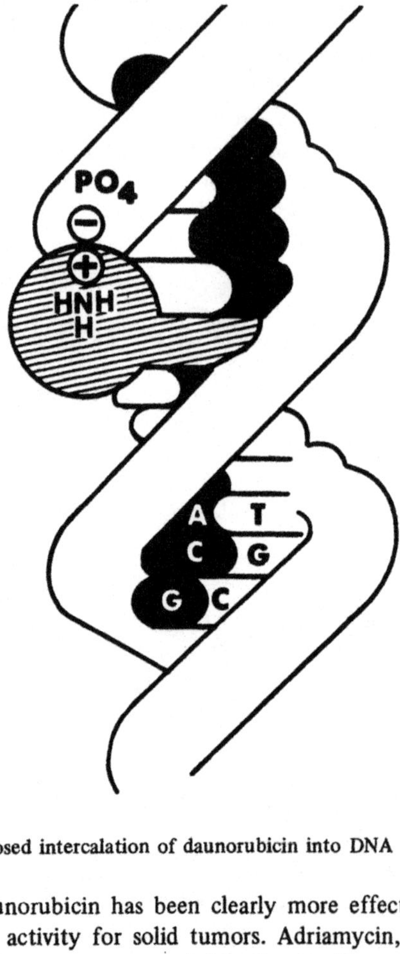

FIG. 2. Proposed intercalation of daunorubicin into DNA double helix.

In clinical usage, daunorubicin has been clearly more effective against hematologic malignancies with lesser activity for solid tumors. Adriamycin, although active against hematologic malignancies, is most remarkable for its "broad specturm" effects on various solid tumors. In addition, differences in potency were ascertained in phase I trials. In animal studies, the therapeutic index of adriamycin was greater than that of daunorubicin.[4]

We have studied the pharmacodynamics of the anthracycline antibiotics and have attempted to correlate clinical observations with properties of the drugs. These studies were the collaborative efforts of Dr. David Huffman, Dr. Delano Meriwether, Mr. Malcolm Gee, Mr. James Cradock and Dr. Merrill Egorin.

Since adriamycin and daunorubicin have different therapeutic indices, we were interested in observing the effects of the drugs on mammalian cells unaffected by the physiologic complexity of the complete animal. We compared the action of these drugs in a tissue culture system. Actively growing mouse leukemia L1210 cells cultured in spinner flasks were incubated with radioactive thymidine or uridine and with different drug concentrations. Both the thymidine incorporation into DNA and the uridine incorporation into RNA were inhibited by the drugs (Table 1).[11] However, daunorubicin was the more potent inhibitor at all three levels of drug tested. The higher activity of daunorubicin was clearly the opposite of previous observations *in vivo*.

TABLE 1. INHIBITION OF PRECURSOR INCORPORATION INTO NUCLEIC ACIDS BY ADRIAMYCIN AND DAUNORUBICIN*

	Inhibitor (% inhibition ± S. E.)		
Precursor	Daunorubicin	Adriamycin	Concn (μM)
	27.4 ± 3.3	16.3 ± 3.1	1.0
Thymidine-methyl-^{3}H	54.9 ± 3.3	31.7 ± 5.8	3.0
	74.3 ± 2.4	58.6 ± 4.1	5.0
	28.7 ± 4.5	12.4 ± 3.6	1.0
Uridine-2-^{14}C	60.0 ± 4.1	35.9 ± 6.3	3.0
	72.7 ± 4.3	56.6 ± 4.4	5.0

*L1210 cells grown in tissue culture were incubated with inhibitor for 1 hr, after which radioactive precursor was added and the incubation continued for 1 additional hr.

Since our findings were the reverse of our expectations, we felt that the differences could result from different delivery rates of drug into the cellular nuclear machinery. That is, the cellular uptake of the drugs may differ. In further experiments with the L1210 cells, we studied drug uptake (Table 2).[11] Both drugs were taken up actively, but daunorubicin clearly entered the L1210 cell both more rapidly and to a greater extent than did adriamycin. At 120 min, the intracellular adriamycin level was less than 1/3 the daunorubicin level, whereas the inhibition of adriamycin at the same extracellular drug level (5 μM) was about 80 per cent of the inhibition caused by daunorubicin. This indicated that adriamycin had a greater specific inhibitory effect than daunorubicin in these cells. Nevertheless, within the confines of these experimental conditions, adriamycin was a less effective inhibitor of nucleic acid metabolism

TABLE 2. ADRIAMYCIN AND DAUNORUBICIN UPTAKE BY L1210 CELLS*

Time (min)	Cellular drug content (nmoles)	
	Adriamycin	Daunorubicin
15	0.20	1.20
30	0.24	1.28
60	0.28	1.53
120	0.55	1.70

*L1210 cells were incubated at 37° in 1 ml buffered electrolyte media with 5 nmoles drug.

in the L1210 cells than daunorubicin. We concluded that this was the result of the lower transport rate of adriamycin into the malignant cells.

In the L1210 cells and in other mammalian cells, the pharmacologic effect of daunorubicin is complicated by the metabolism of daunorubicin in the cell to daunorubicinol (Fig. 3). This reaction catalyzed by the enzyme daunorubicin reductase is the reduction of the carbonyl group at position 13 to an alcohol with NADPH donating the protons.[13,14] The alcohol product, daunorubicinol, is more polar than daunorubicin and is similar to adriamycin in some physical–chemical characteristics. Since the metabolic alteration occurs on the side chain which, according to Pigram's model, should not interfere with the intercalation of the molecule, we felt that daunorubicinol may have pharmacologic activity.

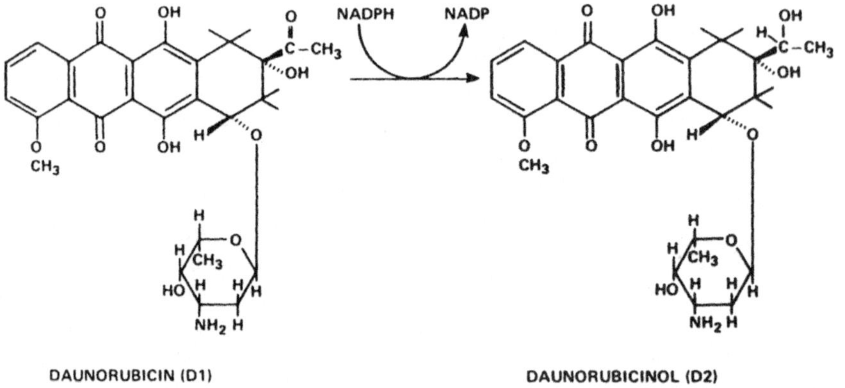

FIG. 3. Daunorubicin reductase reaction.

Among mammalian cells, daunorubicin reductase is nearly ubiquitous, and the activity is easily demonstrated in the soluble fraction of cellular homogenates.[13] The highest activities are in kidney, liver and small intestine (Table 3). Unlike the classical drug-metabolizing enzymes which are primarily in liver microsomes, daunorubicin reductase is found in all tissues, even in rat blood.

Human blood also has daunorubicin reductase in all formed elements, whereas the plasma is devoid of activity (Table 4).[15] After separating the blood cells according to types and testing each type for the reductase, we find that leukocytes and especially the lymphocytes contained higher enzyme levels than the erythrocytes or platelets.

It seemed reasonable to speculate that the activity of daunorubicin against human leukemic cells may be related to the ability of the cell to convert daunorubicin to daunorubicinol. First we determined if daunorubicinol had biochemical activity.

TABLE 3. DAUNORUBICINOL PRODUCTION BY RAT TISSUE SOLUBLE FRACTION*

Tissue	Daunorubicinol (nmoles/mg protein)
Brain	87
Heart	56
Lung	29
Liver	103
Spleen	49
Small intestine	124
Kidney	120
Skeletal muscle	35
Blood	88

*Homogenates of the tissues in 2 vol. of 0.15 M KCl – 0.05 M Tris–Cl, pH 7.4, were centrifuged at 105,000 *g* for 60 min. The supernatant solutions were used for enzyme assay. Reaction mixtures contained 100 μmoles Tris–Cl, pH 7.4, 90 nmoles daunorubicin HCl, 100 nmoles NADPH, and tissue extract and were incubated at 37° for 60 min.

TABLE 4. DAUNORUBICINOL PRODUCTION BY HUMAN BLOOD COMPONENTS*

Preparation	Daunorubicinol (nmoles/mg protein)
Leukocyte homogenate	11
Lymphocyte homogenate	20
Erythrocyte homogenate	2.3
Platelet homogenate	1.7
Bone marrow homogenate	2.2
Plasma	0

*Homogenates of the blood cells were made in 2 vol. of 0.05 M Tris–CL, pH 7.4, and were incubated at 37° for 30 min in a reaction mixture containing 50 μmoles Tris–HCl, pH 7.4, 523 nmoles daunorubicin, and 1000 nmoles NADPH.

We prepared daunorubicinol enzymatically and compared it to daunorubicin in the L1210 cell culture system. At equal concentrations, daunorubicinol was less effective than daunorubicin against DNA and RNA synthesis (Table 5).[16] In fact, daunorubicin was as much as three times more effective than daunorubicinol at the 5 μM level. It would seem that we had a less active metabolite.

To insure that equal levels of test substances were entering the cell, we compared the uptake of daunorubicin with daunorubicinol in L1210 cells (Table 6). Daunorubicin clearly was taken up more rapidly and to a higher level than the metabolite daunorubicinol.

TABLE 5. INHIBITION OF PRECURSOR INCORPORATION INTO NUCLEIC ACIDS BY DAUNORUBICIN AND DAUNORUBICINOL*

	Inhibitor (% inhibition, mean ± S. E.)		
Precursor	Daunorubicin	Daunorubicinol	Conc (μM)
	36.3 ± 9.9	10.3 ± 4.7	1.0
Thymidine-methyl-^{3}H	54.2 ± 9.6	20.9 ± 6.2	3.0
	68.5 ± 3.7	23.8 ± 6.2	5.0
	49.4 ± 7.4	2.6 ± 1.8	1.0
Uridine-2-^{14}C	56.6 ± 8.6	13.3 ± 4.0	3.0
	61.3 ± 4.9	21.8 ± 6.2	5.0

*The same experimental design was used as in Table 1.

TABLE 6. L1210 UPTAKE OF DAUNORUBICIN AND DAUNORUBICINOL*

	Drug content of L1210 cells (nmoles)	
Incubation time (min)	Daunorubicin	Daunorubicinol
15	0.71	0.18
30	0.99	0.39
60	1.41	0.61
120	1.97	0.79

*L1210 cells were incubated at 37° in 1 ml buffered electrolyte media with 5 nmoles drug.

If one compares the inhibition levels with cellular drug concentration, it appears that daunorubicinol has about the same specific inhibitory effect as daunorubicin. That is, equal amounts of daunorubicin and daunorubicinol in the cell will give equal levels of inhibition. Thus, the metabolite is biochemically active, but cannot penetrate the cell membrane as well as the less polar daunorubicin.

Although we have observed a very active enzymatic conversion *in vitro*, there is no guarantee that this occurs *in vivo*. To obtain an idea of the over-all impact of daunorubicin reductase *in vivo*, we determined the daunorubicin and daunorubicinol in rat tissue 8 hr after i.v. injection of drug (Table 7).[17] Daunorubicinol was a major component in most of the tissues analyzed, indicating that daunorubicin reductase is physiologically active.

To ascertain the extent of biotransformation that occurs in the human, we have obtained pharmacokinetic data from leukemic patients who received a single intravenous injection of daunorubicin. After the daunorubicin injection, there was a rapid rise in the plasma level of daunorubicinol, so that by 1 hr the metabolite level exceeded the parent drug level (Fig. 4).[18] By 2 hr after injection, the principal drug

TABLE 7. RAT TISSUE LEVELS OF DAUNORUBICIN AND DAUNORUBICINOL*

Tissue	Daunorubicin	Daunorubicinol
	(nmoles/g tissue wet wt)	
Brain	0.20	0.18
Heart	4.5	8.8
Lung	12.2	6.5
Liver	6.2	6.5
Kidney	7.7	7.3
Spleen	77.1	15.5
Small intestine	5.9	4.4

*Rats injected i.v. with 10 mg/kg of daunorubicin HCl were killed 8 hr later and the indicated tissues were removed, extracted and analyzed for drug and metabolites.

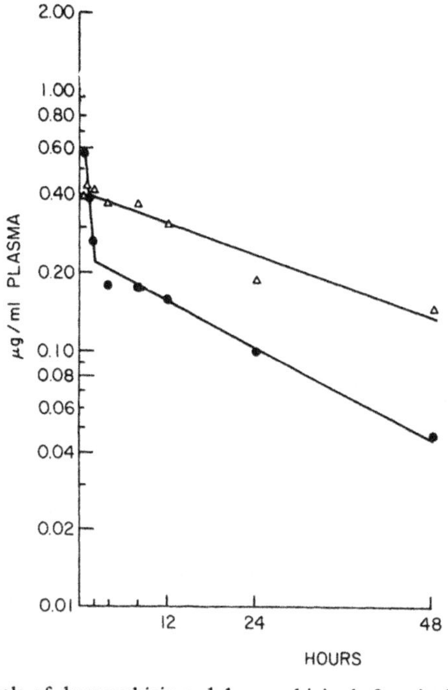

FIG. 4. Human plasma levels of daunorubicin and daunorubicinol after single injection of 180 mg/M² of daunorubicin: ●——●, daunorubicin; △——△, daunorubicinol.

form in the plasma is daunorubicinol. Not only is the plasma level of daunorubicinol high, but also tissues, urine and bile from these patients contain primarily daunorubicinol as the major drug form.

Since daunorubicinol can inhibit nucleic acid synthesis in tumor cells, and since the enzymatic machinery for its formation lies within the target cell, we felt that a reasonable hypothesis for daunorubicin's action should involve the activity of daunorubicin reductase. We propose that daunorubicin readily traverses the cell membrane (Fig. 5). Once inside the cell, it is available for enzymatic manipulation. Depending on the level and activity of daunorubicin reductase in the cell, daunorubicin is converted to daunorubicinol at some rate. In our experiments, the equilibrium of this reaction favors the formation of the alcohol.* Since the alcohol penetrates the cell membrane less readily, it is retained intracellularly and is available for a longer period of time. Daunorubicinol, therefore, has a greater intracellular $C \times T$ than the parent drug. As a pharmacologically active intermediate, daunorubicinol may be of more importance than daunorubicin in both the pharmacologic action as well as the toxicity of this drug–metabolite pair.

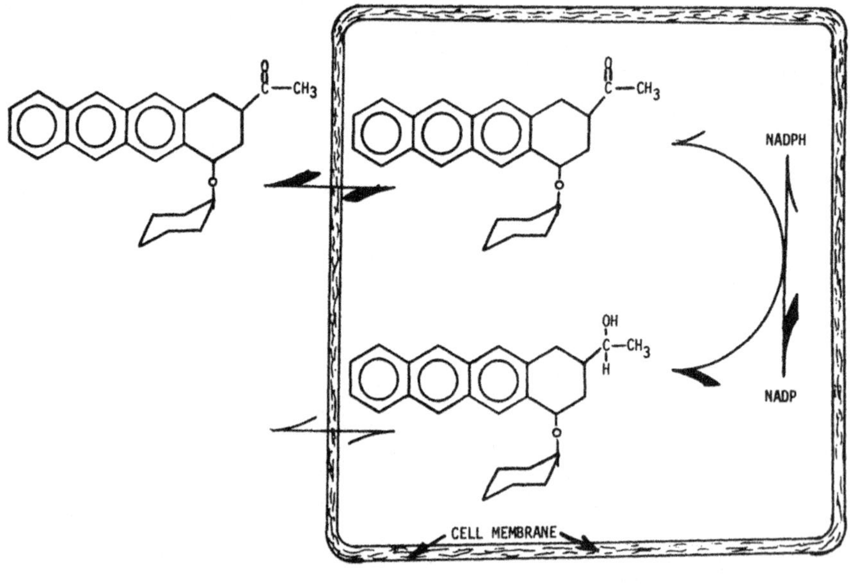

FIG. 5. Cellular pharmacodynamics of daunorubicin–daunorubicinol.

Since we have shown that peripheral human myeloblasts contained high levels of daunorubicin reductase, we studied prospectively the response of patients to daunorubicin and the level of reductase in the peripheral myeloblasts. Thirteen patients were sampled before their treatment with high single dosage daunorubicin, and the reductase levels were determined while their clinical course were assessed. When both information arms were brought together, the myeloblast reductase levels bore an impressive relationship to clinical response (Table 8).[19] In the responding patients, the

*N. R. Bachur and R. Felsted, unpublished observation.

TABLE 8. DAUNORUBICIN REDUCTASE IN NORMAL LEUKOCYTES AND LEUKEMIC MYELOBLASTS*

Clinical status	No. subjects	Daunorubicin reductase (leukocyte/erythrocyte ratio)
Normal subjects	14	5.3
Subleukemic	1	3.2
No response	3	19.5
Died in therapy	4	20.0
Remission	5	46.5

*The same cell preparation and enzyme assay were used as described in Table 4.

enzyme level was high, whereas in nonresponding patients or patients who died during therapy, reductase levels were low. It was also apparent that even in those patients whose therapy failed, the reductase levels in the myeloblasts were much higher than in normal leukocytes. Since this was a small series, we are interested in extending the study to give a clearer estimate of the predictive value of the daunorubicin reductase assay.

Adriamycin reacts differently from daunorubicin both *in vitro* and *in vivo*, and in many situations one does not see the reduced metabolite of adriamycin, i.e. adriamycinol. For example, human blood cells incubated with adriamycin do not produce adriamycinol. However, with purified enzyme preparations, the reduction of adriamycin can occur, although at a very low rate.* Also, in tissue and bile samples from adriamycin-treated patients, adriamycinol is found but not at the level of daunorubicinol. As such, we feel adriamycinol may not play as important a role as the parent drug adriamycin, but this remains to be determined.

In summary, we have shown that adriamycin and daunorubicin both inhibit nucleic acid synthesis, but major differences pertain to the intracellular disposition of the drugs, which may lead to differences in activities. The ubiquitous and active daunorubicin reductase pathway must be considered in evaluations of daunorubicin as a chemotherapeutic agent.

*N. R. Bachur and R. Felsted, unpublished observation.

REFERENCES

1. A. GREIN, C. SPALLA, A. DIMARCO and G. CANEVAZZI, *Gen. Microbiol.* **11**, 109 (1963).
2. A. DIMARCO, M. GAETANI and B. M. SCARPINATO, *Cancer Chemother. Rep.* **53**, 33 (1969).
3. A. DIMARCO, M. GAETANI, L. DORIGOTTI, M. SOLDATI and O. BELLINI, *Tumori* **49**, 203 (1963).
4. J. S. SANDBERG, F. L. HOUSDEN, A. DIMARCO and A. GOLDIN, *Cancer Chemother. Rep.* **54**, 1 (1970).
5. C. L. TAN, H. TASAKA, K. P. YU, L. MURPHEY and D. KARNOFSKY, *Cancer, N.Y.* **20**, 333 (1967).
6. G. BONNADONNA, S. MONFARDINI, M. DELENA, F. FOSSATI-BELLANI and G. BERETTA, *Cancer Res.* **30**, 2572 (1970).
7. E. CALENDI, A. DIMARCO, M. REGGIANI, B. SCARPINATO and L. VALENTINI, *Biochim. biophys. Acta* **103**, 25 (1965).

8. A. DIMARCO, F. ZUNINO, R. SILVESTRINI, C. GAMBARUCCI and R. A. GAMBETTA, *Biochem. Pharmac.* **20**, 1323 (1971).
9. A. RUSCONI and E. CALENDI, *Tumori* **50**, 261 (1964).
10. A. THEOLOGIDES, J. W. YARBRO and B. J. KENNEDY, *Cancer, N.Y.* **21**, 16 (1968).
11. W. D. MERIWETHER and N. R. BACHUR, *Cancer Res.* **32**, 1137 (1972).
12. W. J. PIGRAM, W. FULLER and L. D. HAMILTON, *Nature New Biol.* **235**, 17 (1972).
13. N. R. BACHUR and M. GEE, *J. Pharmac. exp. Ther.* **177**, 567 (1971).
14. N. R. BACHUR, *J. Pharmac. exp. Ther.* **177**, 573 (1971).
15. D. H. HUFFMAN and N. R. BACHUR, *Cancer Res.* **32**, 600 (1972).
16. W. D. MERIWETHER, N. R. BACHUR and M. GEE, *Clin. Res.* **19**, 494 (1971).
17. J. C. CRADOCK, M. J. EGORIN and N. R. BACHUR, *Archs int. Pharmacodyn. Thér.* **202**, 48 (1973).
18. D. H. HUFFMAN, R. S. BENJAMIN and N. R. BACHUR, *Clin. Pharmac. Ther.* **13**, 895 (1972).
19. D. H. HUFFMAN and N. R. BACHUR, *Blood* **39**, 637 (1972).

Pp. 217—223, Supplement Number 2, 1974.
Biochemical Pharmacology. Printed in the U.S.A.

THE VINCA ALKALOIDS

WILLIAM A. CREASEY

Yale University School of Medicine, New Haven, Conn. U.S.A.

THE ANTINEOPLASTIC potential of the source plant of the vinca alkaloids, *Vinca rosea* Linn. or *Catharanthus roseus* G. Don, was discovered by chance during routine screening for hypoglycemic activity.[1,2] Johnson *et al.*[3] have described in detail this and other aspects of early work on these agents. The clinical efficacy of the vinca alkaloids was established a decade ago, long before any significant knowledge of their pharmacological disposition or biochemical mechanism of action was available. Our concern here is to outline briefly what is now known of these aspects of the vinca alkaloids, and how they relate to biological activity. A more complete review of the pharmacology of antimitotic agents may be found elsewhere.[4]

Structure–activity relationships

Four active alkaloids have been isolated from the *Vinca* plant, vinrosidine, vinleurosine, vinblastine and vincristine, of which only the latter two are of proven clinical value. Two semisynthetic derivatives, dihydrovinblastine and vinglycinate, also might have some potential. All the alkaloids possess a dimeric structure based on an indole and a dihydroindole nucleus. Among the structural features necessary for activity are a basic catharanthine indole nitrogen, an acetyl or other acyl function at C_4 of the vindoline moiety, and unsubstituted hydroxyl groups.

Biological actions of the vinca alkaloids

The vinca alkaloids intervene in an extremely wide range of biological processes (Fig. 1). Arrest of mitosis is the first and most characteristic action of this group of compounds,[5] one which is shared by the congeners of colchicine and podophyllotoxin, and by griseofulvin. Commonly termed metaphase arrest or C-mitosis, this phenomenon consists of more than just a fixation of the mitotic apparatus in the metaphase configuration. Rather, it is the spindle that appears to be the target, shrinking and dissolving in drug-dose-related fashion to allow the chromosomes to become eventually disorganized. Chromosome damage where it occurs is a rather minor effect.[6]

Antitumor action has been demonstrated in a range of experimental animal systems as well as in human diseases, especially those such as the lymphomas, acute childhood leukemias, choriocarcinoma and various embryonal or mesenchymal tumors. A point that should be brought out is that, although it may play some part in this antitumor action, mitotic arrest is an essentially reversible process,[7] and has appeared in some studies to be unrelated to cytotoxicity.[8]

The microtubule arrays, such as those found in various cortical areas of the cytoplasm, as well as the neurotubules in the axons, undergo dissolution as a result of

1. MITOTIC ARREST
2. CYTOTOXIC ACTION
3. DISAPPEARANCE OF MICROTUBULES
4. ANTI-INFLAMMATORY EFFECT (GOUT)
5. NEUROLOGICAL TOXICITY
6. CHANGES IN MOTILITY
7. CHANGES IN PHAGOCYTOSIS
8. TERATOGENICITY
9. SUPRESSION OF IMMUNE RESPONSES

FIG. 1. Biological interactions of the vinca alkaloids.

exposure to the vinca alkaloids.[9] In some cells, including human leukocytes and neurones, the material that had comprised the microtubules undergoes a reorganization under the influence of the drugs to form pseudocrystalline aggregates known as microtubule crystals.[10]

Anti-inflammatory activity has been reported for vinblastine when used in patients with gout.[11] This type of anti-inflammatory action is almost certainly related to the suppression of motility and of phagocytotic activity in human polymorphonuclear leukocytes.[12]

Neurological toxicity may be produced by all the alkaloids, as well as by colchicine, but is especially characteristic of vincristine. The neurotoxic lesions that have been encountered include, apart from the microtubule damage, axonal degeneration and demyelination, interference with deep tendon reflexes, inhibition of Schwann cell proliferation, and inhibition of terminal expansion and movement of the undulating membrane of spinal ganglion neurons in culture.[13–15] Among the miscellaneous biological effects are morphological changes in mast cells,[16] teratogenicity[17] and suppression of antibody formation.[18]

Biochemical mechanisms of action

The variety of biological effects of these antimitotic agents may not necessarily reflect corresponding diversity in the underlying biochemical mechanisms. Indeed, it would appear that there are only two major areas of interaction, one involving microtubules, the other biosynthesis of macromolecules. The relation of certain other minor biochemical effects to visible biological changes is unclear.

Microtubule interactions. The microtubule system, consisting of basic units with diameters of about 250Å and lengths up to many microns, is distributed in a wide range of cells and cellular structures. These include the mitotic spindle, flagella and cilia, neuronal processes and cortical cytoplasm. Much of the recent work on cytoplasmic filaments, microtubules and their biological function is summarized in a review by Adelmann *et al.*[19] Study of the nature of the interaction with microtubules was made possible by the availability of tritium-labeled vinblastine and colchicine. Most studies have been undertaken with the latter compound, but the lesser amount of information regarding vinblastine indicates that it behaves similarly. Taylor *et al.*[20–23] have studied the colchicine-binding protein rather intensively. This protein, isolated from brain tissue and sea urchin sperm tails, has a molceular weight of about 120,000 and binds colchicine or vinblastine non-covalently. In general, it is present in the high-speed supernatant fraction of cells. Levels are greater in dividing cells, cilia, brain tissue and the mitotic apparatus, a pattern of distribution resembling that of the microtubules themselves. Similar proteins, able to bind colchicine and vinblastine, have been demonstrated in Sarcoma 180 cells,[24] human leukocytes[25] and grasshopper embryos.[26] Binding of vinblastine by the protein is sensitive to high ionic strength, but not to high concentrations of urea, and is stabilized by colchicine or podophyllotoxin. The explanation for this appears to be that there are two distinct types of binding sites for drugs, one at which colchicine interacts and the other at which vinca alkaloids bind. Each molecule contains one site for colchicine binding and one for attachment of vinca alkaloids. Guanosine triphosphate normally occupies two sites, one of which permits exchange of the nucleotide while the other seems to be non-exchanging.[23] Binding of the antimitotic agents occurs *in vitro* as well as *in vivo*, and in the case of the vinca alkaloids may lead to the precipitation of aggregates that at least in part consist of pseudocrystalline masses like the crystals formed *in vivo.*[27]

At present it appears that the protein is a subunit of the microtubules, which probably serves as a source for spontaneous assembly of these tubules; such a process has been observed *in vitro.*[28] The most probable picture of the dynamic relationship within the system is shown in Fig. 2. Antimitotic agents, by binding to the microtubule protein, may interfere with the equilibria causing dissolution of assembled structures. The protein itself seems to be present in a heterodimeric form, or at least this is the form that reacts with the drugs. Kinetic studies of the binding interaction have been reported,[21,29] but at present the nature of the active sites is unknown.

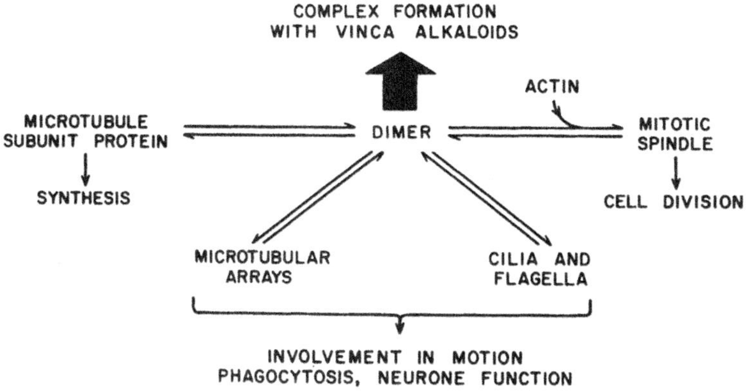

FIG. 2. Interaction of vinca alkaloids with the equilibria of the microtubule system.

Inhibition of nucleic acid synthesis. Starting with Beer,[30] in 1961, who found that DNA synthesis in bone marrow was inhibited, there are many reports that the vinca alkaloids inhibit nucleic acid biosynthesis. Depression of the incorporation of precursors into DNA has been described in rat thymus cells,[31] rat spleen, bone marrow and regenerating liver *in vivo,*[32,33] the protozoan *Tetrahymena pyriformis*[34] and rat Walker tumor.[35] While many of these studies have stressed DNA synthesis as a parameter particularly sensitive to vinca alkaloids, others have found RNA biosynthesis to be more readily affected by these agents. In rat thymus and lymphosarcoma P1798, levels of RNA but not of DNA were reduced after treating animals with vinblastine,[36] while in mice bearing Ehrlich ascites carcinoma, incorporation of uridine into RNA, especially the lower molecular weight fraction, was inhibited in tumor from animals receiving vinblastine, vincristine or colchicine.[37,38] In human leukemic leukocytes, incorporation of precursors into RNA is especially sensitive to vinca alkaloids.[39,40] The neurological toxicity produced by administering vincristine to mice is associated with reduced incorporation of intracranially administered uridine into brain RNA.[41]

As regards the mechanisms involved in inhibition of incorporation of precursors into nucleic acids, several possibilities exist. Interference with uptake of nucleosides by cells does occur, but apparently only ribonucleosides are involved.[42] Vincristine has been reported to cause direct inhibition of RNA polymerase, but rather high drug levels are required.[40] The remaining possibility is that the alkaloids interact with nucleic acids themselves, a process known to occur with the other antimitotic agents, colchicine, podophyllic acid ethyl hydrazide and griseofulvin. Inhibition of nucleic acid biosynthesis might then occur in a manner analogous with that produced by the antitumor antibiotics.

Protein and lipid biosynthesis. Inhibition of protein synthesis occurs in Ehrlich ascites carcinoma cells,[38] and human leukemic[40] and normal[25] leukocyte populations. In some cases, the inhibition is related in time and degree to effects on RNA synthesis, while in others there does not seem to be an obvious relationship. The peculiar antagonism of the effects of the vinca alkaloids by glutamate, reported long ago,[3] may be considered to relate to this area of metabolism. We have found that vinblastine and glutamate compete with each other for uptake by human leukocytes, despite the disparity in chemical structure of the two compounds.[25]

Lipid metabolism is an area that clearly relates to biological damage such as axonal degeneration and demyelination. In both rat gastrocnemius muscle and Sarcoma 180 cells, phospholipid synthesis appears to be sensitive to vincristine and vinleurosine, respectively, whereas neutral lipid formation is but little affected.[42,43] The mechanisms involved in such an action are unknown, but the effect could be mediated through pyrimidine metabolism, as for example the inhibition of uridine uptake produced by the vinca alkaloids, since pyrimidine ribonucleotides are involved in phospholipid metabolism.

Metabolism and distribution of the vinca alkaloids

The vinca alkaloids are cleared relatively rapidly from the plasma of mice,[44] rats,[45] dogs[46] and humans.[47] This is not due to rapid urinary excretion, which occurs only to a very limited extent.[46,48] It would appear that the drugs are rapidly sequestrated by various tissues including blood leukocytes[46] and the platelets,[49] the latter forming, indeed, a major reservoir of circulating drug. Presumably most tissues rich in microtubules would accumulate the drugs, although the nervous system would not appear to be particularly permeable to them. The major route for excretion of the alkaloids is the bile,[46,48] and of this material the larger proportion is in the form of metabolites. While deacetylation at the 4-position is a major catabolic process, knowledge of the over-all degradation of these compounds is currently lacking.

CONCLUSION

As with many other effective cancer chemotherapy agents, the vinca alkaloids undoubtedly have more than one site of action. Interaction with microtubules is clearly the major element, since so many of the biological effects of these drugs point to an underlying disturbance of this system. On the other hand, the inhibition of biosynthesis of macromolecules has been a frequent finding *in vivo*, even if generally unphysiological drug levels are required for these effects to be manifested *in vitro*. It is possible to envisage that inhibition of microtubule protein synthesis could reinforce the effects of depletion of the free pool of this material, thus effecting complementary inhibition.

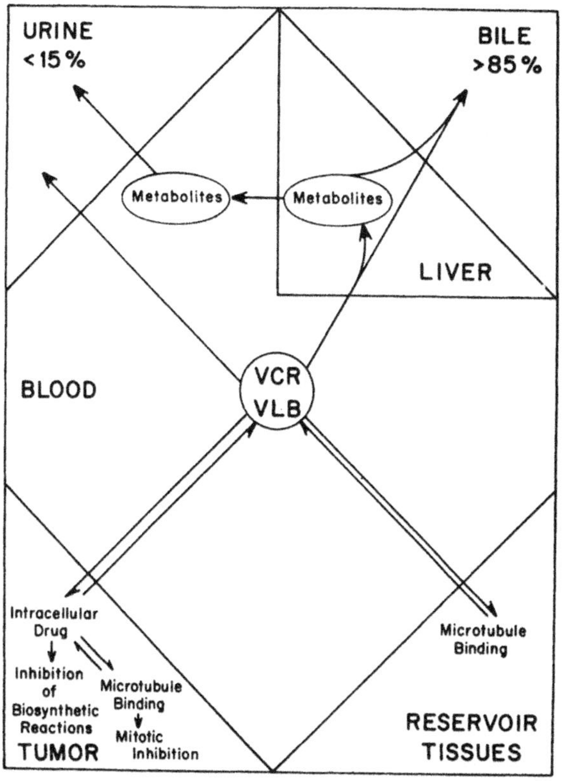

FIG. 3. Distribution and interactions of vinca alkaloids in body compartments.

Finally, the binding of vinca alkaloids within cells, and their relatively slow excretion, are of clinical relevance. They provide a basis for empirical clinical findings that more frequent administration of these agents, for example daily treatments, is accompanied by unacceptable increments in host toxicity. Figure 3 presents in summary form many of the topics covered in this article.

Acknowledgements – I am indebted to Mrs. Dorene Mohammad, Miss Carolyn Chomiak and Mr. Bartlett Toftness for their invaluable assistance in the experiments carried out in my laboratory. Financial support has been derived from the American Cancer Society (ACS-ET-14G) and USPHS (CA-12317, CA 08341).

REFERENCES

1. C. T. BEER, *Br. Emp. Cancer Campaign* **33**, 487 (1955).
2. I. S. JOHNSON, H. F. WRIGHT and G. H. SVOBODA, *J. Lab. clin. Med.* **54**, 830 (1959).
3. I. S. JOHNSON, J. G. ARMSTRONG, M. GORMAN and J. P. BURNETT, JR., *Cancer Res.* **23**, 1390 (1963).
4. W. A. CREASEY, in *Handbook of Experimental Pharmacology* (Eds. A. C. SARTORELLI and D. J. JOHNS), Vol. 38 p. 670 Springer, Berlin (1973).
5. G. CARDINALI, G. CARDINALI, A. H. HANDLER and M. F. AGRIFOGLIO, *Proc. Soc. exp. Biol. Med.* **107**, 891 (1961).
6. P. SENTEIN, *C. r. hebd. Séanc. Acad. Sci., Paris* **258**, 4854 (1964).
7. A. KRISHAN, *J. natn. Cancer Inst.* **41**, 581 (1968).
8. E. FREII, III, J. WHANG, R. B. SCOGGINS, E. J. VAN SCOTT, D. P. RALL and M. BEN, *Cancer Res.* **24**, 1918 (1964).
9. E. ROBBINS and N. K. GONATAS, *J. Histochem. Cytochem.* **2**, 704 (1964).
10. K. G. BENSCH and S. E. MALAWISTA, *J. Cell Biol.* **40**, 95 (1969).
11. I. H. KRAKOFF, *Arthritis Rheum.* **8**, 760 (1965).
12. S. E. MALAWISTA, *Arthritis Rheum.* **11**, 108 (1968).
13. Q. L. UY, T. H. MOEN, R. J. JOHNS and A. H. OWENS, JR., *Johns Hopkins med. J.* **121**, 349 (1967).
14. W. E. TOBIN and S. G. SANDLER, *Nature, Lond.* **212**, 90 (1966).
15. A. BARASA, V. MACCOTTA, G. FILOGAMO and B. CANAVESE, *Boll. Soc. ital. Biol. sper.* **46**, 860 (1970).
16. J. PADAWER, *Ann. N.Y. Acad. Sci.* **103**, 87 (1963).
17. V. H. FERM, *Science, N.Y.* **141**, 426 (1963).
18. A. C. AISENBERG, *Nature, Lond.* **200**, 484 (1963).
19. M. R. ADELMANN, G. G. BORISY, M. L. SHELANSKI, R. C. WEISENBERG and E. W. TAYLOR, *Fedn. Proc.* **27**, 1186 (1968).
20. G. G. BORISY and E. W. TAYLOR, *J. Cell Biol.* **34**, 525 (1967).
21. G. G. BORISY and E. W. TAYLOR, *J. Cell Biol.* **34**, 535 (1967).
22. M. L. SHELANSKI and E. W. TAYLOR, *J. Cell Biol.* **34**, 549 (1967).
23. R. C. WEISENBERG, G. G. BORISY and E. W. TAYLOR, *Biochemistry, N.Y.* **7**, 4466 (1968).
24. W. A. CREASEY, *Pharmacologist* **9**, 192 (1967).
25. W. A. CREASEY, K. G. BENSCH and S. E. MALAWISTA, *Biochem. Pharmac.* **20**, 1579 (1971).
26. L. WILSON and M. FRIEDKIN, *Biochemistry, N.Y.* **6**, 3126 (1967).
27. R. MARANTZ, M. VENTILIA and M. SHELANSKI, *Science, N.Y.* **165**, 498 (1969).
28. R. E. STEPHENS, *J. molec. Biol.* **33**, 517 (1968).
29. J. BRYAN, *Biochemistry, N.Y.* **11**, 2611 (1972).
30. C. T. BEER, *Can. Cancer Conf.* **4**, 355 (1961).
31. J. F. RICHARDS, R. G. W. JONES and C. T. BEER, *Cancer Res.* **26**, 876 (1966).
32. J. L. VAN LANCKER, A. L. FLANGAS and J. ALLEN, *Lab. Invest.* **15**, 1291 (1966).
33. A. LUYCKX and J. L. VAN LANCKER, *Lab. Invest.* **15**, 1301 (1966).
34. I. J. SLOTNICK, M. DOUGHERTY and D. H. JAMES, JR., *Cancer Res.* **26**, 673 (1966).
35. R. DESJARDINS, D. E. GROGAN, J. P. ARENDELL and H. BUSCH, *Cancer Res.* **27**, 159 (1967).
36. P. H. WIERNIK and R. M. MCLEOD, *Proc. Soc. exp. Biol. Med.* **119**, 118 (1965).
37. W. A. CREASEY and M. E. MARKIW, *Biochem. Pharmac.* **13**, 135 (1964).

38. W. A. CREASEY and M. E. MARKIW, *Biochim. biophys. Acta* **87**, 601 (1964).
39. W. A. CREASEY, *Cancer Chemother. Rep.* **52**, 501 (1968).
40. M. J. CLINE, *Br. J. Haemat.* **14**, 21 (1968).
41. B. M. AUGUSTIN and W. A. CREASEY, *Nature, Lond.* **215**, 965 (1967).
42. W. A. CREASEY, *Biochem. Pharmac.* **18**, 227 (1969).
43. G. L. A. GRAFF, C. GUEUNING and J. HILDEBRAND, *C. r. Séanc. Soc. Biol.* **161**, 2645 (1967).
44. R. J. OWELLEN and D. W. DONIGIAN, *J. med. chem.* **15**, 894 (1972).
45. R. L. NOBLE, *Can. Cancer Conf.* **4**, 333 (1961).
46. W. A. CREASEY and J. C. MARSH, *Proc. Am. Ass. Cancer Res.* **14**, 57 (1973).
47. C. G. SMITH, J. E. GRADY and F. P. KUPIECKI, *Cancer Res.* **25**, 241 (1965).
48. C. T. BEER, M. L. WILSON and J. BELL, *Can. J. Physiol. Pharmac.* **42**, 368 (1964).
49. H. F. HEBDEN, J. R. HADFIELD and C. T. BEER, *Cancer Res.* **30**, 1417 (1970).

Pp. 225—232, Supplement Number 2, 1974.
Biochemical Pharmacology. Printed in the U.S.A.

REACTIONS AND EFFECTS OF NITROSOUREAS*

GLYNN P. WHEELER

Southern Research Institute, Birmingham, Ala. 35209, U.S.A.

A GENRALIZED formula that shows the structure and the mode of decomposition of 1,3-disubstituted-1-nitrosoureas is given below:

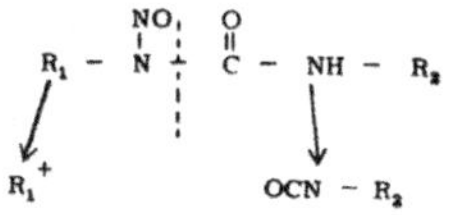

R_1 AND R_2 may be the same or different, and for significant therapeutic effectiveness it is necessary to have a proton on N-3.[1,2] Decomposition at physiological conditions occurs by scission at the locus indicated by the dashed line to yield a carbonium ion, R_1^+, and an isocyanate, R_2NCO. R_1 and R_2 together determine the stability and solubility of the parent compound. R_1 determines the reactivity of the generated carbonium ion, and R_2 determines the reactivity of the generated isocyanate. Testing of a number of these nitrosoureas against murine leukemia L1210 led to the conclusion that the best therapeutic activity is obtained with compounds in which R_1 is a 2-haloethyl group, preferably 2-chloroethyl or 2-fluoroethyl.[3] Therefore a large number of compounds bearing one of these two groups as R_1 and a wide variety of groups as R_2 were synthesized and tested. Three of these compounds have progressed to the stage of clinical testing and have yielded some therapeutic benefit. These compounds are 1,3-bis(2-chloroethyl)-1-nitrosourea (BCNU; NSC 409962), 1-(2-chloroethyl)-3-cyclohexyl-1-nitrosourea (CCNU; NSC 79037), and 1-(2-chloroethyl)-3-(*trans*-4-methylcyclohexyl)-1-nitrosourea (MeCCNU; NSC 95441).

The details of the decomposition of BCNU (I) in buffer at pH 7.4 and 37° are shown below:[4]

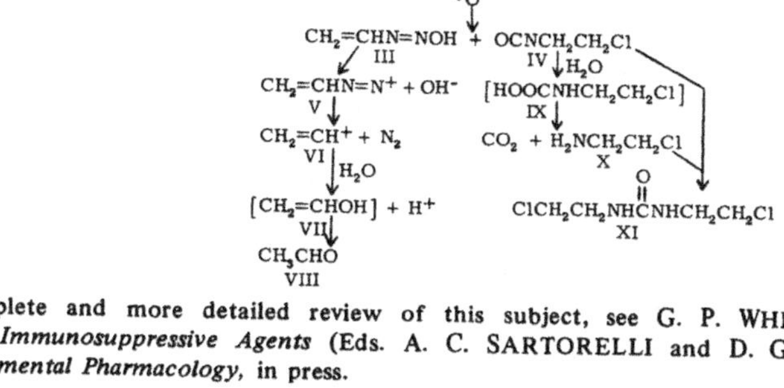

*For a more complete and more detailed review of this subject, see G. P. WHEELER, in *Antineoplastic and Immunosuppressive Agents* (Eds. A. C. SARTORELLI and D. G. JOHNS), *Handbook of Experimental Pharmacology*, in press.

Chemical evidence[4] indicates that elimination of a chloride ion and formation of an intermediate cyclic compound (II) precede scission of the molecule between N-1 and the carbonyl group. Scission yields vinyl diazohydroxide (III) and 2-chloroethyl isocyanate (IV). Ionization of the vinyl diazohydroxide yields a diaxonium ion (V), which loses nitrogen to form a vinyl carbonium ion (VI). This ion reacts with water to form vinyl alcohol (VII), which rearranges to give acetaldehyde (VIII). The 2-chloroethyl isocyanate reacts with water to give the unstable carbamic acid (IX), which decomposes to give carbon dioxide and 2-chloroethylamine (X). The 2-chloroethylamine can act as an alkylating agent (perhaps after conversion to ethylenimine),[5] and it can react with newly generated 2-chloroethyl isocyanate (IV) to give 1,3-bis(2-chloroethyl)urea (XI).

Through an analogous series of reactions, decomposition of CCNU yields acetaldehyde, cyclohexylamine and 1,3-dicyclohexylurea.[4] The cyclohexylamine differs from the 2-chloroethylamine in that the former has no potential alkylating activity, and this difference might account partially for some of the different biological effects of BCNU and CCNU. The decomposition of MeCCNU is assumed to be analogous to that for CCNU. If other compounds with nucleophilic centers are present when the nitrosourea decomposes, they will compete with the water for the generated carbonium ion, and alkylation of these compounds may occur. In intact cells a major site of alkylation is the nucleic acids, particularly the DNA, and a lesser extent of alkylation of protein occurs.[6] If compounds bearing active hydrogen atoms are present, they may react with the generated isocyanate to yield carbamoyl compounds. In intact cells carbamoylation of proteins occurs much more extensively than carbamoylation of nucleic acid,[6] although the latter may occur to some extent.[7,8] Carbamoylation probably accounts for a large part of the binding to blood proteins, as Oliverio *et al.* have reported,[9] and the binding is probably primarily with the ϵ-amino groups of the lysine moieties.[10,11]

There is evidence[12] that both alkylation and carbamoylation contribute to the biological effects of these agents. It would be expected that alkylation of DNA and RNA might cause cytotoxicity, mutagenicity and carcinogenicity, while carbamoylation of proteins might contribute primarily to cytotoxicity.

Perhaps as a result of reactions with nucleic acids or proteins or both, these agents alter the rates of synthesis of nucleic acids. Administration of BCNU to mice bearing subcutaneously implanted solid L1210 lymphoma and to hamsters bearing subcutaneously implanted plasmacytomas inhibited the incorporation of ^{14}C of formate-^{14}C and of adenine-8-^{14}C into both the RNA and DNA of the tumors; the inhibition was greater for DNA than for RNA, and the inhibition of the incorporation of ^{14}C from formate-^{14}C was greater than that from adenine-8-^{14}C.[13] With elevated doses of BCNU there was inhibition of the *de novo* synthesis of purine ribonucleotides but not of the conversion of adenine-8-^{14}C to purine nucleotides; there was a small inhibition of the incorporation of DL-leucine-4,5-^{3}H into protein. Other investigators have also reported inhibition of the synthesis of nucleic acids by BCNU in host tissues and murine sarcoma 180[14] and in Ehrlich ascites cells,[15] and by 1-propyl-1-nitrosourea in Ehrlich ascites cells and a murine hepatoma.[16] Stimulation of synthesis of nucleic acids, particularly RNA, after low doses of the agents or at short times after larger doses of the agents, was observed in several of these investigations. Maximum inhibition of the synthesis of RNA and DNA in L1210 solid tumor,[13] murine Lewis lung carcinoma[41] and hamster plasmacytoma,[41] and of DNA in murine sarcoma 180[14] occurred 16–24 hr after a single dose of nitrosourea. Delayed inhibition of the synthesis of DNA also occurred in several host tissues, but these host tissues recovered their normal rates of synthesis of DNA much more quickly than did the neoplasms. Incubation of crude cell-free preparations from L1210 ascites cells with BCNU or CCNU caused decreases in the DNA nucleotidyltransferase activity of these preparations, but incubation of commercial DNA with BCNU did not significantly alter its activity as a primer or template for the DNA nucleotidyltransferase system.[17] Since 2-chloroethyl isocyanate decreased the nucleotidyltransferase activity as much as BCNU or CCNU, it was concluded that the decreases were probably caused by carbamoylation of the enzymes. Treatment of L1210 cells *in vivo* or *in vitro* with selected concentrations of BCNU caused inhibition of the synthesis of DNA by the intact cells without decreasing the DNA nucleotidyltransferase activity of cell-free preparations derived from these treated cells. It was concluded that, although under certain conditions BCNU can cause decreases in the DNA nucleotidyltransferase activity, deactivation of this enzyme is probably not the cause of decreased synthesis of DNA *in vivo*. Such a conclusion is consistent with the possibility that the DNA nucleotidyltransferase that is measured in this assay system is a repair enzyme rather than an enzyme for normal replication of DNA. It is still unclear whether the inhibitions of the synthesis of nucleic acids are causes or effects of cytotoxicity.

The effects of nitrosoureas upon the synthesis of nucleic acids are also reflected in the effects of these agents upon the progression of cells through the cell cycle. The labeling of cultured cells initially in S at the time of exposure to BCNU was partially inhibited,[18] and the progression of cells from G_1 into S was delayed.[18,19] Progression of cells from S to mitosis was also delayed,[18,19] and evidence for the lengthening of the S phase without decreasing the labeling index of L1210 cells *in vivo* by the administration of BCNU[20–22] and CCNU[22] has been presented. At low concentrations BCNU prevented cultured cells in the first half of G_2 from proceeding to mitosis,[18] and at higher concentrations it delayed cells in all parts of G_2 from reaching mitosis.[18,19] 2-Chloroethylamine caused effects upon the progression of cultured cells similar to those caused by BCNU,[18] and cyclohexyl isocyanate increased the length of the S phase of L1210 cells *in vivo* similarly to CCNU.[22] These results indicate that both alkylation and carbamoylation can interfere with the progression of cells through the cycle.

Dose–response data and the kinetics of cell kill indicate that the nitrosoureas kill cells in all phases of the cell cycle,[18,19,23–27] but studies with certain lines of cultured mammalian cells show that the cells are most sensitive at the G_1/S boundary[26] or in mid-S phase.[19] There is also evidence that proliferating lymphoma cells are more sensitive to nitrosoureas than nonproliferating stem cells,[24] but exposure of cultured L1210 cells to BCNU in buffer under conditions not conducive to proliferation of the cells resulted in killing the cells.[28]

Knowledge of these effects of the nitrosoureas upon cell kinetics and cell survival in conjunction with knowledge of the cell kinetics of host tissues and tumors, make possible some rationality in planning cancer chemotherapy.

It was stated above that the substituents on N-1 and N-3 determine the degree of stability of the nitrosoureas. The chemical half-lives in phosphate buffer, pH 7.4, at 37° of eleven 1,3-disubstituted-1-nitrosoureas that have either a 2-chloroethyl group or a 2-fluoroethyl group on N-1 fall within the range of 19–68 min. Table 1 gives the chemical half-lives of BCNU, CCNU and MeCCNU.[12] These half-lives are rather short, and hence periods of exposure of tissues to the active agents will be rather short. Biological half-lives of the compounds[29–31] are also given in Table 1. These data show that the parent compound disappears from the plasma and the cerebrospinal fluid more rapidly than it decomposes, and therefore a sizable portion of the parent compound is evidently delivered to various tissues before it decomposes. Consideration of these half-lives is important for planning dosage regimens and in considering the product of concentration multiplied by time of exposure.

TABLE 1. HALF-LIVES OF NITROSOUREAS

	Time (min)	Reference
Chemical (phosphate buffer, pH 7.4, 37°)		
BCNU	43	12
CCNU	53	12
MeCCNU	53	12
Biological		
BCNU		
Mouse	*ca* 15	29
Dog		
Plasma	< 15	30
Cerebrospinal fluid	< 15	29
Monkey		
Cerebrospinal fluid	< 15	29
Man		
Cerebrospinal fluid	< 15	29
CCNU		
Mouse		
Plasma	*ca* 5	9
Dog		
Plasma	*ca* 5	9
Cerebrospinal fluid	*ca* 5	9
MeCCNU		
Man		
Plasma	< 10	31
Cerebrospinal fluid	< 10	31
Urine	< 10	31

TABLE 2. SOME VALUES OF P (n-OCTANOL/H_2O)*

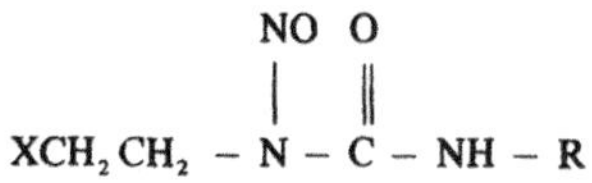

X	R	P
Cl	$-CH_2CH_2Cl$	34
F	$-CH_2CH_2F$	2
Cl	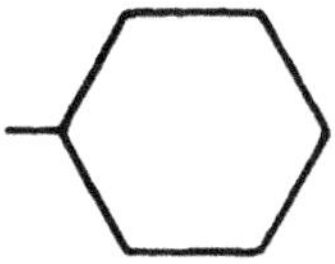	676
F	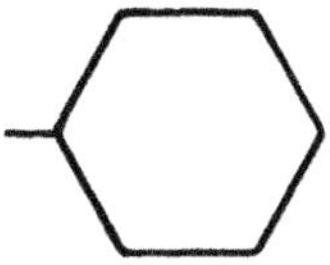	169
Cl	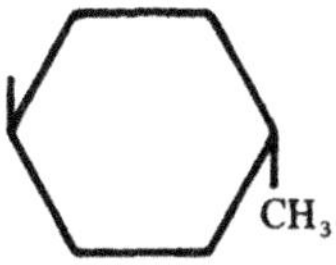	1995
F	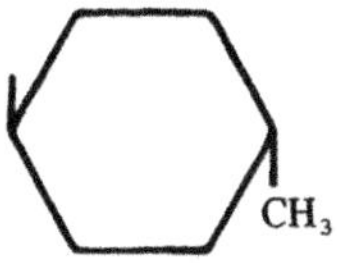	501

*Data of Hansch *et al.*[32]

The substituents on N-1 and N-3 also determine the solubility of the nitrosoureas. Table 2 contains the values of the distribution coefficients of a few compounds for the *n*-octanol–water system, which Hansch *et al.*[32] have experimentally determined or calculated, along with those for a number of other nitrosoureas. It is evident that both the halogen atom on the ethyl group and the group on N-3 influence the solubility. Hansch *et al.*[32] have concluded that for significant therapeutic activity the distribution coefficients must fall within a certain range of values; compounds with coefficients that are either above or below this range will be less effective or completely ineffective. This is not surprising, because the solubility of the compound is important

TABLE 3. CROSS-RESISTANCE AND RETAINED SENSITIVITY

Test system	Cross-resistant to	Sensitive to	Reference
E. coli/BCNU	Mitomycin, porfiromycin, nitrogen mustard, myleran, azaserine, 6-dizao-6-oxo-L-norleucine, u.v.		35
E. coli/mitomycin	BCNU		35
E. coli/porfiromycin	BCNU		35
E. coli/nitrogen mustard	BCNU		35
E. coli/azaserine	BCNU		35
E. coli/BCNU (BB)		CCNU	*
E. coli/CCNU (BB)		BCNU	*
E. coli/MeCCNU (BB)	CCNU (partially)	BCNU	*
Plasmacytoma/BCNU	cyclophosphamide, triethylenemelamine		36
Plasmacytoma/ cyclophosphamide		BCNU	37
L1210/BCNU	CCNU	Cyclophosphamide	37†
Lewis lung carcinoma/ MeCCNU		Cyclophosphamide	‡
L1210/BIC	BCNU, CCNU, streptozotocin, DIC	Phenylalanine mustard, cyclophosphamide, thio-TEPA, nitrogen mustard	38
L1210/DIC		BCNU, CCNU, BIC, nitrogen mustard, triethylenemelamine	39

*G. P. Wheeler, B. J. Bowdon and J. A. Grimsley, unpublished observations.
†W. R. Laster, unpublished observations.
‡J. G. Mayo, unpublished observations.

in preparing formulations of the drugs and in the drug's crossing the cell membranes and the "blood–brain barrier." I know of no evidence for or against the active transport of nitrosoureas across cell membranes, and therefore solubility would be quite important for passive diffusion of these agents. Solubility is also quite important in determining whether agents cross the blood–brain barrier and are effective against neoplasms of the central nervous system.

It is recognized that natural and acquired resistances are clinical problems that must be faced. It is well known that all types of clinical or experimental neoplasms do not respond equally to a single or to a variety of alkylating agents, and a tumor that has become resistant to one alkylating agent may[33] or may not[34] respond to a second alkylating agent. Since the nitrosoureas can act as both alkylating and carbamoylating agents, one is interested in whether the phenomenon of cross-resistance of neoplasms to nitrosoureas and other types of alkylating agents exists. Table 3 lists instances of cross-resistance and retained sensitivity in several experimental systems in which a drug-resistant line was selected by repeated exposure of the parent drug-sensitive line to increasing concentrations or dosages of the compound. This list shows that one cannot make a general statement about cross-resistance between nitrosoureas and several other types of alkylating agents. The biochemical reasons and the possible relevance of carbamoylation for these varied results are not presently known. This present unpredictability of development of cross-resistance is problematical for the clinician. Therefore, perhaps it would behoove him to choose a dosage regimen that would minimize the likelihood of the development of any resistance, such as the administration of a single large dose of a nitrosourea, either alone or in combination with other agents including other alkylating agents. Schabel[40] has reported the successful use of such regimens in experimental systems.

Knowledge of the reactions and effects of nitrosoureas that have been discussed above should be useful as one plans for the treatment of primary neoplasms and metastases, including those of the central nervous system, for designing dosage regimens, and for choosing combinations of drugs that might have synergistic effects and/or prevent the development of drug resistance.

REFERENCES

1. J. A. MONTGOMERY, T. P. JOHNSTON and Y. F. SHEALY, in *Medicinal Chemistry*, (Ed. A. BURGER), third edn, part I pp. 680–783. Wiley-Interscience, New York (1970).
2. T. P. JOHNSTON, *Cancer Chemother. Rep.* **3**, 50 (1972).
3. T. P. JOHNSTON, G. S. MCCALEB, P. S. OPLIGER, W. R. LASTER and J. A. MONTGOMERY, *J. med. Chem.* **14**, 600 (1971).
4. J. A. MONTGOMERY, R. JAMES, G. S. MCCALEB and T. P. JOHNSTON, *J. med. Chem.* **10**, 668 (1967).
5. P. L. LEVINS and Z. B. PAPANASTASSIOU, *J. Am. chem. Soc.* **87**, 826 (1965).
6. C. J. CHENG, S. FUJIMURA, D. GRUNBERGER and I. B. WEINSTEIN, *Cancer Res.* **32**, 22 (1972).
7. A. M. SEREBRYANYI, M. A. SMOTRYAEVA, K. E. KRUGLYAKOVA and R. G. KOSTYANOVSKII, *Dokl. Akad. Nauk SSSR* **185**, 847 (1969).
8. A. M. SEREBRYANYI and R. M. MNATSAKANYAN, *FEBS Lett.* **28**, 191 (1972).
9. V. T. OLIVERIO, W. M. VIETZKE, M. K. WILLIAMS and R. H. ADAMSON, *Cancer Res.* **30**, 1330 (1970).
10. B. J. BOWDON and G. P. WHEELER, *Proc. Am. Ass. Cancer Res.* **12**, 67 (1971).
11. B. SCHMALL, C. -J. CHENG, S. FUJIMURA, D. GRUNBERGER and I. B. WEINSTEIN, *Proc. Am. Ass. Cancer Res.* **13**, 65 (1972).
12. G. P. WHEELER, B. J. BOWDON, J. A. GRIMSLEY and H. H. LLOYD, *Cancer Res.* **34**, 194 (1974).

13. G. P. WHEELER and B. J. BOWDON, *Cancer Res.* **25**, 1770 (1965).
14. N. S. MIZUNO and E. W. HUMPHREY, *Cancer Chemother. Rep.* **53**, 215 (1969).
15. G. R. GALE, *Biochem. Pharmac.* **14**, 1707 (1965).
16. L. B. GORBACHEVA and G. V. KUKUSHKINA, *Biochem. Pharmac.* **19**, 1561 (1970).
17. G. P. WHEELER and B. J. BOWDON, *Cancer Res.* **28**, 52 (1968).
18. G. P. WHEELER, B. J. BOWDON, D. J. ADAMSON and M. H. VAIL, *Cancer Res.* **30**, 1817 (1970).
19. S. C. BARRANCO and R. M. HUMPHREY, *Cancer Res.* **31**, 191 (1971).
20. R. C. YOUNG and V. T. DEVITA, *Cancer Res.* **30**, 1789 (1970).
21. S. SHIRAKAWA and E. FREI, III, *Cancer Res.* **30**, 2173 (1970).
22. D. A. BRAY, V. T. DEVITA, R. H. ADAMSON and V. T. OLIVERIO, *Cancer Chemother. Rep.* **55**, 215 (1971).
23. L. J. WILKOFF, G. J. DIXON, E. A. DULMADGE and F. M. SCHABEL, JR., *Cancer Chemother. Rep.* **51**, 7 (1967).
24. W. R. BRUCE and F. A. VALERIOTE, in *The Proliferation and Spread of Neoplastic Cells*, pp. 409–420. Williams & Wilkins, Baltimore (1968).
25. B. K. BHUYAN, L. G. SCHEIDT and T. J. FRASER, *Proc. Am. Ass. Cancer Res.* **11**, 8 (1970).
26. B. K. BHUYAN, L. G. SCHEIDT and T. J. FRASER, *Cancer Res.* **32**, 398 (1972).
27. B. DREWINKO, J. K. NOVAK and S. C. BARRANCO, *Cancer Res.* **32**, 1206 (1972).
28. F. M. SCHABEL, JR., H. E. SKIPPER, M. W. TRADER and W. S. WILCOX, *Cancer Chemother. Rep.* **48**, 17 (1965).
29. V. T. DEVITA, C. DENHAM, J. D. DAVIDSON and V. T. OLIVERIO, *Clin. Pharmac. Ther.* **8**, 566 (1967).
30. T. L. LOO, R. L. DION, R. L. DIXON and D. P. RALL, *J. pharmac. Sci.* **55**, 492 (1966).
31. R. W. SPONZO, V. H. BONO and V. T. OLIVERIO, *Proc. Am. Ass. Cancer Res.* **13**, 33 (1972).
32. C. HANSCH, N. SMITH, R. ENGLE and H. WOOD, *Cancer Chemother. Rep.* **56**, 443 (1972).
33. D. E. BERGSAGEL, D. H. COWAN and R. HASSELBACK, *Can. med. Ass. J.* **107**, 851 (1972).
34. E. BOESEN and W. DAVIS, *Cytotoxic Drugs in the Treatment of Cancer*, pp. 40–42. Edward Arnold, London (1969).
35. R. F. PITTILLO, A. J. NARKATES and J. BURNS, *Cancer Res.* **24**, 1222 (1964).
36. H. E. SKIPPER, D. J. HUTCHINSON, F. M. SCHABEL, JR., L. H. SCHMIDT, A. GOLDIN, R. W. BROCKMAN, J. M. VENDITTI and I. WODINSKY, *Cancer Chemother. Rep.* **56**, 493 (1972).
37. F. M. SCHABEL, JR., in *Proc. Chemotherapy Conference on the Chemotherapy of Solid Tumors: An Appraisal of 5-Fluorouracil and BCNU* (Ed. S. K. CARTER), pp. 159–180. Cancer Therapy Evaluation Branch, National Cancer Institute, Bethesda, Md., (1970).
38. D. D. TYRER, I. KLINE, M. GANG, A. GOLDIN and J. M. VENDITTI, *Cancer Chemother. Rep.* **53**, 229 (1969).
39. I. KLINE, R. J. WOODMAN, M. GANG and J. M. VENDITTI, *Cancer Chemother. Rep.* **55**, 9 (1971).
40. F. M. SCHABEL, JR., in *Proc. Fifth Int. Congr. Chemotherapy, Symp. B-110, Cancer Chemother.* (Eds. T. C. HALL and K. KARRER), pp. 65–82. Verlag der Wiener Medizinischen Akademie, Vienna (1968).
41. G. P. WHEELER and J. A. ALEXANDER, *Cancer Res.* **34**, 1957 (1974).

Pp. 233—236, Supplement Number 2, 1974.
Biochemical Pharmacology. Printed in the U.S.A.

CONCLUDING REMARKS

ALAN C. SARTORELLI

THE ATTAINMENT of optimal therapeutic mileage from any given cancer chemotherapeutic agent is strongly aided by a knowledge of the pharmacological factors influencing drug action. The first session of this conference was dedicated to a discussion of these factors. Absorption, protein binding, distribution and excretion of any given chemical agent in part dictate the concentration of drug, as well as the duration and intensity of its effect, both at the target site(s) within neoplastic cells and at the locus or loci in normal tissues responsible for the rate limiting host toxicity. Dr. Oliverio has presented these principles of pharmacology as they influence drug action using methotrexate as a model agent. The other important consideration in drug action is its susceptibility to biotransformation, which may play a major role in both the activation and inactivation of cancer chemotherapeutic agents. This feature was discussed by Dr. Garattini, who described the role of the microsomal enzyme system of the liver in metabolic alterations and implicated the presence of a tumor in changing the capacity of the microsomal system to metabolize foreign agents.

The intensity of the cytotoxicity of a drug is dependent upon the concentration of the active agent at the site of action within the susceptible neoplastic cell and the duration of exposure of the target site. This relationship, expressed as a constant described by the drug concentration and time ($C \times T$), to cell lethality was discussed by Dr. Mellet who related findings in cells in culture, in tumor-bearing animals and in the clinical situation. The importance of the availability of pharmacokinetic models based upon anatomically discrete compartments to the optimization of therapy was convincingly outlined, using methotrexate as the model, by Dr. Zaharko.

Since the majority of clinically useful antineoplastic agents act at sites within neoplastic cells, the permeation of cellular membranes by these drugs is critical to their activity. Dr. Kessel has outlined the factors involved in the transport of a variety of anticancer agents and the importance of drug transport as a mechanism of acquired insensitivity. He has also summarized results demonstrating biochemical changes in the plasma membranes of drug-resistant mutants associated with decreased drug transport. Evidence is available to suggest that the permeability of the capillaries of both normal and neoplastic tissue of the central nervous system limits the delivery of chemotherapeutic agents to the brain; thus, this compartment (i.e. the central nervous system) has been termed a pharmacologic sanctuary for neoplastic cells. The parameters involved in the distribution of antineoplastic agents in the central nervous system, the cerebrospinal fluid and the meninges were discussed by Dr. Fenstermacher with particular relation to the therapy of central nervous system tumors.

A knowledge of the components influencing drug selectivity – and it is important for me to stress that selectivity does exist for clinically useful cancer chemotherapeutic agents – also may provide opportunity for further exploitation of relevant differences in the biology and biochemistry of neoplastic and normal tissues. The contributions of these two scientific disciplines to selective toxicity were discussed by Dr. Steel, who related the theoretical means of manipulating population kinetics to gain therapeutic advantage, and by Dr. Henderson, who summarized the balance of enzymatic activation and inactivation as it affects tissue selectivity of drugs.

To delineate the mechanisms by which neoplastic cells acquire drug resistance and possibly to select mixtures of potential synergists, it is critical to have an understanding of the pharmacological and biochemical features that dictate cytotoxic potency in neoplastic cells. For these reasons, a session of this Symposium was devoted to a discussion of the mechanism of action of some relatively new and important clinically useful anticancer drugs. Bleomycin appears to be a particularly promising antibiotic because its clinical toxicity differs from that of many of the standard cancer chemotherapeutic agents, making bleomycin a prime candidate for combination therapy. Dr. Pietsch described studies using a mercury staining technique to localize the intracellular binding sites of the antibiotic molecule with a view toward the development of a possible test to predict susceptibility of cancer cells to this drug.

Adriamycin ranks as perhaps the most promising drug presently available for the treatment of solid tumors in man. Dr. Bachur has compared the degree of inhibition of nucleic acid biosynthesis by this agent with that of daunorubicin, and has related the differences in the metabolism of these two antibiotics, a factor which may be of importance in determining their specificity against malignant diseases. The clinical utility of the vinca alkaloids has been firmly established, with vincristine being particularly useful in combination therapy because its primary central nervous system toxicity differs from that of most anticancer drugs and toxicity of mixtures containing this alkaloid can thereby be spread over a number of normal tissues. Dr. Creasey has summarized existing knowledge on the action of this class of agents; he has stressed that, like most effective cancer chemotherapeutic drugs, they have more than one site of action. The microtubules would appear to be the major locus, but inhibition of macromolecular synthesis also appears to be involved.

The nitrosoureas are representative of a class which is clearly a triumph for the principles of drug design, with structure–activity relationships leading to a relatively large family of active agents. Dr. Wheeler has effectively reviewed the evidence implicating both alkylation and carbamoylation in the biological action of these agents, as well as studies on the effects of these reactive derivatives on nucleic acid biosynthesis.

One of the major limitations to the continued effectiveness of clinically active anticancer drugs is the relatively rapid acquisition of insensitivity by neoplastic cells. Because of the importance of this phenomenon to the ultimate attainment of cures, a number of papers on the mechanisms by which cancers of man achieve resistance were included. A general survey of biochemical mechanisms involved in the acquisition of drug insensitivity for many of the clinically important carcinostatic agents was presented by Dr. Lane. This was followed by several reports on important classes of drugs. The development of resistance to alkylating agents was characterized by Dr. Connors as often being a slower process than that occurring with other classes of cytotoxic drugs and that a number of biochemical changes may be responsible for acquired tumor insensitivity. These included small changes in thiol content and in permeability of resistant variants, as well as the acquisition of efficient DNA repair enzymes. Dr. Bertino has indicated that the loss of susceptibility to folic acid antagonists can be due to increased levels of the target enzyme dihydrofolate reductase, an altered dihydrofolate reductase with a decreased affinity for folic acid analogs, or impared transport of the folate antagonists. The purine analogs, particularly the 6-thiopurines, were described by Dr. Brockman. With these agents, evidence is available to implicate the following mechanisms: (a) a decreased capacity for conversion of the drugs to their active nucleotide forms, (b) increased breakdown of the drug itself or of the nucleotide forms of the purine analogs, (c) decreased sensitivity of target sites, and (d) failure of the analogs to gain entry into insensitive cells. Dr. Hall has described similar biochemical alterations as being involved in the attainment of clinical resistance to arabinosylcytosine and 5-fluorouracil, which are the two most important pyrimidine derivatives available today for the treatment of neoplasia in man.

Means of circumventing resistance, both natural and acquired, are, therefore, of major importance to the successful long-term treatment of many patients with inoperable cancer. One of the possible ways in which this can be achieved is by the use of combination chemotherapy. This conclusion is based upon the finding that the ability of cells to attain resistance to two active drugs simultaneously is the product of the individual mutation frequencies of each agent employed alone. For this reason, coupled with the fact that the use of mixtures of drugs has gained great importance in the treatment of human cancer, considerable discussion was given to combination chemotherapy. Dr. Sartorelli stressed that, at present, biochemical and pharmacological approaches have contributed minimally to the therapeutic management of cancer in man, but outlined the great potential of these disciplines for optimizing patient care. Dr. Venditti described several examples of therapeutic synergism in the mouse leukemia L1210 system. The lack of additive toxicity was presented as a reasonable basis for expecting therapeutic advantage from a drug mixture, as was the use of an agent designed to protect the host selectively from the toxic effects of the chemotherapeutic drug. A specific example of a drug combination, methotrexate and asparaginase, which can produce either synergism or antagonism depending upon the schedule of administration, was provided by Dr. Capizzi. The potential exploitation of such knowledge for the development of an effective strategy for administration of this combination in man was stressed. Dr. Schabel then described several new synergistic drug mixtures in animal systems; he stressed the principle of employing drugs which interact with DNA in combination with other active antineoplastic agents in the selection of combinations of agents with clinical potential.

The success of mixtures of drugs in man was exemplified by three different investigators who described new combinations of great potential employed in patients with generally unresponsive diseases. Dr. Averette reported on the application of cell kinetics to fashion a mixture consisting of methotrexate, hydroxyurea and vincristine for treating gynecologic cancer. Dr. Bodey discussed the rationale for the development and application of a four-drug regimen consisting of vincristine, bleomycin, cyclophosphamide and 1-(2-chloroethyl)-3-(*trans*-4-methylcyclohexyl)-1-nitrosourea (methyl CCNU) for the treatment of oat cell and epidermoid cancer of the lung. The employment of three-drug (i.e. adriamycin, vincristine and dimethyl triazeno imidazole carboxamide) and four-drug (i.e. adriamycin, vincristine, dimethyl triazeno imidazole carboxamide and cyclophosphamide) mixtures in the chemotherapy of metastatic sarcomas with encouraging results was presented by Dr. Gottlieb.

Thus, it seems clear that new approaches are leading to the development of potentially useful therapies for cancer in man.

I wish to conclude this conference by thanking the Clinical Investigations Branch of the National Cancer Institute and the Cancer Clinical Investigation Review Committee for their sponsorship of this Symposium and the speakers who have made a convincing case for the utilization of the tools of pharmacology and biochemistry to attain optimal therapeutic advantage from existing chemotherapeutic agents.

The International Encyclopedia of Pharmacology and Therapeutics sponsored by the International Union of Pharmacology

To be published in journal form commencing July 1, 1975 under the title

PHARMACOLOGY & THERAPEUTICS

Part A - Chemotherapy
Part B - General and Systematic Pharmacology
Part C - Clinical Pharmacology and Therapeutics

Editorial and Publishing Developments

Both the international Editorial Board and the Publisher are aware of the need to increase the usefulness of the encyclopedia to research workers by improving the speed of dissemination of the results of all research areas in pharmacology and therapeutics. The present formula of commissioning multiauthored monographs has proved unwieldy and delays in publication have resulted from the late submission of contributions. For this reason it has been decided to publish contributions in journal form, as they are received.

The aims and scope of Pharmacology and Therapeutics are to present lucid, critical and authoritative surveys of the currently important topics in their respective fields, specially commissioned as invited contributions. Particular attention will be paid to new subjects not yet amenable to book treatment. The text will be discursive and fully illustrated to ensure clarity to exposition. Publication time will be less than six months after acceptance of manuscripts for publication.

Editorial Board

D Bovet - *Rome*	C Radouco-Thomas, *Quebec*
A S V Burgen - *London*	H Raskova - *Prague*
J Cheymol - *Paris*	A C Sartorelli - *New Haven*
G B Koelle - *Philadelphia*	J M Walker - *Oxford*
M J Michelson - *Leningrad*	V V Zakusov - *Moscow*

Some of the contributors and their contributions to be published in the early issues of the journal:

BARER	*Sheffield*	Physiology of the pulmonary circulation and methods of study
COOPER & GUNTHER	*Calgary*	Respiratory effects of drugs acting on metabolism and temperature control
CURZON	*London*	Metals and melanins
DANIEL & JANIS	*Alberta*	Calcium regulation in the uterus
KOCHAKIAN	*Alabama*	Definition of androgens and protein anabolic steroids
LERNER	*Milan*	Androgen antagonists
NEFF	*Washington*	Turnover of striatal monoamines
PROCTOR	*Baltimore*	Physiology and pharmacology of nasal mucus: decongestants
SHUTE & LEWIS	*Cambridge*	Cholinergic pathways
VANSTEENKISTE	*Ghent*	The use of computer in biostatistics
VAUGHAN WILLIAMS	*Oxford*	Classification of antidysrhythmic drugs
WIDDICOMBE	*London*	Physiology of the nervous control of breathing
WILLIAMS & VANE	*Bristol*	Inhibition of uterine motility: the possible role of the prostaglandins

Number of pages to be published in 1975 approximately 2,500

Subscription price for all 3 parts US $250.00, or individual parts US$100.00 each

PERGAMON PRESS

Maxwell House, Fairview Park, Elmsford, New York 10523
Headington Hill Hall, Oxford OX3 OBW, England

BEYOND DRUGS

by Stanley Einstein

The major goal of Dr. Einstein's book is to help people, young and old, go beyond drug issues and drug problems to a life based on celebration rather than pro- or anti-chemical adaptation. Those who will permit themselves to travel the paths of this book will discover or rediscover many facts, issues, and problems, but they will be secondary to their being asked to think out the available options, rules, rights, and responsibilities that they can choose from as they adapt to a world of more people and more chemicals.

About the book . . .

- Offers useful insights to those concerned about the increasing drug problem.
- Challenges numerous drug abuse myths and untested assumptions.
- Thoroughly discusses the implications of the wide-spread use of alcohol and tobacco, as well as narcotics and hallucinogens.
- Serves as a catalyst which cuts through much of the hopelessness and despair concerning drug abuse.
- Offers viable alternatives in place of the usual black and white reactions to a whole spectrum of colorful private and public behavior.
- Offers some guidelines and criteria that may prove personally useful in evaluating the consequences of dependence upon specific treatment, educational, preventional, and detectional techniques and programs.
- Points out the various roles that the use and misuse of all kinds of drugs have and continue to have in our daily lives.
- Challenges readers to weigh the non-drug alternatives that already exist in their own lives or are within reach.

1974 ISBN 0-08-017767-0 $12.00
ISBN 0-08-017768-9 pbk. $ 7.00

pergamon

Printed in Dunstable, United Kingdom

91338433R00141